ETHICAL &
LEGAL ISSUES

IN CANADIAN NURSING

SECOND EDITION

Margaret Keatings, RN, MHSc

O'Neil B. Smith, BA, LLB
(of the Ontario Bar)

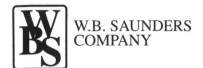

W.B. SAUNDERS
COMPANY

A Harcourt Canada Health Sciences Company

Toronto Montreal Fort Worth New York Orlando
Philadelphia San Diego London Sydney Tokyo

Canadian Cataloguing in Publication Data
Keatings, Margaret
  Ethical and legal issues in Canadian nursing

2nd ed.
Includes bibliographical references and index.
ISBN 0-920513-36-0

1. Nursing ethics—Canada. 2. Nursing—Law and legislation—Canada.
I. Smith, O'Neil B. (O'Neil Brian), 1962–   . II. Title.

RT85.K43 2000   174'.2   C99-930787-8

NEW EDITIONS EDITOR: Liz Radojkovic
PRODUCTION COORDINATOR: Cheryl Tiongson
COPY EDITOR/PRODUCTION EDITOR: Francine Geraci
COVER AND INTERIOR DESIGN: Jack Steiner Graphic Design
TYPESETTING AND ASSEMBLY: Jack Steiner Graphic Design
PRINTING AND BINDING: Transcontinental Printing Inc.
COVER ART: Greg Stott/Masterfile

Harcourt Canada
55 Horner Avenue, Toronto, ON, Canada M8Z 4X6
Customer Service
Toll-Free Tel.: 1-800-387-7278
Toll-Free Fax: 1-800-665-7307

This book was printed in Canada.
  3 4 5   03 02 01

Since the first edition of this book was published, debate has continued within and outside the nursing profession on the ethical issues surrounding withdrawal of treatment, euthanasia, assisted suicide, and human reproductive technology. This edition traces some of the changes that have occurred since the first edition. It also discusses some new issues that have grown in prominence in recent years.

As with the first edition, *Ethical and Legal Issues in Canadian Nursing* is by no means a comprehensive or exhaustive text. Chapters are arranged to facilitate both class discussion and individual study. Point-form Learning Objectives guide the reader through the material; each chapter Summary reiterates and reinforces the key points. Many more case studies have been added to explore the issues raised and to encourage class discussion. Additional cases appear at the end of each chapter to encourage critical thinking, discussion, and debate among students or practitioners and their colleagues. Following the case studies are questions for discussion, which are intended to integrate the chapter's key concepts.

Chapter One contains a brief background and introductory discussion. Chapters Two, Three, and Four have been rearranged to reflect the fact that ethical theory, rather than law, is often the point of departure in many courses on nursing ethics and law. Chapter Two describes various facets of ethical theory and thought; Chapter Three, the fundamentals of the Canadian legal system and the differences between the common law and civil law traditions. Chapter Four reviews the provincial regulatory systems that govern the nursing profession; the chapter concludes with a discussion (including case-study examples) of the values expounded in the CNA's *Code of Ethics for Registered Nurses* (1997).

The remainder of the book examines the ethical and legal aspects of prominent issues facing nurses and health practitioners today. In addition to the issues discussed in the first edition, material has been included on human reproductive technologies and the use of foetal tissue for transplantation.

Our goal throughout has been to explain current ethical and legal concepts in Canadian nursing in as lucid a style as possible. To this end, tables and figures have been added to illustrate pertinent concepts. Key terms are highlighted in bold type and are further defined and explained in the Glossary, which has been expanded for this edition.

We continue to regard *Ethical and Legal Issues in Canadian Nursing* as a work in progress. Many of the issues discussed continue to be debated in Parliament, provincial legislatures, the courts, and health care institutions. We welcome suggestions, criticism, and comments from readers in our continuing effort to improve this work.

The second edition of *Ethical and Legal Issues in Canadian Nursing* states the law as it stood in July 1998. While every attempt has been made to ensure the accuracy of the information given, the authors and publisher emphasize that they are not engaged in providing medical, legal, or other professional advice. Those desiring such advice are encouraged to seek the assistance of appropriate professionals.

ACKNOWLEDGEMENTS

The challenge of preparing a second edition of this book was no less difficult than writing the first edition. During preparation of the manuscript, we relied upon the help, support, and encouragement of people too numerous to mention.

We wish to thank Liz Radojkovic at W.B. Saunders Canada for her patience and understanding. We also acknowledge and thank those who reviewed the manuscript and provided helpful comments, constructive criticism, and suggestions for improvements.

We wish to thank those nurses who shared their stories with us so that the case studies would more accurately reflect real practice situations. In particular, Margaret would like to acknowledge her family members, whose experiences in the health care system are captured in many of the case studies, and whose stories added a new dimension to her appreciation of what constitutes ethical nursing practice.

Finally, we wish to thank members of our families for their patience and understanding during the many hours spent away from them during the preparation of this edition. Their sacrifice has not gone unnoticed, and their immense support has made this difficult work a good deal easier.

Margaret Keatings, RN, MHSc
O'Neil B. Smith, BA, LLB
February 1999

CONTENTS

Introduction to Nursing Law and Ethics

LEARNING OBJECTIVES

The purpose of this chapter is to enable you to:
- identify the reasons why nurses must be familiar with the law and ethics
- clarify the knowledge required to practise according to ethical and legal standards
- articulate the role of professionals in serving the public interest
- understand how and why the field of ethics has grown over recent years
- appreciate the challenges faced by nurses when dealing with complex legal and ethical issues.

Introduction

Nurses must be familiar with the law, ethics, ethical theory, and the workings of Canada's legal system as these pertain to their profession. Like other professionals, nurses operate within a framework of legal and ethical rules and guidelines. These are aimed at ensuring consistency, quality, competency, and safety to consumers of health services, while preserving respect for individual rights and human dignity.

As part of their professional role, nurses must make and act on decisions that relate to both independent practice and collaborative roles and relationships. For all these decisions and actions, the nurse as a professional is held accountable to individual patients, their families, health care team members, employers, the profession, and society as a whole. This process of decision making and action requires a sound knowledge base, practical and reasoning skills, and a willingness both to take risks and to be accountable. Frequently, our decisions and subsequent actions relate to, or are influenced by, law and ethics. They are thus guided by a set of rules (the law) and our individual and collective values and beliefs (ethics).

Nursing, the Law, and Ethics

Members of professional groups have an obligation to serve the public interest and the common good because their roles, missions, and ethical foundations focus not only on the individuals they serve, but on society as a whole. Professionals have this authority, and therefore this responsibility, because of their unique body of knowledge, skills, and expertise. Our society has traditionally depended on professionals as custodians of such fields as knowledge, health, law, and education. Professionals are therefore placed in a position of respect, and they are accordingly given the power and authority to engage in decisions that influence and shape public policy, law, and societal norms. As technology advances and society becomes more complex, professionals become more specialized. Hence, they acquire new power, and correspondingly greater ethical responsibility.[1]

Why Study Ethics and the Law?

In recent years, the field of ethics in health care has grown to meet the increasing complexity and volume of ethical dilemmas. This increase is primarily due to the growing sophistication of medical science and advanced technology. The rise in ethical dilemmas has contributed to caregiver stress, uncertainty, and value conflict. There is also a growing awareness of patients' rights and a greater emphasis on respect for individual autonomy. Consequently, a growing number of advocacy groups have been created to represent the interests of various patient constituencies.

As medical science and technology advance, traditional norms and values are challenged by questions about what health professionals do, how and why they do these things, and whether they ought to be doing them in the first place. New technology has made it possible for us to affect various life processes in ways that pose moral and legal problems for health professionals, patients, and society alike.

Nurses, in particular, have been challenged by this increase in ethical and legal dilemmas and concerns. As they confront and experience each new issue, they may be confused by the often conflicting interplay of ethics and law. They are forced to deal with these dilemmas and conflicts within the context of a health system strained by limited funds and resources as they continue to face the challenge of providing quality ethical care to patients.

Nurses must therefore have a high level of awareness of the ethical and legal issues they face. More than any other health professional, they are in sustained contact with patients in the home, in the community, and in the institutional setting. Nurses must fulfil the important task of supporting patients and their families, as well as intervening or lobbying on behalf of those patients when necessary. Their role involves professional and trusting relationships with people throughout the life continuum from birth to death. These relationships require knowledge, skill, and sensitivity with regard to health care issues as well as their ethical and legal dimensions.

Nurses must have knowledge of ethics in order to guide the difficult decisions they make. Chapter Two explores theories, principles, and decisional frameworks that guide ethical choices by nurses. This material is not exhaustive, and is intended only to provide nurses with a foundation in ethics. It will begin the process of lifelong professional learning in this area, and provide a framework for the specific ethical themes discussed in later chapters.

The situations nurses face as health professionals may involve clear institutional rules and procedures, or straightforward legal rules and statutes. Yet, many situations are more complicated and require nurses to decide, from many possible alternative courses of action, the morally correct thing to do. At times, conflicts may arise in situations where what we believe to be the most morally correct course of action may not necessarily be supported in law.

Since society holds nurses to high standards of professional, moral, and ethical competence, it also affords them certain rights and privileges. The law strives to keep these competing interests in constant balance. It regulates the education and licensing of nurses; the conditions of their employment; their collective bargaining rights; their rights, duties, and responsibilities towards patients, physicians, other health professionals, the public, and each other; and a host of other matters. Furthermore, the legal system provides a forum for resolving disputes and conflicts, which inevitably arise when these divergent interests clash.

Thus, for example, a nurse who is being made to work in conditions that are unsafe or even dangerous has recourse against the employer under occupational health and safety legislation in force in some provinces. Likewise, a patient who has suffered injury or harm as a result of the negligence of a nurse may commence a civil suit in the courts against that nurse and the hospital for damages.

There are many other reasons why nurses should be familiar with the law and have a basic understanding of Canada's legal system. Firstly, the Canadian Nurses Association's *Code of Ethics for Registered Nurses*[2] and each provincial regulatory body impose certain requirements with respect to nurses' level of professional knowledge and skill. Failure to meet these requirements, or undertaking the practice of nursing without adequate education, leaves the nurse open to disciplinary action from his or her provincial professional governing body and, if the conduct is serious enough, perhaps the courts. Chapter Three outlines the principles of Canada's legal system in order to provide nurses with a basic understanding of what often seems an obscure and confusing institution. The roles of the courts, legislatures, and executive branches of government are discussed, as well as some of the legal concepts and principles applicable to nursing law. These provide a framework for the chapters that follow. Chapter Four describes the structure, role, and workings of various provincial professional regulatory bodies and institutions. Against this background, nurses can begin to appreciate how their profession is regulated, and in particular, how the concept of self-government is integrated into this regulatory structure, and into professional codes of ethics. Like the chapters that follow, Chapter Four includes one or more case studies, providing factual situations and ample material for further exploration.

A second reason for understanding the law is that nurses have access to drugs that are heavily regulated by legislation and hospital procedures governing their use, dispensation, and handling. An understanding of the legal system, and of the law and rules of negligence, underscores the importance of following such procedures and regulations when administering any medication. Not only civil, but also criminal consequences can flow from a breach of such laws. Chapter Five deals with issues of negligence and standards of care in the nursing profession. It describes how nurses' conduct and professionalism in carrying out their duties are measured in relation to tort law and current ethical standards.

Thirdly, the everyday actions and decisions made by nurses affect the basic rights of their patients. These actions and decisions may involve going beyond the usual consensual barriers. For instance, a patient who needs an injection may readily consent by holding out an arm to the nurse who administers it. However, in cases where a patient is unable to consent to a procedure owing to physical or mental incapacity, the nurse bears the onus of ensuring that any action undertaken or treatment administered is in the patient's best interests and is consistent with that patient's wishes. Failure to do so leaves the nurse open to the risk of a civil suit for damages from the non-consenting patient or the next-of-kin. Further, health professionals are under a positive duty to ensure that the patient understands the nature of the illness, the need for treatment, and all the attendant risks and benefits of such treatment, if that patient is to give as fully informed a consent as the law requires. Issues of consent to treatment and the many subissues arising from this area are treated in Chapter Six.

Chapter Seven discusses the life–death continuum and current subjects such as euthanasia, assisted suicide, human reproductive technologies, and organ donation—subjects that have gained public prominence in recent years and hold profound implications for nurses. Recent, extraordinary advances in medical technology have made it possible both to manipulate the reproductive process at one end of the life continuum and, at the other, to extend life in cases where death would once have been certain. New reproductive and genetic technologies now exist that not only attempt to overcome infertility but have the capacity to identify genetic anomalies and to control the characteristics of the children produced. This overwhelming power to manipulate the creation of life has the potential to reshape our society and to redefine future generations. Further, our fear of death has led to an emphasis on finding ways to extend life at all costs. Yet, there is a heavy cost when extending someone's life also diminishes the quality and dignity that give life its meaning. As ways of dealing with death and the dying process change, nursing is challenged to find new ways to preserve the person's human values, autonomy, and dignity.

Often, these issues arise before laws can be made to deal with them. Knowledge of the legal system gives the nurse a better appreciation of the fact that the law often is not an exhaustive source of guidance and direction in such matters, and also that it is slow to adapt legal solutions to them. As well, the nurse will see that the law is, not infrequently, out of step with current societal values. Law is usually perceived as a "black and white" proposition, while ethical situations—such as euthanasia and physician-assisted suicide—are vastly more complicated by shades of grey. Today, the single biggest challenge facing the law and our legal system is the attempt to come to terms with the grey areas and to provide more realistic and practical guidelines for dealing with ethical dilemmas.

A further reason for studying the law as it applies to nursing is that nurses have access to confidential information about individual patients. They have both legal and ethical obligations to keep all such information confidential and not to divulge it without the patient's consent. In cases where that consent cannot be obtained, they may reveal only as much as is absolutely necessary in the interests of the patient. They may disclose information only to persons whose participation in the patient's treatment is necessary. There may be cases where nurses are required to divulge such information in court in the form of testimony. Knowledge of the workings of the law, the rules of evidence, ethics, and the judicial system provides a framework when determining whether to disclose sensitive and confidential information about a particular patient. Ill or injured patients are in a vulnerable state and are not always able to protect their rights as citizens. In order to ensure that the interests of their patients or clients are represented, nurses must understand the rights of their clients and their professional obligations to protect or respect these rights. These issues are explored in Chapter Eight.

Ensuring a high standard of documentation is important in maintaining effective communication, which is key to professional nursing practice. The nurse's assessment and progress notes monitor, on a continuing basis, the course of a patient's treatment and the effect of interventions. Inadequate documentation or failure to review client information and history have a negative influence on the quality of care. Given that multiple caregivers may be involved, it is impossible to achieve effective communication and continuity of care without accurate documentation. Thus, Chapter Nine explores the legal, ethical, and practical aspects of proper documentation.

If nurses have obligations to their clients, they also have rights regarding what they can expect as professionals. Like all other Canadians, under the *Charter of Rights and Freedoms* nurses have the right to privacy and respect, and to freedom of expression—the right to think, say, write, or otherwise act in accordance with their beliefs. However, these rights must be considered in the context of nurses' responsibilities as professionals and of their obligations to patients and clients. Chapter Ten focusses on the balance between these rights and obligations.

Summary

Clearly, the impact of the law and ethics on the nursing profession is widespread and significant. An understanding of the law's structures, terminology, and mechanisms is essential to the nurse's ability to operate within society's expectations and standards. In order to practise within a framework that supports high standards of ethical care to patients and clients, nurses must be guided by the values and ethical standards of their profession. The authors have tried to lay the basis for such an understanding in the chapters that follow.

The key points introduced in this chapter include:

- the reasons why nurses must be familiar with the law and ethics
- the knowledge required to practise according to ethical and legal standards
- the role of professionals in serving the public interest
- the reasons why the field of ethics has grown in recent years
- the challenges faced by nurses when dealing with complex legal and ethical issues.

Critical Thinking

QUESTIONS FOR DISCUSSION

1. Why did you decide to enter the nursing profession?
2. What personal values do you share with the nursing profession?
3. Have you or your family had an experience with the health care system? What did you most like about this experience? What did you least like about it?
4. In your opinion, what are the most significant legal issues that nurses may face? What would be the significant ethical issues?

5. If you were a patient today, what would you expect from the nurses caring for you? If a member of your family were a patient today, what would you expect? As a nurse or a student, do you meet these expectations with your own patients or clients?

References

1. Jennings, B., Callaghan, D., Wolf, S.M. (1987, February). The professions: Public interest and common good. *Hastings Center Report* (pp. 3–4).
2. Canadian Nurses Association (CNA). (1997). *Code of Ethics for Registered Nurses*. Ottawa: Author. (See Appendix A.)

CHAPTER Two

Ethical Theoretical Perspectives

LEARNING OBJECTIVES

The purpose of this chapter is to enable you to:
- understand the importance of having knowledge of ethics
- appreciate the complexity of ethical choices nurses make
- understand the influence of values on ethical decision making
- realize the relevance of a solid understanding of ethical theory
- develop a basic understanding of ethical theory and principles
- apply theory and principles in practice
- utilize tools and processes to assist in identifying, understanding, and working through ethical challenges
- know when and how to utilize hospital ethics committees.

Introduction

Nurses enjoy a position of extraordinary responsibility in our society. The decisions we make every day influence the quality of life and death of sick, vulnerable people who hold us in their trust. We must believe that our choices are the best we can make. As professionals we must be able to clarify, and justify, our decisions and actions to patients/clients, colleagues, our profession, the organizations in which we are employed, the justice system, and society as a whole. To do this effectively we need to have knowledge about ethics and the skills and tools to support our positions.

The nature of our responsibilities requires us at times to make difficult decisions about complex issues. Often, we must choose our course of action from among several alternatives. The relative merit of these choices may be unclear, and we may have to choose the least wrong (or only slighter better) option. How, then, do we make choices that ensure an optimal level of care? How do we determine whether the decisions we make and actions we take are the right ones? How do we identify ethical dilemmas and violations? Do we even know when we are confronted with an ethical dilemma, or that our choices are indeed ethical in nature? When are ethical violations the result of poor communication, inadequate system support and resources, or substandard patient care processes?

This chapter will show that the process of making and supporting ethical choices can be facilitated through a solid understanding of ethical theory and principles. It will conclude with one framework that may guide ethical discussion and decision making, and an overview of the role of clinical ethics committees.

Why Should Nurses Study Ethics?

Nurses function within a health care team and interact with many other health professionals. Today, nurses practise in many different contexts beyond the traditional health care settings: in the community or the home; in continuing care or rehabilitation; in business or industry, and in the insurance setting. In some situations, nurses may interact with other professionals who do not share the same perspective or understanding about nursing or health care in general. Each member of the team may have a different perspective on an ethical issue, or may share a similar position. However, similarities—as well as differences—must be clarified. Without discussion and clarification, on occasion others may interpret some decisions and actions undertaken by members of the team as wrong. If the reasons, values, and perspectives behind these decisions and actions are explained, they may more readily be understood and respected, if not accepted, by others.

Within health care, choices are often not easy; it may be difficult to determine, from among many alternatives, which is best. Consider, for example, a situation in which the medical team may be aggressively treating a terminally ill patient in an Intensive Care Unit. Some nurses involved with the person's care may consider this approach wrong because they believe that it will only diminish the quality of the patient's remaining life. If the medical staff were to clarify their position—say, at a team conference—the dissenting nurses might discover that the team's actions were based on a belief in the sanctity of life, and the view that the role of the physician is to preserve life at all costs. Possibly, on an earlier occasion, the patient may have asked the doctor to try anything that would save his life. Or, perhaps, the physician has more knowledge about the patient's story. Perhaps the patient has a particular religious or cultural perspective that requires every effort to be taken to sustain life. Perhaps there was an advance directive stating this; or perhaps the family was awaiting a beloved relative's arrival from out of town so that final good-byes could be said. Though the views of some nurses may not change, they may come to a better understanding of the reasons behind the physicians' actions. Such discussion would reduce the moral conflict and distress experienced by some nurses, and ensure better relationships among members of the team.

It is imperative that patients/clients, families, physicians, nurses, and other team members discuss such issues together, and attempt to reach agreement on a course of action. Since most ethical dilemmas do not have clear-cut answers, collaboration and effective communication can enhance the resolution process. The communication that is necessary to clarify and justify our moral actions and choices to our professional colleagues is improved through a shared language grounded in a solid foundation of ethical theory. The entire process should be grounded in respect for one another's values and beliefs.

The study of ethics provides nurses with some tools to be better able to manage and contribute to this process. Knowledge of abstract philosophical theories and terminologies does not always provide solutions to ethical problems; however, such knowledge can serve to help us better understand the moral context and the values and beliefs of ourselves and others.

As nurses, we face ethical choices every day in our practice. The issues do not always make headlines. We may deal with important choices in the areas of pain control, patient comfort, restraints, patient choice, and family involvement in care. Ethics is involved when we decide how to allocate time and nursing care to patients; when we decide whose needs are to be met first; and when we show respect to our patients, their families, one another, and to ourselves.

Nurses are involved not only in the ethical context of the individual nurse–patient/client relationship; they are also affected by, and are in a position to influence, the wider context of health care and the health system. A rapidly changing environment influences the volume and content of the issues they face. Ethical issues arise as new technology is introduced, especially as that technology distances us further from the people we serve. Further, during times of downsizing and restructuring, as resources are diminished or as different delivery models are introduced, greater ethical challenges and complexities arise.

For example, advances in the area of organ transplantation and reproductive technology force questions about how we allocate these scarce resources, and indeed, whether we should be providing this technology at all. The growth of the consumer movement, the proliferation of special interest groups, and the occupational issues that arise from collective bargaining and unionization all influence the context of health care today, and hence nurses' ethical choices. The effect of budget cuts on the nurse–client ratio poses additional challenges relative to how nurses allocate their time and services. Further, the role of the nurse is expanding: nurses are being given more autonomy and with that, more authority and responsibility.

Every-day Ethical Issues Nurses Face

As nurses, we have the opportunity to defend and protect patient rights, to promote compassionate care, and to enhance the dignity and autonomy of our patients or clients. As suggested earlier in this chapter, nurses are often required to choose from among a number of good or least wrong alternatives, and to assess and defend the choices or actions taken. We may not even be aware of the ethical nature of the choices we make. Since many choices are not always clear, how do we decide what is the right thing to do?

Within the context of a health system strained by limited funds and resources, nurses frequently face the challenge of providing high-quality and ethical care to patients. The following scenarios are not uncommon.

An infant in a paediatric centre has been diagnosed with a malignant cerebral tumour. The infant is comatose and non-responsive, and on life support systems. There is nothing the team can do to halt the progress of this terminal disease. They believe it would be in the child's best interest to discontinue life support and to allow the child to die a natural death. The parents disagree and want all measures taken to save their child's life.

Who decides the best interests of this child? Do patients or families have the right to expensive, futile health care? How do the nurses support the parents through this crisis and their ultimate loss? How do we ensure quality care for this child throughout the dying process?

Joe, a 20-year-old man diagnosed with schizophrenia since the age of 16, is admitted to the psychiatric unit of a community hospital. He is agitated and expresses a wish to "end all this pain." He refuses all medications to deal with his symptoms. He wants to go home.

What rights does Joe have in this situation? Is there meaning behind Joe's wish to "end all this pain," or is this merely a symptom of his disease process?

A man with end-stage cancer of the liver is at home receiving palliative care. His wife and children, with some support from home care and community nurses, are his primary caregivers. As his condition deteriorates, his symptoms become more difficult to manage. As his family tires, they question whether he might be better off in hospital. The patient, however, has always stated his preference is to die at home.

How does the community nurse manage the conflicting interests of this patient and his family? What is society's role in ensuring adequate resources to address the needs of the dying patient at home?

A 40-year-old single man is recovering from surgery to his lower back. Though he is still in pain and continues to have difficulty with mobility, the hospital needs the bed, and he has reached his expected length of stay. The hospital nurse discusses his transition to the community with the home care case managers, who determine that he does not qualify for home-maker support. He does not have family or friends to support him at home.

How do these nurses ensure this man a safe transition home? How do they deal with the rules that limit needed resources in the community?

An occupational health nurse in an industrial setting is managing the case of a worker who was injured at work. He has recovered and is functionally able to return to his former work. Management is eager to have him return as soon as possible. However, the worker confides to the nurse that his front-line manager constantly harasses him and his co-workers; he believes that it was this stressful environment that led to his accident in the first place. He asks the nurse to keep this information confidential, as he fears further repercussions.

How does the nurse balance responsibility to ensure this worker's safe return to work—and concern for the safety of other workers in this hostile environment—with the obligation to honour the worker's request for confidentiality?

An elderly patient in a geriatric unit is confused and agitated. The use of physical restraints is considered.

How do we balance the risks and benefits of this option and still respect the patient's wishes?

It is the middle of an evening shift on a busy medical unit. A patient is dying; family and friends are not around.

Do we let this patient die alone?

These are only a few of the complex and difficult situations faced by nurses on a daily basis. Furthermore, it is not uncommon for nurses to be confronted with a number of these ethical issues and questions simultaneously. Limited understanding of ethical theory, lack of awareness that we are facing ethical issues, lack of knowledge and skill required to address them, and lack of appropriate system supports often lead to avoidance of the issues. How can nurses ensure that the best care is provided to patients without identifying the ethical issues and dilemmas, and acting towards their resolution?

Before proceeding with the rest of this chapter, take some time now to reflect on the above scenarios. What choices would you make? What are your reasons for making them? Is your rationale consistent across each scenario, or does your approach vary depending on the situation or your past experience? Are you able to defend your approach to your colleagues?

As you review the theoretical perspectives below, reflect back on these scenarios. Was your approach to these problems consistent with any of these theories? Did your views change as you read? Did these perspectives provide you with arguments to assist in defending your position? Are you better able to identify the ethical issues in these scenarios? Do they help you decide on a course of action?

Ethical Theory

A number of factors influence how we determine right and wrong. These factors may include the norms and beliefs of society, the context of the particular situation, previous experiences with similar situations, the potential outcomes or consequences of actions, the relationship of the individuals involved, and professional and individual values and beliefs.

Over the centuries, many philosophers have attempted to uncover the foundations of morality in an attempt to understand the key moral principles that guide our decisions regarding right and wrong. Believing that decisions about morality transcend our emotions and feelings, they developed theories and identified principles grounded in a "reasoned" or "rational" approach to ethical decision making.

Definitions

Ethics, the philosophical study of morality, is the systematic exploration of questions about what is morally right and morally wrong. The study of ethics enables us to evaluate the variables that influence our moral decisions, obligations, character, responsibility, social justice, and the nature of the good life.[1] **Ethical theory** is the study of the nature and justification of general ethical principles that can be applied to moral problems,[2] and attempts to provides a more rigorous and systematic approach to how we make decisions about what is right and wrong. The field of **biomedical ethics** explores ethical questions and moral issues associated with health care. **Nursing ethics** focusses on the moral questions within the sphere of nursing practice and the nurse–patient/client relationship.

Morality is the tradition of beliefs and norms within a culture or society about right and wrong human conduct. Morality within a social tradition or culture has historical roots and is guided by explicit codes of conduct and rules governing right and wrong behaviour. A well-known example is the "golden rule": "Do unto others as you would have them do unto you." As children grow up within particular societies and cultures, they are taught these moral rules along with other mores and social norms.[3]

There are two approaches to the study of morality, non-normative and normative. *Non-normative* approaches to ethics involve the analysis of morality, without taking a moral position, whereas *normative* ethics focusses on the analysis of what is right and what is wrong.[4]

Non-normative studies include the fields of descriptive ethics and metaethics. **Descriptive ethics** encompasses factual descriptions and explanations of moral behaviour and beliefs. By looking at a wide range of moral beliefs and behaviours, this field of study attempts to explain how moral attitudes, codes, and beliefs differ from person to person and across societies and cultures. **Metaethics** analyzes the meaning of key terms such as "right," "obligation," "good," and "virtue," and attempts to distinguish between what is moral and what is not—for example, the difference between a moral rule and a social rule. Further, metaethics analyzes the structure or logic of moral reasoning and justification,[5,6] and explores the nature of morality and the meanings and interrelationships of the fundamental concepts of moral language. For example, in metaethics the following questions are pursued:

- How is a moral principle different from a non-moral one?
- What do we mean when we say an act is right?
- What does it mean to have "free will" or to be "morally responsible"?[7]

In normative ethics, attempts are made to identify the basic principles and virtues that guide morality and to provide coherent, systematic and justifiable answers to moral questions.[8] Through the development of ethical theory, normative ethics provides a system of moral principles or virtues, and provides reasons to guide decisions regarding what is right and what is wrong.[9]

Applied ethics is that field of ethics in which these theories and principles are applied to actual moral problems, for example, in health care.[10]

Ethical dilemmas arise when the best course of action is unclear, when strong moral reasons support each position (whenever good reasons for mutually exclusive alternatives can be cited),[11] and when we must choose between the most right or the least wrong. Resolution to ethical dilemmas may often be facilitated simply by obtaining all the facts and information concerning the areas of moral controversy.[12] This is why it is important for members of the health care team, the patient, and the family to work together to address difficult ethical issues. The first step is to ensure that we have all the relevant information and that the issues and alternatives are clearly understood by all. Health care providers rarely face these challenges alone. However, members of a multidisciplinary health care team must be able to communicate about ethical issues with colleagues, patients, and families. **Moral distress** results when we are not able to face these issues and deal effectively with them. Moral distress may contribute to feelings of guilt, discomfort and dissatisfaction in not being able to do what we think is best.

Ethical theories provide a framework of **principles** and guidelines to help identify ethical issues and reconcile dilemmas or conflicts. While the answers to these questions may not always be clear, the questions themselves can guide the decision process. Thus, it is important that nurses have a deeper understanding of normative ethics and the many theories and principles available to guide ethical reflection and discussion. If these theories and principles are not able, in every circumstance, to help resolve an ethical conflict, they yet serve as a template or guide to assist us in justifying our moral position to others.

Moral Justification

Persons involved in the field of ethics draw upon ethical theories and principles not only to select an ethical approach to an issue, but also to justify and defend their position to others. Points of view, especially in controversial areas, are open to criticism and debate and require justification. To justify a moral point of view requires an argued defence of one's perspective. Using theories and principles of ethics can provide clear relationships between reasons and conclusions. Claims are justified through reasoned arguments and evidence, and are subject to criticism and counter-examples. Arguments can be disguised by rhetoric, irrelevancies, redundancies, and subtle connections with other arguments, and can mislead those not comfortable with ethical language and theory.[13] As the extent of moral problems in the health care environment increase in volume and intensity, it becomes increasingly important for nurses to have knowledge of ethical theory and some skill in justifying and defending a point of view to others.

Table 2.1 sets out the *deductive* (hierarchical) process for the development of a moral argument. An ethical point of view, opinion, or decision is supported by rules that, in turn, are grounded in ethical principles evolved from various theoretical perspectives. Some of these theories and principles will be described later in this chapter.

Values

Before we describe the more common ethical theories that are available to assist nurses in ethical decision making, it is important to clarify the influence of values, not only on ethical theory but on the norms, rules, and laws of our society. Since Canada comprises a mosaic of cultural and religious perspectives, nurses care for patients and families whose basic value systems—and hence beliefs, rituals, and customs—may differ from their own. Therefore, an understanding of values helps to ensure respect for differences.

For example, cultural values may influence the beliefs that a particular group or society holds about treatment of the body after death. These beliefs may influence the rituals and behaviours associated with death and dying.

TABLE 2.1 *Levels of Justification in Moral Argument*[14]	
Moral Judgement	Expresses a decision, verdict, or conclusion about a particular action or character trait. Justified by rules.
Moral Rule	Guides decision, asserts what ought or ought not be done. Justified by principles.
Moral Principles	More general and fundamental; justifies reasons for accepting rules. Justified by ethical theories.
Ethical Theories	Bodies of principles and rules that are more or less systematically related.

Nurses who understand these values and differences can then clarify their own role and enrich their relationship with patients, clients, and families.

Dealing with differences can be stressful for nurses. Enhanced understanding minimizes stress and contributes to role clarity and satisfaction. Further, when our behaviours are not congruent with our own values, internal conflicts can arise. It is therefore important for us to understand and respect the values that ground our own ethical perspectives. The *Code of Ethics for Registered Nurses* of the Canadian Nurses Association, described in Chapter Four, articulates value statements to guide the ethical behaviour of nurses and the profession.[15]

Influence of Values on Ethical Decision Making

Our individual values influence how we respond to ethical issues and the decisions we make. A **value** is an ideal that has significant meaning or importance to an individual, a group, or a society. For example, in Canadian society we value individual freedom, health, fairness, honesty, and integrity. We see evidence of these values in our laws, our country's *Charter of Rights and Freedoms,* and our individual and collective actions and behaviours. The structure of the Canadian health system demonstrates how we value equality, individual rights, health and well-being, quality of life, and human dignity. This is evident in the principle of universality, that is, the attempt to provide equal access to health and illness care to all Canadians, regardless of where they live and their socio-economic status.

Values influence our beliefs, our view of others, and our opinions in such areas as literature, art, objectives, and ideals. Our behaviours, rituals, symbols, structures, rules, and laws represent the collective values and beliefs of our society. Because Canadian nurses work with and care for patients who represent a broad spectrum of cultural and religious perspectives, we must strive to clarify our own values, and respect and learn to understand those of others.

Values may shift over time within a culture. For example, in recent years Canadian society has become more sensitive to the meaning and quality of life versus prolonging life at all costs. This is evident in current debates over euthanasia and assisted suicide. Health practices in the area of palliative care reinforce this growing concern for quality and dignity within the dying process. Respect for individual rights and freedoms is a modern concept that has emerged only over the past couple of centuries and is more prevalent in western societies.

We develop our values through our life experiences. Values emerge through our associations with others: our families, classmates, friends, teachers, colleagues, personal relationships, religious experiences, and the environment we live in. In recent times, the media and television have also had a strong influence on value development. Gender is also said to affect the development of values in individuals and groups.[16] Though changing, the nursing profession has been and continues to be dominated by women. As members of a primarily female profession, nurses have traditionally related to physicians, a male-dominated group (though this is changing) whose values may have developed differently from those of nurses. Our respective values may influence the perspectives that nurses, physicians, and other health professionals bring to the ethical issues and dilemmas we share.

Professional values build on and expand our personal values, and emerge as we are socialized into the nursing profession. Sometimes there is a struggle between personal beliefs and professional responsibilities. As health professionals, nurses face life-and-death situations, joy, pain, and sorrow that may alter our perspective and reshape and reorder our values.

Value conflicts arise in situations where our actions conflict with our beliefs, and this results in stress for health professionals. Value conflict is evident when we hold different views of how a particular ethical dispute should be managed (e.g., withdrawal of treatment, abortion, euthanasia, patient restraint). Our duty as professionals and as members of a health care team requires that we understand and respect the values of other members of that team. Since conflict in values can result in moral distress, it is imperative that we understand our own values, articulate and clarify them to one another, and establish processes whereby this can be done.

Value Clarification

Nurses do not function in isolation. We work within a team that includes patients/clients and their families. The team's focus is the recovery, well-being and optimal health, not only of the individual patient, but also of society as a whole. Since team members come together with different experiences, cultural and religious perspectives, it is important that we understand one another's values before we attempt to decide our best course of action.

Value clarification is an ongoing process that occurs through each individual interaction and team discussion or case conference. It is a process through which individuals come to understand the values they hold and the importance of these values relative to others. It thus facilitates mutual understanding. This process requires open discussion, communication, active listening, understanding, and mutual respect. It is enhanced if we share the same language and terminology in relation to ethical issues. A focus on specific situations and case studies helps nurses to identify values, evaluate various responses to specific situations, and hence come to understand the various perspectives on the issues.

Frequently, the demands of high workload in health care restrict the time available for discussion. However, structuring our time to allow such dialogue is a worthwhile investment. The rewards include improved communication and collaboration among professional groups, a reduction in moral distress, and subsequent improvement in patient care as ethical problems are addressed and action plans identified.

Relativism

Prior to reviewing some of the best known ethical theories, we should note that not all thinkers and philosophers agree on a single, correct, and objective framework for morality.[17,18] Some consider individual and group responses to morality to be relative to the norms and values of that particular culture or society, or to the situation presenting itself. This view is labelled **cultural** or **normative relativism.**

Relativists consider morality to be more a matter of cultural differences and taste, an arbitrary notion of what one believes or feels, and not based on some deeper set of objectively justifiable principles.[19,20] Proponents of relativism believe that moral beliefs and principles relate only to individual cultures or persons, and that the values of one person or one culture do not govern the conduct of others. What is morally right and morally wrong, they believe, varies from place to place. There are no absolute or universal moral standards that can apply to all persons at all times.[21] Concepts of rightness and wrongness are therefore meaningless apart from the specific contexts in which they arise. Relativists note that what is deemed worthy of moral approval or disapproval in one society varies from standards in other societies, even though all possess a moral conscience or general sense of right and wrong. A moral standard is a historical product, sanctioned by custom over time, and moral beliefs of individuals vary according to historical, environmental, and familial differences. The particular actions, motives, and rules that are praised or blamed vary greatly from culture to culture;[22] therefore, according to relativists, there are no universal norms.

Opponents to this view argue that despite apparent differences in conclusions, there is a "universal structure of human nature, or at least a universal set of human needs which leads to the adoption of similar or even identical principles in all cultures."[23] It does not follow that there is disagreement regarding moral standards or principles just because individuals or groups disagree about the ethics of a particular situation or practice.[24] Universalists argue that conflicts between moral beliefs across cultures are not basic or fundamental; disagreements over critical facts or concepts are usually the underlying source of moral diversity. A society may agree on ideals of individual liberty and general happiness, yet disagree on when society has the right to make people happy in spite of themselves. They may agree on principles but disagree on their range of application. For example, consider the historical practice of the Inuit to leave elderly family members to die. This practice was based on respect for the elderly and the belief that one's status in the afterlife reflected that person's condition at the end of life on earth. Therefore, from the Inuit perspective, it was better to die when one's mental and physical capabilities were more or less intact. As a second example, the dietary prohibitions of Jews and Muslims regarding pork were founded originally on safety concerns.

Normative Ethical Theories

Over the centuries, many philosophers and thinkers have attempted to define morality and to provide a framework of universal rules and principles to guide right action.

Various ethical theories offer approaches to the analysis of ethical issues. The following discussion is not intended to be an exhaustive presentation of ethical theories, but a review of some better-known theoretical perspectives.

Ethical theories can be used to develop decision-making tools for application in the clinical setting. One example of such a tool is described at the end of this chapter.

Background

In the discipline of philosophy, decisions about what is right and wrong have traditionally required a reasoning process based on an ethical theory or the principles and rules derived from those theories. Opinions without arguments or reasons to support them were discouraged. Emotive responses were devalued, although (as will be seen later in this chapter) our emotional reactions are today considered by some thinkers as important indicators of what is right or wrong.

Theories are meant to assist in this reasoning process. It is important for nurses to be familiar with the fundamentals of the major ethical theories and the principles and frameworks that can guide and help to communicate ethical decisions.

Normative ethical theories are intended to provide frameworks and rules to guide decisions about what is right and wrong with respect to actions and behaviours. They provide a system of principles by which to determine what ought and ought not be done. Two traditional categories of ethical theory are deontology (derived from the Greek *deontor,* "duty") and teleology (derived from the Greek *teleos,* "end").[25] *Deontological* theories make explicit those duties and principles that should guide our actions, whereas *teleological* theories focus on the ends or outcomes and consequences of what we do. Teleologists look ahead to the consequences of action; deontologists look back at the nature of the act itself, evaluating it in terms of duties and obligations one has, either by virtue of being a human being or by the virtues of the specific person and his or her social relationships.[26]

Utilitarian Theories

Those who espouse **utilitarianism** believe that the ethical choice is the one with the best consequences, outcomes, or results. They believe that an "action or practice is right (when compared to any alternative action or practice) if it leads to the greatest possible balance of good consequences or to the least possible balance of bad consequences in the world as a whole."[27] In utilitarian theories there are no absolute principles, moral codes, duties, or rules; rather, there is the assumption that good can be quantified, and that we can calculate the relative good or harm that would result from our actions.[28] One acts best by increasing the greatest good and the least amount of harm for the greatest number of people. Essentially, the consequences of an act consist of the sum total of differences which that act will make in the world.

Utilitarian theories provide us with evaluative standards for assessing and ordering consequences. One may choose to evaluate the moral value of an act based on outcomes that may be related to happiness, welfare, pleasure, pain, risk, or costs and benefits. The consequences of an act are measured in their totality. For example, in a situation where withdrawal of treatment is being considered, the consequences of this action would be evaluated not only in relation to the patient, but also to the family, the health professionals involved, and society as a whole. Immediate and long-term consequences would also be considered.

Mill's Utilitarianism

Utilitarianism, one of the best-known normative theories, was formulated by John Stuart Mill (1806–1873) based on the earlier work of Jeremy Bentham (1748–1832).[29] The theory articulated by Mill is founded on the principle of utility (the greatest happiness for the greatest number of people). Mill's utilitarianism had both a normative and psychological foundation: normative in the principle of utility, and psychological in Mill's views of human nature. Key to the validity of his theory was his belief that most people desire unity and harmony with one another, and essentially wish to benefit others.[30] These basic goals—to benefit others and to control harm—ensure, Mill believed, a commitment from all rational beings to strive to do their best. Mill saw a moral framework as a means not only to fulfil individuals' needs, but also to facilitate the achievement of broad social goals.[31]

From a normative perspective, Mill argued that the principle of utility is grounded in the pursuit of pleasure and the avoidance of pain, which he believed to be the main goals of life. In fact our actions, he argued, have even greater moral significance when they have a greater effect on the pleasure or pain of others.[32] Mill believed that actions are right when they promote happiness, wrong if they produce the reverse. In choosing among alternatives, he believed an act to be right if and only if its utility is higher than the utility of any other act the person could have done instead.[33] Out of our desire for unity and harmony with others, it would follow that our actions produce the greatest happiness for the greatest number. In order to evaluate happiness and to prioritize consequences, Mill argued that we should rely on our common sense, our habits, and our past experiences. Based on these factors, we could then reasonably predict what would produce the most happiness and, therefore, the best consequences.[34]

A Theory of Value

An important component of a utilitarian theory is its dependence on some theory of value or intrinsic good; on the outcome or consequence of right actions worth seeking. Debate among utilitarians focusses on what result has the greatest utility or value—what is the ultimate intrinsic good. Many differences in views relate to the distinction between what is instrumentally good (good because of its consequences) and intrinsically good (good in and of itself).

Bentham and Mill fall within the category of hedonistic utilitarians in that they saw utility in terms of pleasure or happiness. They argued that the ultimate intrinsic good is happiness, and that all other goods are instrumental towards this end. Happiness, to Mill, was not merely defined as "pleasurable excitement" but was a "realistic appraisal of the pleasurable moments afforded in life, whether they take the form of tranquillity or passion."[35] He argued that pleasure and freedom from pain can be measured and compared from one alternative to another. Thus, the moral value of an action is determined by adding the total happiness produced, and subtracting the pain involved. The balance is the moral value of that act.[36]

Utilitarians do not always agree on these goals and values, whose goals count, or why. Pluralistic utilitarians, for example, believe that no single goal or state constitutes the good. They accept many values—such as friendship, love, devotion, welfare, health, beauty, and moral qualities such as fairness—as having intrinsic worth. They consider this total range of intrinsic values as important products of a good action, not pleasure alone. The greatest aggregate good is achieved when these multiple intrinsic goods are considered in the analysis of right and wrong actions.[37]

Act and Rule Utilitarianism

There are two approaches to utilitarian theory: one considers particular acts in relation to particular circumstances; the other formulates rules of conduct that determine what is right and wrong in general. In *act utilitarianism,* each act is judged on its consequences ("What good and evil consequences will result directly from this action in this circumstance?").[38] In *rule utilitarianism,* one considers the utility of general patterns of behaviour rather than specific actions ("What good and evil consequences will result generally from this sort of action?").[39] A rule is correct provided that more utility would be produced by people following it, rather than by any other rule that would apply to the situation or act. (Some argue that this approach is similar to Kant's notion of universality, which will be discussed later in this chapter.)

In practice, then, a person might list the alternative actions available, consider the possible consequences or outcomes of each act, then quantify the consequences in relation to the "good," whether that be utility, pleasure, or happiness. The right alternative or rule would be the one that produced the most utility, the greatest good, or the least harm for the greatest number of people.

Rule utilitarians hold that rules have a central position in morality and cannot be compromised by the demands of a particular situation. The effectiveness of a rule is judged by determining that its observance would, in theory, maximize social utility[40] better than any possible substitute rule, or no rule. Theoretically, utilitarian rules are firm and protective of all classes of individuals, independent of factors of social convenience and momentary need.[41]

Critics of rule utilitarianism question how one resolves conflict among moral rules in particular circumstances or situations. They argue that ranking of rules is almost impossible; therefore, in circumstances of conflict, the principle of utility decides and the theory is reduced to act utilitarianism.[42] Rule utilitarians argue that every moral theory "has certain practical limitations in cases of conflict,"[43] but that in the majority of circumstances, the rules make sense.

Criticism of Utilitarianism

Critics of utilitarianism argue that it is impossible and impractical to use this theory in determining what one ought to do in daily life. They suggest that the model is relatively useless for purposes of objectively quantifying widely different interests in order to determine where maximal value—and therefore right action—lies.[44] Further, given the focus on pleasure as the desired end, critics have concerns about individuals who might have morally unacceptable preferences and use these in their calculations. Supporters argue that we must rely on common sense, our habits, and our past experiences in quantifying consequences. We need to be only reasonably predictive, recognizing that it is not always possible to be error-free. Further, they suggest, most people are not perverse; if they were, then their actions would result in great unhappiness in society and would be wrong, thus demonstrating the validity of the theory.[45]

Other critics suggest that "good" cannot be measured and comparatively weighed. In response, utilitarians argue that we make crude, rough-and-ready comparisons of values every day. What is important is to be morally conscientious and serious in our analysis.[46]

One of the more serious judgements against utilitarianism is that it can lead to injustice. Critics argue that the greatest balance of value for the greatest number may bring harm to a minority, thus failing to consider issues of distributive justice.[47]

Utilitarians respond that "considerations of social utility and the basic rules of justice determined by these calculations set a limit or the risk of harm that can be permitted."[48] In other words, considerations regarding justice and social utility are part of the calculations considered in the short- and long-term evaluation of the rightness of a particular act or rule under utilitarian theory. Rule utilitarians deny that single cost–benefit determinations ought to be accepted. General rules of justice should constrain the use of cost–benefit analysis in all cases and ensure that standards of distributive justice are included in the analysis.[49]

Application to Health Care

In order to evaluate the application of utilitarian theory to day-to-day practice, consider the following scenario:

> Mary is the charge nurse on evening shift in an Intensive Care Unit in a major city hospital. It is a busy night: Frank, a 27-year-old male, is dying, having sustained major head injuries in a motor vehicle accident. Another patient, who received a lung transplant earlier in the day, has just gone into cardiac arrest. Meanwhile, the nurses are preparing for an admission from the Emergency Department, and because it is dinnertime, they are relieving one another.
>
> Members of Frank's family have just arrived from out of town and wish to spend time with him. On this unit, two visitors at a time are permitted for 10 min/h. That maximum has already been met, yet two brothers and two sisters are still waiting. Frank's relief nurse is also involved in preparing for the new admission. She informs the family of the rules, stating that it is "just too busy" to have visitors at this time. The family complains to Mary, who sympathizes, especially as she doesn't believe Frank will survive the shift. When approached, Frank's relief nurse cites unit policy and suggests that her priority is helping the new patient who, unlike Frank, still has a chance. How can she do her job effectively if Frank's family is in the way?

Is there an ethical dilemma in this case? Would a utilitarian ethical theory help Mary to identify the dilemma and resolve the issue? How? On what grounds would the hospital have based its visiting policy? Are these grounds justified? What position would an act utilitarian take in this circumstance? What are the relevant ethical considerations?

Would a utilitarian theory assist you in justifying your position on this case? Would this theory assist you in your day-to-day practice?

Deontological Theory

In deontological theory, rules are established to determine what is right or wrong based on one's obligations and duties. These obligations and duties are based on unchanging or absolute principles that are derived from universally shared values.[50] Deontologists believe that these standards for moral behaviour exist independently of means or ends.[51] Consequences, they argue, are irrelevant to moral evaluation. An act or rule is right if it satisfies the demands of some overriding principle or principles of duty. Further, they argue, our duties to others are complex, and vary according to our relationships in society, as, for example, the duties and obligations a parent has to a child, or the responsibilities physicians and nurses have to patients.[52]

Deontologists attempt to identify the source of these moral standards and the extent of duties and obligations upon which they are founded. There are various deontological perspectives on the foundation of duty—for example, the will of God, reason, intuition, universality, or the social contract.[53]

As with utilitarianism, there are two types of deontological theory, act and rule. The *act deontologist* believes that an individual in any situation should grasp immediately what ought to be done without the need to rely on rules. Act deontologists emphasize the particular and changing features of the moral experience and value the intuitive response to situations or circumstances.[54]

Rule deontologists promote that acts are right or wrong relative to their "conformity or nonconformity to one or more principles or rules," independent of their consequences.[55] Further, there are two types of rule deontologists: monistic, who hold that there is one supreme principle, and pluralistic, who believe that there are many principles to guide moral conduct. The monistic deontologist argues the existence of one fundamental principle that provides "the source from which other more specific moral rules can be derived"—for example, the golden rule ("Do unto others...").[56]

Rule deontologists argue that rules facilitate decision making. Further, they suggest that act theories present problems for cooperation and trust, and reduce morality to "rules of thumb." Moral rules, they say, should be binding.[57]

Immanuel Kant (1724–1804) formulated the best-known rule-oriented deontological theory.

Kantian Ethics

Kant believed that the ordinary person needed no guidance in determining right from wrong; this would be clear to every decent human being.[58] The challenge, he believed, was for people to maintain the self-control to do what was right. He set out to establish a comprehensive theory of the nature of morality, in order to explain how morality was both possible and rational.[59] He rejected the utilitarian notion of happiness and the maximization of human desire as the basis for morality. People, he said, do not derive their dignity or worth from desiring happiness; rather, morality must be based on the values of rationality and freedom. He argued that one could not be acting morally while justifying one's actions by an appeal to human desires.[60] Further, a focus on the principle of utility would lead to grave injustices, there being no assurance that the distribution of happiness would be fair. Kant placed great emphasis on justice and individual liberty.[61]

Kant developed two distinct theories of morality—a theory of moral obligation and a theory of moral value. The theory of moral obligation focussed on how we decide an act is right, whereas the theory of moral value considered how we decide when a person is morally good or has a good character.[62]

Theory of Moral Value

How do we determine whether a person is morally good or has a good character? According to Kant, it is insufficient to look only at actions and the consequences of those actions, without also looking at the person's motives and intentions. Actions alone do not give the complete picture of one's moral character, since a bad person may do the right thing for the wrong reasons. The only moral motive, a sign of good character, is the motive of conscientiousness (acting from duty). A morally good person is one with good will, that is, one who acts from duty.[63] For example, a person tells the truth because of the duty to tell the truth regardless of the consequences.

The notion of justice is fundamental to Kant's theory of moral value, and is tied to notions of freedom and rationality. Kant considered individuals as rational, moral agents who have the right to make their own choices, unless those choices interfere with the freedom of others. He believed that morality presupposed the existence of free will and that we have the choice to act from good will or not.[64] An action, behaviour, or decision, chosen in accordance with one's duty or good will, is therefore right. If an act and one's motivation to do that act is right, then it is intrinsically good; that is, it is good in and of itself. If an act is intrinsically good, then it has moral value.[65]

Kant placed great emphasis on performance of one's duty for its own sake. While it is possible to engage in right actions for many reasons—for example, fear or self-interest—Kant considered such actions morally praiseworthy only if they are performed out of duty.[66] Thus, to be moral, an individual must demonstrate good will or good intention by doing what he or she ought to do, rather than acting from inclination or self-interest.[67]

Some actions based on inclination or self-interest may be worthy of praise; they may also happen to be in accordance with duty. But these do not have "moral" value.[68] For example, a rich benefactor may donate a million dollars to a health care agency in order to have the agency renamed in his honour. This act, then, might be praiseworthy and in accordance with duty, but it would not have moral value. Alternatively, an individual recently unemployed who continues to contribute weekly to his church is acting from a sense of duty, and hence his actions have moral worth or value. Actions with true moral worth, when they are evaluated, stand alone, independently of other motives. Thus, an act performed from duty has moral worth because of the principle guiding that act; the worth does not spring from the act's results or outcomes.

Kant emphasized duty as the prominent feature of moral consciousness. Duty accords with moral law, the essential characteristic of which is universality, discussed in the next section.[69]

Theory of Moral Obligation

Kant's theory of moral obligation is focussed on how those principles and rules that guide duty should be determined.

Kant tried to establish the ultimate foundation for the validity of moral rules in pure reason, not on intuition, conscience, or utility. Morality, he argued, should provide a rational and universal framework of principles and moral rules that constrain and guide everyone, regardless of personal goals and interests.[70] The moral worth of an individual's action depends only on the moral acceptability of the rule upon which that person is acting.[71] As discussed earlier, a person's act has moral worth when performed with good will, present when one *knowingly* governs oneself in accordance with universally valid moral principles."[72]

Kant believed that valid moral and ethical principles are based on an abstract, *a priori* foundation, that is, independent of empirical reality and morally obligatory. Hence, he argued, morality is objectively and universally binding; it is absolute. If something is right, it is always right, and not dependent on circumstance or outcome.[73] For example, if telling the truth is morally correct, then one must always tell the truth, regardless of the context of the situation or the consequences.

Kant believed that we are able to isolate these a priori, or absolute, elements that ground morality through reasoning. He claimed that the universal basis of morality lies in an individual's rational nature rather than in human desires and inclinations, because rationality is the same for everyone.[74] (Later in this chapter, when we discuss feminist views, we will describe a different perspective.)

Kant identified one supreme principle that a law of morality must follow, and called this the **categorical imperative;** categorical, in that Kant admits of no exceptions to the rule that is absolutely binding, and imperative, in that it gives instructions about how one must act.[75] Kant set out some guidelines, or *maxims,* for determining rules of conduct based on the categorical imperative. He stated that an act is morally right if and only if its maxim is universalizable.

The categorical imperative is fundamental to Kant's theory on how to identify the rules or principles that guide our actions and moral decisions, and is independent of our goals or desires. Kant expresses the categorical imperative, or moral law, in a number of formulations:

> I am never to act otherwise than so that I could also will that my maxim should become a universal law.[76]

> We must be able to will that the maxim of our action should become a universal law.... Since you would not want others to behave in the way you propose to behave, you should not behave in that way.[77]

> So act as to treat humanity whether in thine own person or in that of any other, in every case as an end withal, never as means only.[78]

According to Kant, we must determine the implications of universalizing the rules that guide our actions. For example, would we be able to establish a rule that lying is morally correct? What would happen if everyone lied? Whom would we be able to trust? Could we establish a rule that only doctors may decide on treatment options for patients? What would a society be like if we were denied the freedom to decide about our own health care? What if it were permissible to cross an intersection on a red light? A rule must undergo such scrutiny. If it can be applied universally, then it is what we "ought" to do. If not, then it is morally wrong.

One formulation of the categorical imperative (the third quotation from Kant, above) requires us to treat each human being or person as an end, never as a means to any other end. This is based in Kant's view that the existence of humanity has in itself absolute worth. Therefore, all human beings should be respected.[79]

For example, Kant would argue that we have a duty to tell the truth, since persons ought to be respected and not used as a means to some other desired end (such as keeping the truth from someone to protect our own interests). Even if lying were to produce some desired outcome for the person being lied to, the act would still be disrespectful. It would constitute using a person as a means to a desired end and therefore should not be tolerated. However, Kant did not say that, as persons, we would never be used as means—for example, for some instrumental good. But if we are used as an instrument towards some other good, we must also be regarded as ends in ourselves. Hence, for example, the notion of informed consent: Kant would probably agree that it was morally acceptable to use persons for research or organ donation, but only if our right to self-determination was respected.

To summarize: according to Kant, a rule, principle, or maxim is a fundamental, objective moral law grounded in pure practical reasoning, upon which all people would act if we were purely rational, moral agents.

Criticism of Kant

There are a number of criticisms of Kant's theory, particularly related to its application in everyday practice. For example, how is duty to be determined when two or more duties are in conflict? What happens if, in order to protect someone from harm, we have to lie or withhold the truth? (Consider a situation in which someone provides protection to a woman who is being abused by her husband, and the husband arrives asking about her whereabouts.) Kant's theory seems to demand that both relevant duties be fulfilled: the duty to tell the truth and the duty to protect the woman from harm. Kant does not provide a means to deal with this type of dilemma; he indicates only that we have the duty to do both.[80]

Critics also argue that the categorical imperative is ultimately reduced to a determination of consequences. That is, in looking at the universal application of an action, one is actually looking at the overall consequences of that act. If the universal performance of a certain type of action is undesirable overall, then it is wrong.[81] In response, Kantians argue that consequences are not totally disregarded; the features of making something right are not dependent on any outcome alone.[82]

Application to Health Care

In order to evaluate the application of Kantian theory to day-to-day practice, consider the following scenario:

> *Joanne is a public health nurse in a rural community in northern Alberta who is following the care of a new mother and her two-week-old daughter. Joanne finds the mother, Margaret, more stressed than most new mothers she has worked with. During a recent visit, Joanne observes that Margaret has been crying. As nurse and patient have developed a good relationship, Margaret soon reveals the source of her distress.*
>
> *Margaret and her husband had experienced some difficulties about a year earlier. At that time, she took a vacation with a woman friend. While away, she had sexual relations with a man who lives somewhere in the United States. She has no idea how to contact him, and he knows nothing about her whereabouts. After Margaret returned from vacation, the situation with her husband improved, and she decided not to reveal her indiscretion. She strongly suspects the baby is not her husband's, and asks Joanne to keep her confidence.*
>
> *A few weeks later, Margaret's husband asks Joanne to explain how their daughter has red hair. He can't think of anyone on either side of the family with that hair colour.*

What are the ethical issues and problems related to this case? What conflicting obligations does Joanne have? What should she do, and why? What guidance would Kantian ethics provide? What position would a utilitarian take in this circumstance? What are the relevant ethical considerations?

Would Kantian theory assist you in your day-to-day practice?

The Deontology of W.D. Ross

W.D. Ross, a British philosopher of the early 20th century, developed a pluralistic, rule-oriented deontological theory that attempts to resolve the problem of conflict of duties. Ross identified **prima facie duties,** that is, those duties that one must always act upon unless they conflict with those of equal or stronger obligation.[83] The stronger duty is determined by an examination of the respective weights of the competing prima facie duties. Ross accepts that prima facie duties are not absolute, since they can be overridden. Instead, he argues they have greater moral significance than mere rules of thumb.[84]

Sometimes moral rules or principles conflict. When one is faced with a number of alternatives, the "right" alternative is the one consistent with all the rules. If a number of alternatives are consistent with the rules, then the choice is one of preference. When each choice is consistent with one rule but in conflict with another, then one attempts to appeal to the higher rule to resolve the conflict. For example, sanctity of life would have priority over the rule of veracity or truth telling.

In response to criticisms that it is not always possible to evaluate the respective weights of principles in conflict, Ross also reduced his argument to a claim that no moral system is free of conflicts and exceptions.[85]

Would the deontological approach formulated by Ross be easier to apply to Margaret's case? How? What are the ethical principles? Which ones have greater priority?

Ethical Principles

Ethical principles are derived from moral theory and serve as rules to guide moral conduct, and to assist us in taking consistent positions on specific and related issues.[86] As a framework for ethical decision making, they are the most familiar to health professionals and constitute a popular approach to health care ethics. Ethical principles are expressed in many professional codes of ethics.

The use of biomedical ethical principles as a guide for ethical decision making in health care was introduced by Beauchamp and Childress (1983) in *Principles of Biomedical Ethics*.[87] The important principles commonly applied to health care issues and dilemmas include sanctity of life, autonomy, non-maleficence, beneficence, justice, fidelity, and veracity. Ethical principles are considered prima facie—that is, their application may be relative to another principle that may have more weight or priority in a given situation. However, some individuals may consider particular principles to be a priori, or binding. For example, some people advocate sanctity of life in all forms and at all costs, while others believe that quality of life may override sanctity of life in some circumstances.

Autonomy

The principle of **autonomy** (Greek: *autos*, "self"; *nomos*, "rule") asserts that a capable and competent individual is free to determine, and to act in accordance with, a self-chosen plan.[88] Autonomy, founded on respect for persons, is based on the notion that human beings have worth and moral dignity not possessed by other creatures. To respect persons is to recognize them, without condition, as worthy agents who should not be treated as mere means to any other end. To treat persons as a means to an end is to treat them as if they were not moral agents, and would be disrespectful.[89] Thus, persons—who possess moral dignity—can rightfully decide their own destiny and should be allowed to make their own evaluations, choices, and actions, so long as these do not harm nor interfere with the liberty or freedom of others.[90] Respect for autonomy also means granting individuals the right to privacy and confidentiality. Confidentiality is important in the health care environment, in which patients and clients must trust health professionals with private information in order to receive safe and competent care. Patients have the right to expect that such information will remain confidential unless there is a risk to self or others, or unless disclosure is required by law.

This principle supports the Kantian view that individuals be respected as ends in and of themselves, and never as means to some other end. As discussed earlier in this chapter, this view is based in Kant's belief that humanity itself has absolute worth. Therefore, all human beings should be respected.[91]

This principle is also consistent with Mill's utilitarian ethics, which states that autonomy maximizes the benefits of all concerned, and that social and political control over individual action is legitimate only if it is necessary to prevent harm to others.[92]

The legal doctrine of **informed consent** is based on respect for the principle of autonomy and an individual's right to the information required to make decisions about one's own health care. Failure to provide a patient with adequate information limits that person's autonomy and interferes with his or her rights. (The elements of informed consent will be discussed in Chapter Six.) The concept of the autonomous individual gives rise to the duty of respecting a person's values and choices. Autonomy assumes the person is competent; has the ability to decide rationally, rather than impulsively; and has the ability to act upon those decisions and choices.[93]

In order to be autonomous, a person must be free of external control and be able to take action to control his or her own affairs.[94] Even if it is believed that clients' evaluations or decisions are wrong, or even potentially harmful to themselves, as long as those actions pose no threat of serious harm to others, then the principle of autonomy demands they be respected. On occasion, autonomy conflicts with other principles, such as beneficence—for example, when a patient refuses treatment that the nurse and health care team firmly believe is in the patient's best interest. As nurses know, illness puts limits on individual autonomy. The hospital environment further limits the patient's control. The views of the health care team may be readily apparent to the patient, leading to subtle forms of coercion in relation to choices the patient must make. Patients may experience anxiety and stress, and even be overwhelmed by uncertainty with regard to their future and prognosis. It is the duty of the nurse to support the patient through this process, ensure that he or she has the information required to make choices, and give him or her time to reflect on these choices to determine the best course of action.

Some philosophers believe autonomy to be the primary moral principle, which takes precedence over all other moral considerations.[95] The challenge, particularly for health professionals, is to ensure that clients have the ability to act autonomously—that is, they are making decisions with a full understanding of the facts, issues, and consequences of that decision. Some persons are unable to act autonomously owing to immaturity, incapacity, lack of information, or coercion. A person of diminished autonomy is highly dependent on others and, to some degree, is unable to choose a plan on the basis of controlled deliberations. Young children and the mentally ill fall into this category of individuals whose rights may need to be protected by others.

Since autonomy is a prima facie principle, it may at times conflict with another principle of higher moral weight in a particular circumstance. For example, a person with a terminal disease who is in constant pain may, after careful deliberation, freely decide that assisted suicide is his preferred option. Even if his decision has the support of his family and friends, the principle of **sanctity of life** continues to have more weight in Canadian society than respect for autonomy in this circumstance.

Another important principle that is derived from the principle of autonomy is the principle of **veracity,** the duty to tell the truth.

Veracity, or truth telling, is central to ensuring and maintaining trust within the nurse–patient/client relationship. An individual's right to the truth is linked to respect for persons, since the principle of autonomy acknowledges the dignity of each human being. Patients have the right to expect that the nurses caring for them will provide honest responses to their questions and communicate truthfully to them about the nature of their condition and the care they receive.

Conflicts associated with our obligation to the principle of veracity arise when the truth may result in harm. For example, consider a patient who is dying of a terminal disease. How should caregivers respond to questions associated with the outcome of a particular treatment when the likelihood for success is poor, but they still wish to communicate some sense of hope? How does one balance the need to share relevant information with a client while ensuring that the information is shared in a respectful and benevolent manner? How and when to communicate bad news, for example, is a critical ethical issue. One cannot appeal to the principle of veracity as justification for revealing bad news to a patient without considering the timing and manner of communication, and the need for follow-up care and support.

Truth telling is fundamental to the establishment and maintenance of trusting relationships. Key to the relationship of trust between nurses and patients is the ability to care, to provide comfort, and to maintain honest and truthful communication while continuing to convey a sense of hope and purpose.

Non-Maleficence

The principle of **non-maleficence** is associated with the Latin maxim, *primum non nocere:* "above all (or first), do no harm." This is expressed in many professional codes of ethics and in the Hippocratic Oath: "I will use treatment to help the sick according to my ability and judgement, but I will never use it to injure or wrong them." This principle obliges us to act in such a way that we prevent or remove harm.[96] All members of society are obliged by law to respect this principle.

In nursing, professional practice standards express the competencies that nurses must have to ensure the provision of safe patient care. Often, the actions of nurses may produce some temporary harm (e.g., the administration of medication by injection, restraining patients, painful procedures such as dressings or intravenous insertion). This temporary harm is justified if it is a means towards producing a good and if the principle of autonomy is respected.

There are four hierarchical elements related to non-maleficence.[97] These move from a minimal to a higher standard of obligation. The first three represent adherence to the principle of non-maleficence, whereas the higher standard expressed in the fourth relates to the principle of beneficence, described next.

(1) One ought not to inflict evil or harm.
(2) One ought to prevent evil or harm.
(3) One ought to remove evil or harm.
(4) One ought to do or promote good.[98]

Beneficence

The principle of **beneficence** sets a higher standard than non-maleficence in that one must make a positive move to produce some good or benefit for another. It asserts a positive obligation to come to the assistance of those in need. Beneficence asserts a duty or obligation to help others to further their important and legitimate interests.[99] Many thinkers argue that it is the ideal to be beneficent, but that we are not morally obliged to take positive action to benefit others. Indeed the law in Canada, except for the Province of Quebec, does not require us to assist others, for example in emergencies. This differs from "good Samaritan" laws in force in some European countries. In France, individuals can face criminal charges for failing to provide assistance in emergencies; in Quebec, a person who fails to render assistance can be sued by the injured person for such failure.

As professionals, nurses have the duty to act in such a manner that not only protects patients from harm but also produces some good or benefit. Failure to do this may violate professional duties and obligations.

At times, the principle of beneficence may conflict with that of autonomy. This is often a source of distress for health professionals when we know a particular intervention is likely to benefit a patient yet the patient refuses consent. Health professionals have an obligation to ensure that patients are provided with the information, support, and time to make decisions that are truly in their best interests. Fear, lack of understanding, and previous negative experiences may play a role in a patient's decision.

Paternalism

Traditionally, but less so in recent years, health professionals may have acted in a paternalistic ("father knows best") way towards patients, in an effort to protect them from the potentially harmful consequences of their choices. That is, out of a desire to be beneficent, physicians and nurses may have given that principle priority over others (autonomy, truth telling) in an effort to do what they think is best for the patient.

Paternalism restricts the liberty of individuals. Treatment may be given or withheld without the client's consent; the justification for such action is either the prevention of some harm they might do to themselves or the production of some benefit they might not otherwise secure.[100] In the past, some health professionals went so far as to withhold information from patients with a terminal illness in order to protect them from the "pain" of knowing their death was imminent. (Of course, patients may choose to have information withheld from them, in such circumstances.) Others would fail to disclose all the side effects or consequences of major surgery in order to secure consent. Examples of paternalism that are considered justified in Canadian society today include involuntary committal to a mental health facility, preventing the suicide of a competent person, resuscitation without consent, denial of innovative treatment, and the requirements to use bike helmets, seat belts, and immunization against disease.

Fidelity

The principle of **fidelity** is the foundation of the nurse–patient relationship. This rule is about loyalty, keeping promises, truth telling (veracity), and being faithful to those entrusted to our care.[101] Fidelity comes into play when we uphold our commitment to provide adequate pain control, when we provide quality care, comfort and support when needed, when we represent the interests of our clients and when we tell the truth. This principle is challenged when nurses are placed in situations where being loyal to a patient may compromise their own ethical principles, as when a terminally ill patient requests assistance to die when pain cannot be controlled and life has lost its dignity. Even if the nurse understands the patient's physical and emotional pain, and agrees that this action would demonstrate care and compassion, he or she is restricted by law (and perhaps by the nurse's own beliefs) from helping the patient in this circumstance.

Justice

The principle of **justice** is based on the notion of fairness. In particular, theories of justice focus on how we treat individuals and groups within society, how we distribute benefits (e.g., health care) and burdens (e.g., taxes) in an equitable way, and how we compensate those who have been unfairly burdened or harmed. In health care, justice is fundamental to issues associated with the allocation of resources and rationing, in times of scarcity or diminishing resources. There are two forms of justice relevant to health care: distributive justice and compensatory justice.

Distributive justice is described as the proper distribution of both social benefits and burdens across society.[102] Unfortunately, most perspectives on justice describe the concept theoretically, but fail to provide effective tools to determine equality or proportion, leaving distribution open to differences in interpretation.

Different perspectives on distributive justice apply the following divergent principles. In determining equitable distribution of resources, decisions may be based on one of several considerations:[103]

- To each person an equal share.
- To each person according to individual need.
- To each person according to that person's rights.
- To each person according to individual effort.
- To each person according to societal contribution.
- To each person according to merit.

Questions of how to distribute resources equitably are a challenge when resources are scarce, as they increasingly are in health care. Nurses have to deal with such questions as to how financial resources are distributed; which programs are funded; how staff are allocated; how patient assignments are organized; who gets the scarce organ for transplantation, and many others. Recently, major restructuring in a number of Canadian hospitals has led to the introduction of different models of care that include various levels or categories of care providers. These models add a new dimension to resource allocation from a nursing perspective in that there is a further requirement to evaluate the care needs of patients relative to the type of provider competent to provide that care.

Rationing is a method of allocating resources when these are scarce and one has to decide who will most benefit. For example, although in Canada we have decided that health care will be provided to all citizens, rationing challenges exist when a particular health care resource is scarce and cannot be provided to everyone in need of it. A well-known example of rationing is in the area of organ donation. Even if all the health care dollars necessary were available to perform all the transplants needed, there is still a scarcity of donor organs. Thus, transplant programs must determine how this limited resource will be distributed. Should an organ be given to the person waiting the longest, to the person with the best chance for survival, to the sickest, to the one with the greatest need, or to the person who "deserves" it the most (e.g., the liver transplant recipient who has never consumed alcohol or the lung transplant recipient who has never smoked)?

Macro resource allocation decisions are made at the policy level. Administrators or legislators decide which programs will be funded. For example, do we increase the number of cardiac surgical procedures performed annually, or do we invest in a program of prevention? Individual nurses face

micro resource allocation decisions on a daily basis. Which patient gets admitted to the one remaining intensive care bed? How much home care do we
provide to a dying patient? How do we allocate the time we spend with the
eight home care patients we have to visit today? If we are short of staff and
can't provide all the care needed today, what do we eliminate?

Compensatory justice involves providing compensation or payment for
harm that has been done to an individual or group. Compensation is commonly provided to individuals or groups as a result of a successful suit for
negligence or malpractice. Recently, large groups in Canada have been compensated for harm that resulted from problems with the blood system.
Federal and provincial governments compensated victims of HIV and hepati-
tis C who contracted their diseases through blood transfusions.

Application to Health Care

In order to evaluate the application of ethical principles to day-to-day practice, consider the following scenario:

> *John is 16 years old. Two years ago he was diagnosed with a sarcoma (bone
> cancer) in his right foot. At that time he received aggressive chemotherapy
> and had his foot amputated. He has done well since, though he had been
> unable to participate in the contact sports he loves. Now the cancer has
> recurred in John's right tibia. The planned treatment involves an above-the-
> knee amputation and more chemotherapy.*
>
> *Since John's first round of chemotherapy, treatment approaches and out-
> comes have improved dramatically. However, John refuses this treatment. He
> does not believe his doctor's optimistic projections and states he cannot go
> through chemotherapy again, nor does he want to lose his leg. He maintains
> his refusal even when informed of its consequences and the pain he will expe-
> rience without the surgery.*
>
> *John's parents are very distressed. They ask if he can be forced to accept
> the treatment.*

What are the relevant ethical principles in this case? Are any of these
principles in conflict? Which have priority? Would a review of ethical principles assist John's team and the family in developing a plan? What plan
would you propose? How would you justify your approach?

Feminist and Feminine Perspectives on Ethics

In recent years, feminine and feminist perspectives on ethics have emerged
that offer alternatives to traditional ethical theories which, by and large, have
been developed or formulated by men. As we have seen, the deontological

and utilitarian theories of morality place a strong emphasis on rationality and notions of justice. If (as Carol Gilligan's[104] study on moral development argues) the moral development of women differs from that of men, then these approaches can be problematic for women. Gilligan challenged the notion that there is one superior way to think about moral problems—that is, in terms of abstract and general notions of justice and rights. Given the patriarchal power structures within health care, and the fact that nursing continues to be dominated by women, nurses need to understand these alternative perspectives, which can play a significant role in influencing our thinking on the ethical challenges we face.

Feminine and feminist theorists resist the model of traditional rationalistic ethics, believing instead that ethical analysis must make sense in the real world, and cannot be based primarily on abstract notions.[105] Feminist thinkers believe there is more to ethics than abstract reasoning: there is the context of the situation, and the relationships and unique interest of all the individuals involved.

Feminine and feminist perspectives are critical of the traditional ethical theories they claim are based on male perspectives, standards, biases, and experiences. They argue that traditional ethics searches for a "systematic approach to evaluate the standards or justifications" of morality; the interest is in "determining which rules ideally should be followed."[106] Such rules, they suggest, may fail to fit the moral experience and intuitions of many women and fail to address the unique perspective of the individual.[107] The different experiences of women, feminists argue, may be ignored or downplayed in traditional theories. Further, the emphasis on reason and justice offers little help in explaining our moral duties to children, the ill, or other vulnerable people who have traditionally been cared for by women, rather than men.

The term "feminist ethics" refers to a wide range of feminist-related moral issues. The goal of feminist ethics is to create a plan or ideology that will end the social and political oppression of women. Traditional morality is male-oriented, feminists believe, and there is a unique female perspective of the world that can be shaped into an important and relevant theory.[108]

Feminist Theory[109]

To provide a context for a discussion on a feminine and feminist approach to ethics, it is important to describe briefly the feminist theories upon which they are based. Two premises are accepted as key to feminist thinking:[110]

- Female and male experiences/bodies/socialization are not identical.
- Male perspectives are (currently and historically) dominant, and female perspectives are often marginalized, muted, or simply unrecognized.

A feminist is described as anyone who acts to give voice to these different female perspectives, attempts to balance or integrate male and female perspectives, or who promotes feminine over masculine perspectives. Feminist work considers gender and sex to be important analytic categories, and seeks to understand their operation in the world. The major focus is on the effort to change the distribution and use of power and to stop the oppression of women.[111] While all feminists agree that women are oppressed and that oppression is wrong, different feminists characterize oppression differently and stress different approaches to overcoming it.

Liberal Feminism

This branch of feminism is concerned with the equality of women and the equitable distribution of wealth, position, and power. Though not critical of the "traditional" role of woman as wife and mother, liberal feminists are concerned about the social, political, and economic forces that channel women into these roles. Liberal feminists affirm individual choice and urge equal rights for women and the reform of systems to ensure the inclusion of women.[112] The liberal tradition emphasizes rights and freedoms, and seeks to replace a patriarchal protection of male freedoms and limitations with equal rights for women. For example, since men can father children well into their later years, a liberal feminist might argue that women should have right of access to post-menopausal infertility treatment.[113]

The liberal feminist agenda, then, is to influence the social and political forces that will overcome oppression and provide women with the same rights and opportunities as men. Some strategies include providing greater educational opportunities for women, ensuring women have access to male-dominated professions (such as medicine and engineering), and implementing legislation that ensures equality for women.[114]

From the liberal feminist perspective, the Kantian autonomous-agent model might be acceptable, but both women and men should be able to act as free, rational agents unless their actions constrain the equal rights of others. The problem for the liberal feminist is that women's freedoms are unfairly constrained.

Social Feminism

Social feminists examine the cultural institutions that contribute to the oppression of women and the relationship between the private sphere of the home and the public domain of productive work. They focus primarily on the role of economic oppression in women's lives.[115] They argue that equity will never be attained until changes are made to structures such as the patriarchal family, motherhood, housework, and consumerism, since they influence the distribution of power, wealth, and privilege. Further, they believe that the social and political structures must change so that women's responsibilities within the home, and traditional female professions such as nursing, are valued to the same extent as those of men.[116]

To help distinguish between social feminism and a liberal feminist perspective, consider the different responses to the suggestion supporting in vitro fertilization (IVF) for fertile women in their 20s to allow them to finish their education, launch careers and have children later in life with reduced risks of birth defects. A social feminist would respond that the educational and business institutions are not structured in ways that allow women to work and have families at the healthiest time in their life cycle, and so the institution should be restructured instead. The liberal feminist is more likely to assert rights to both, as the woman herself sees fit.[117]

Radical Feminism

Radical feminists view women-centred perspectives and institutions as the only or primary ones, thus inverting, not just challenging, the current patriarchy. They argue that women's oppression cannot be explained in economic terms alone and that gender oppression is the crucial variable. They challenge concepts and frameworks of traditional philosophical and scientific inquiry. This perspective challenges the patriarchal underpinnings of our society, since radical feminists seek to analyze and value women's experiences from the perspective of female rather than male standards and biases.[118]

The focus is on the development of women-defined thought, culture, and systems; in order for these to evolve, gender discrimination and sexual stereotyping need to be eliminated. Though the childbearing role of women and values such as nurturance are considered important, radical feminists also see them as the historical basis of oppression towards women. There is a greater (not universal) tendency to blame men for oppressing women, not merely to acknowledge that structures in a society are problematic.[119] An implicit, or explicit, recommendation is that men should be removed from their position of dominance and replaced by women. Thus, the liberal feminist goal of economic and political equality with men is perceived as aiming too low.[120]

While the role of childbearing and child rearing in oppression may be a concern within all forms of feminism, for the radical feminist the role of pregnancy is central. All feminists tend to want women, not men, to control the means of reproduction and to have at least an equal voice in reproductive policies. They may argue that that voice should be dominant, since woman are more greatly affected by pregnancy and reproductive interventions than men are. The liberal feminist wants greater reproductive liberty and thus is more likely to want minimal restrictions on surrogacy, egg selling, and other means of reproductive choice. The social feminist not only wants to change the institutions that limit women's choices so that women can thrive whether or not they choose to have families, but challenges the values we place on reproduction and family life. (Thus, social feminists may wish to reject some practices, such as surrogacy or egg selling, as exploitative of women and children.) The radical feminist is more likely to characterize a reproductive intervention as a plot to control the bodies of women.[121]

Although these three perspectives embrace a broad range of feminist thought and practice, all share the following themes:

- recognition of the oppression of women,
- support for equal rights and opportunities for women, and
- an orientation to initiating change.[122]

Feminist theory is complex, as are the ethical perspectives it raises. Nurses can benefit through increased awareness of, and interest in, the ethical views that feminist theory offers.

Feminist Ethics

Feminist approaches to bioethics have historically attempted to expose the ways in which medical practices contribute to the oppression of women. Challenging the paradigms of bioethics, they reject liberal assumptions about autonomous individuals.[123] Humans, they argue, are fundamentally relational, and this is in itself is morally significant.[124] Of key interest to feminists in the area of bioethics is the debate over abortion, surrogate motherhood, maternal–fetal relations, use of fetal tissue, and medical conditions affecting women that have hitherto been ignored.

In feminist ethics, the oppression of women is felt to be an issue of utmost moral concern. It is derived from the "explicitly political perspective of feminism, wherein the oppression of women is seen to be morally and politically unacceptable."[125] Feminist ethics is committed to "eliminating the subordination of women."[126] In all contexts of ethical decision making, the question is asked, "What does this mean for women?" The focus is on changing the status quo, empowering women, and eliminating oppression.[127] Without such changes, feminists believe a truly ethical reality is not possible.

Feminine Ethics

Feminine ethics as recognized by Carol Gilligan, a feminist thinker, has become a focal point in philosophy. Gilligan suggests that women and men make ethical choices based on different sets of values, perceptions, and concerns.[128] Feminine views give significance to the nature of the relationships within a particular ethical context. Gilligan argues that when faced with a moral issue, women use an empathetic form of reasoning[129] and tend to seek out innovative solutions that will ensure that the needs of all parties are met, whereas men tend to seek the dominant rule, even when someone else's interests are sacrificed.[130] An example might be the various approaches to visiting-hour rules in hospitals. One could treat all visitors the same and impose strict time limits, or recognize the special needs of individual patients and families, allowing a more open, client-directed approach.

Those with a feminine view of ethics argue that traditional theories are overly concerned with rational, logical, and objective thinking and acting. In contrast, the feminine view focusses on values, feelings, and desires. There is a greater emphasis on presence, listening, taking feelings seriously, searching for meaning, and seeing the person and the world from a more holistic perspective.[131] Ethical situations are seen to have more than one dimension, and can encompass many principles and theories.

An Ethic of Care

Some feminists who accept Gilligan's assertion that women think differently than men argue for an "ethic of care."[132] Critical of the dominance of principles, and of the historical preference in traditional theories for abstract rules that reinforce a deductive reasoning process, they argue instead for an *inductive* process in which the starting point is the individual's circumstances or personal story. This approach, they suggest, more accurately depicts real life and ensures that all dimensions of the situation are addressed.[133] Reasoning from abstract rules and principles governed by requirements for universality and impartiality, they argue, overlooks the importance of partiality, context, and relationships. The ethics of care is relational, contextual, and empathetic, as opposed to an abstract, universalized, and principled approach of an ethic of justice.[134] An ethic of care is suggested as a new approach to reason that values feelings and emotions, empathy, and care—all important components of our ethical responses. Further, it recognizes the demands of relationships and the particular situations we face.

This view of feminine ethics places greater importance on our emotive responses to ethical choices.[135] Historically, emotion has played a diminished role in ethical decision making, but given the caring nature of the nursing profession, and the intensity of the nurse–client relationship, it is important that we consider this influence.

Using woman's experience as a model for moral theory, an ethic of care advocates spontaneous caring for others as would be appropriate to each unique circumstance. The agent becomes part of the situation, in contrast to the "mechanical actor" who performs a duty but is distant from and unaffected by the situation.[136]

Feminine ethical decision making is based on the desire to respond to each person as an individual. The focus is on caring rather than on justice. Rather than treating all people alike in the name of fairness, it is recognized that some people need and want to be treated differently. Out of interest and concern for each individual's personal context, a focus on caring requires us to examine all dynamics of a situation. In this view, we enter another's world in order to see things as that person sees them.[137] Thus, we can better understand the values and beliefs of others.

The emphasis is on the process of self-understanding, whereby one offers explanations, rather than justifications, for choices. The sharing of unique perspectives facilitates a greater understanding of the dynamics of a situation and therefore provides greater insights to guide our choices. This approach is not limited to the nurse's relationship with the patient. It is recommended as a means of understanding and respecting the various views and life experiences of all members of the health care team.[138]

Not all feminists agree that caring should supplant justice; some worry that it is a "compassion trap" that will keep women in their traditional roles.[139] Some radical feminists have concerns about the feminine notion of caring, which they view as a gender trait and a survival skill of an oppressed group.[140] Too much emphasis on the welfare of others, they believe, can drain the resources and energy of women. These feminists do not reject the relevance of caring, but instead attempt to identify criteria for determining when it should be offered and when not.

Social feminists would agree that feelings play a role in ethical decision making, but that these need to be balanced in relation to social justice.[141] When dealing with ethical issues, there is also the need to consider our experiences, the morally relevant features and responsibilities of the relationships involved, and the context of the situation.[142]

Yarling, McElmurry, and Noddings also focus on an "ethic of care."[143] Noddings, in fact, suggests that caring, which women take more into consideration because of their traditional role within the family, is the only moral consideration.[144] This view has been criticized, since it suggests the exclusion of women who do not share familial responsibilities for caring, and males, from the possibility of such caring and nurturing.[145] Noddings argues that an ethic of care is a quest for new virtues based on traditional women's practices, and that the traditional female role as nurturer can be shaped into an ethic of care.

Other thinkers have argued that it is not only women who offer a caring perspective within their ethical framework. Tschudin and Marks-Maran, who build on the work of Richard Niebuhr (1963), maintain that people function primarily through relationships as responsive, creative beings.[146] Within the context of an ethical discussion, they start with the question, "What is happening?" and emphasize a person's response to a context or situation. Assuming that the wish to do the right thing is an inborn human urge, then a person's response (feeling, emotional reaction, "gut" reaction) is the key indicator of morality.

Application to Health Care

In order to evaluate the application of feminist/feminine theory to day-to-day practice, consider the following scenario:

> Jan is a 40-year-old single woman who works as an accountant with a major consulting firm. She lives in Halifax, though she sometimes travels in her job. Jan has two brothers who moved to Vancouver some years ago.
>
> Jan's mother died about a year ago; her 82-year-old father continues to live alone in the family home. He has done well, but recently was admitted to hospital with pneumonia. He is recovering, and the hospital team would like to discharge him with home care. The home care resources are limited, so they inform Jan that her father will need 24-h assistance from her for at least two to three weeks. Jan has already taken her vacation for the year, and this is audit time for her clients.

How would feminists evaluate this scenario? How would feminist concerns enter into the deliberations of the health care team planning the discharge for Jan's father? Are these concerns ever discussed in your practice?

An Ethical Decision-making Process

This chapter has attempted to introduce the theories, principles, rules, and codes that guide ethical decision making. The following framework is offered as a guide for ethical discussion within the context of health care practice. This framework provides the opportunity to incorporate one or more of the various theories, principles, and codes into the decision-making process. As well, it ensures the proper collection of the data relevant to that process, and that all aspects of the situation are considered. Decision-making frameworks provide a process or approach to guide ethical decision making. They serve as useful guides that assist individuals or groups to focus on the relevant questions and issues.

(1) Describe the Problem

Determine whether the situation constitutes an ethical dilemma, an ethical violation, or whether some significant gap in the care process, such as a breakdown in communication, has led to this problem.

(2) Gather the Facts

What is the patient's diagnosis? Prognosis? Age? What is the patient's cultural background and religion? Are there family or significant others? What is their relationship? Who is involved in the patient's care? Is the patient competent? Has a proxy decision maker been appointed? Is there a living will?

(3) Clarify Values

What are your beliefs about the situation? What are the values of other members of the team? Of the patient and family? Will the cultural and religious background influence what is happening and who should be involved in dealing with this problem?

(4) Note Reactions

How is everyone responding in this situation? What are their behaviours? Are there any emotive reactions? What is everybody feeling? Do they have a gut reaction to what is happening?

(5) Identify Ethical Principles

Which principles apply to this situation? Are any of these principles in conflict? Does one principle (or more) have priority over the others?

(6) Clarify Legal Rules

Are there any legal rules that govern this situation (as in release of confidential information)?

(7) Explore Options and Alternatives

How many options are available? Evaluate each in relation to ethical theories and principles. What are the potential consequences of each alternative? Are there rules that apply to these alternatives? Are they in conflict? How do they apply to the CNA's *Code of Ethics for Registered Nurses*?

(8) Decide the Course of Action

Is one course of action more consistent with ethical theories, principles, and rules? Is there one consistent with your own values and beliefs? How do you feel about making this choice? Do you have a gut reaction to this decision? Can you live with the consequences of this decision?

(9) Develop an Action Plan

Once the choice has been made, how will it be carried out? How will the choice and the reasons behind it be communicated to others? Who will be involved? What are the responsibilities of the patient, the family, the nurse, and the health care team?

(10) Evaluate the Plan

Review the situation regularly. Modify the plan or strategy as required. In retrospect, is there anything you would have done differently? How might you improve this process next time? Is there anything in this process that should be incorporated into a guideline that could help others deal with a similar situation in the future?

Ethics Committees

Ideally, most ethical issues and dilemmas are resolved, and most decisions are made, by the patient, the family, and the health care providers most involved in that patient's care. However, these participants need education, guidelines, and supports to assist them. Sometimes the issues they face are complex and not easily resolved; or, they may have larger implications for the agency, the community, or society. Ethics committees exist to provide education, guidelines, advice, and support with respect to these issues.

The growth in number and complexity of ethical issues in health care has led to the growth in number of ethics committees in Canadian hospitals. Surveys of Canadian hospitals completed in 1984, 1989, and 1991 provide evidence of this growth.[147,148] A poll of 215 Canadian hospitals with more than 300 beds conducted in 1984 found that 36 (26 English, 10 French) of the 196 who responded had ethics committees.[149] A similar study of 142 English-language hospitals having more than 300 beds indicated that 70 of the 120 (84.5%) who responded had an ethics committee.[150] In 1991 in Quebec, 60 institutions surveyed had some form of clinical ethics committee, while 144 did not. The busier hospitals seemed more likely to have a committee, and 77% of those who did had more than 400 beds. The majority of these ethics committees were instituted between 1985 and 1990.[151]

Clinical Ethics Committees

A clinical ethics committee is defined as "any committee that is recognized as being primarily involved in ethical issues regarding patient care."[152] Unlike research ethics committees, who have the function of reviewing the ethical aspects of research proposals, clinical ethics committees deal primarily with the ethical perspectives of patient care. The roles of clinical ethics committees vary and may include one or more of the following functions.

Consultation

Rarely are ethics committees in Canada involved in decisions regarding patient care. Rather, they offer advice about how a situation may be approached, or they assist those seeking help in working through the decision process. Essentially, it is the patient, the family, and the caregivers who must make decisions and act on them, but they can obtain support and assistance from ethics committees. Patients, families, physicians, nurses, other caregivers, and administrators can make referrals to ethics committees.

Education

Most clinical ethics committees play a role in the education of staff. In fact, this is their most important function, given the increased need for staff to be knowledgeable about these issues. Education is provided through interest sessions or in-services, workshops, case presentations, and internal publications.

Policy

Ethics committees may have the responsibility of establishing policies or guidelines to assist staff in dealing with complex issues, or to help clarify the ethical values and duties within an organization or agency. These may include policies on confidentiality, and guidelines respecting resuscitation, withdrawal of treatment, use of reproductive technologies, and consent. Guidelines developed by ethics committees can also serve as educational tools for staff if the ethical rules and principles involved in developing the guidelines are made explicit.

Research

Ethics committees may also conduct research on ethical issues. For example, a committee may survey provider attitudes on withdrawal of treatment or organ donation in order to develop guidelines in these areas, or they may be interested in determining the extent of ethical problems that caregivers face and the decision processes they use.

Composition of Ethics Committees

Most ethics committees have representation from physicians, nurses, chaplains, lawyers, administrators, social workers, and other care providers. Some also have ethicists, board members, and community representatives on the committee. Ethics committees tend to report either to the board of directors of the hospital or to the medical advisory committee.

Implications for Nurses

Surprisingly, it was demonstrated in a pilot study by Storch et al. (1990) that nurses in general had limited awareness of, and experience with, ethics committees. This phenomenon has been linked to the power structures within hospitals and the narrow focus of nurses at the bedside.[153]

Nurses, more than any other health professional, have prolonged exposure to the patient. Consequently, they are likely to understand more than other members of the health care team how the patient feels. Their knowledge of the patient is critical when making ethical decisions. Further, nurses are involved in the outcomes of these decisions. For example, when treatment is withdrawn, or when "no CPR" orders are written, nurses implement these decisions and participate in their consequences.

Nurses are aware of the extent of ethical problems and violations because they face them daily. Therefore, nurses must be involved in ethics committees. They must pursue their issues or concerns. Though due process should be followed, nurses need to be aware that when satisfaction is not achieved they have access to ethics committees. Furthermore, as professionals who are held accountable for their practice, nurses have the right (and often the responsibility) to go directly to ethics committees for advice and consultation. These committees can also support nurses in determining the most appropriate process to follow, and can provide the information or knowledge required. Representatives from ethics committees may also be invited to participate in discussions with other care providers, patients, and families in direct care environments.

Summary

In this chapter we have introduced the theories, principles, codes and decision frameworks that can guide ethical decision making by nurses. In recent years the field of ethics has grown in response to the growing ethical challenges faced by health care providers. The material covered in this chapter is intended to provide nurses with a foundation in ethics that will launch the beginning of a lifelong learning process.

Nurses' commitment and allegiance to the individuals they serve may at times conflict with the interest of society and the common good, and this conflict may emerge in many everyday, practical decisions that nurses face. Such decisions may relate to standards of care, quality of life, and indeed to the very ethic of caring within the nursing profession and the health system.

Technology has altered the boundaries between living and dying. The irony is that major advances in health care delivery have brought caregivers not a sense of greater control, but rather, increased feelings of powerlessness. This has become a predominant theme in discussions among health care providers. We can extend life, but at what cost? We can influence the creation of life, but should we?

At the same time that technological advances are challenging the ethical choices we make, nurses are faced daily with the consequences of downsizing and restructuring the health system. Budget cuts and increased ratios of nurses to patients threaten the standard of care we are able to provide as these technological advances in care are realized.

Nurses must have knowledge of ethics in order to guide the difficult decisions they make and to understand the issues they face.

The key points introduced in this chapter include:

- the complexity of ethical choices nurses make
- the influence of values on ethical decision making
- the relevance of a solid understanding of ethical theory
- a basic introduction to ethical theory and principles
- the tools and process to assist in identifying, understanding, and working through ethical challenges
- when and how to utilize hospital ethics committees.

Critical Thinking

QUESTIONS FOR DISCUSSION

1. Are any of the ethical approaches described in this chapter used when discussing ethical issues in your practice environment?

2. What are the limitations of these theories in applied practice?
3. Compare and contrast utilitarian and deontological approaches. Though feminists are critical of these traditional approaches, are there any areas of similarity with feminism?
4. Is there a theory more consistent with your values? Why?
5. What trends in health care and nursing reinforce the value of a more rigorous ethical reasoning processes?
6. Do you think it is possible to develop an ethical theory that will assist in resolving the major ethical dilemmas faced in health care and nursing?
7. Does use of a theory to resolve an issue necessarily lead to consensus on the solution to a dilemma or problem? Why or why not?

References

1. Grassian, V. (1981). *Moral reasoning: Ethical theory and some contemporary moral problems* (p. 3). New Jersey: Prentice-Hall.
2. Beauchamp, T.L. (1982). *Contemporary issues in bioethics* (2nd ed., p. 1). California: Wadsworth.
3. Ibid.
4. Ibid.
5. Ibid., p. 2.
6. Grassian, supra footnote 1, p. 4.
7. Ibid.
8. Ibid., p. 4.
9. Ibid.
10. Beauchamp, supra footnote 2, p. 2.
11. Ibid., p. 3.
12. Ibid., p. 4.
13. Ibid., p. 11.
14. Ibid., p. 12.
15. The Code is reproduced in Appendix A, page 323.
16. Gilligan, C. (1988). *In a different voice* (pp. 5–23). Cambridge: Harvard University Press.
17. Grassian, supra footnote 1, p. 28.
18. Beauchamp, supra footnote 2, p. 7.
19. Ibid.
20. Grassian, supra footnote 1, p. 28.
21. Beauchamp, supra footnote 2, p. 7.
22. Ibid., p. 8.
23. Ibid.
24. Ibid.
25. Beauchamp, T.L., & Childress, J.F. (1983). *Principles of biomedical ethics* (p. 19). New York: Oxford University Press.
26. Grassian, supra footnote 1, p. 25.
27. Beauchamp, supra footnote 2, p. 13.
28. Ibid.
29. Mill, J.S. (1987). On liberty and considerations on representative government. In *Utilitarianism*. London: Everyman.
30. Beauchamp, supra footnote 2, p. 13.
31. Ibid.
32. Ibid.

33. Mill, J.S. (1993). *On liberty and utilitarianism* (pp. 145–148). New York: Bantam.
34. Ibid.
35. Beauchamp, supra footnote 2, p. 15.
36. Ibid.
37. Ibid.
38. Ibid., p. 15.
39. Ibid.
40. Ibid., p. 16.
41. Ibid.
42. Ibid.
43. Ibid.
44. Ibid., p. 15.
45. Ibid.
46. Ibid.
47. Ibid., p. 19.
48. Ibid.
49. Ibid.
50. Ibid.
51. Ibid.
52. Ibid.
53. Ibid., p. 20.
54. Ibid.
55. Ibid.
56. Ibid.
57. Ibid.
58. Grassian, supra footnote 1, p. 72.
59. Ibid., p. 73.
60. Ibid., p. 74.
61. Ibid.
62. Ibid., p. 79.
63. Ibid., p. 75.
64. Ibid., p. 79.
65. Albert, E., Denise, T., & Peterfreund, S. (1975). *Great traditions in ethics* (pp. 210–212). New York: Van Nostrand.
66. Grassian, supra footnote 1, p. 75.
67. Albert et al., supra footnote 65, p. 207.
68. Ibid., pp. 210–212.
69. Ibid., pp. 215–216.
70. Beauchamp, supra footnote 2, p. 21.
71. Ibid.
72. Ibid.
73. Albert et al., supra footnote 65, pp. 204–207.
74. Ibid., p. 205.
75. Ibid.
76. Ibid., p. 215.
77. Ibid., p. 216.
78. Ibid., p. 223.
79. Grassian, supra footnote 1, p. 79.
80. Beauchamp, supra footnote 2, p. 23.
81. Ibid., p. 25.
82. Ibid.
83. Ibid., p. 23.
84. Ibid.
85. Ibid.
86. Ibid., p. 26.

87. Beauchamp & Childress, supra footnote 25.
88. Ibid., p. 59.
89. Beauchamp, supra footnote 2, p. 26.
90. Ibid., p. 27.
91. Beauchamp & Childress, supra footnote 25, p. 59.
92. Ibid., pp. 59–61.
93. Beauchamp, supra footnote 2, p. 27.
94. Ibid.
95. Ibid.
96. Beauchamp & Childress, supra footnote 25, pp. 106–107.
97. Beauchamp, supra footnote 2, p. 26.
98. Ibid., p. 28.
99. Beauchamp & Childress, supra footnote 25, p. 148.
100. Beauchamp, supra footnote 2, p. 38.
101. Beauchamp & Childress, supra footnote 25, p. 237.
102. Beauchamp, supra footnote 2, p. 30.
103. Beauchamp & Childress, supra footnote 25, p. 187.
104. Gilligan, supra footnote 2.
105. Sherwin, S. (1992). *No longer patient* (p. 55). Philadelphia: Temple University Press.
106. Ibid., p. 35.
107. Ibid., p. 42.
108. Reich, W.T., Ed.(1995) *Encyclopedia of bioethics* (p. 810). New York: Simon & Schuster/Macmillan.
109. For the following précis of feminist theories, the authors are indebted to P.E. Valentine, "A female profession: A feminist management perspective," Chapter 20 in J.M. Hibberd & M.E. Kyle (Eds.), *Nursing management in Canada* (Toronto: W.B. Saunders, 1994).
110. Personal communication. Laura Shanner, March 29, 1995.
111. Wolf, S.M. (Ed.). (1996). *Feminism and bioethics: Beyond reproduction* (p. 8.). New York: Oxford University Press.
112. Reich, supra footnote 108, p. 808
113. Shanner, supra footnote 110.
114. Valentine, supra footnote 109.
115. Reich, supra footnote 108, p. 808.
116. Valentine, supra footnote 109.
117. Dawson, K., Singer, P. (1988). Australian developments in reproductive technology. *Hastings Center Report, 18*(2), 4.
118. Valentine, supra footnote 109.
119. Shanner, supra footnote 110.
120. Ibid.
121. Ibid.
122. Adamson, N., Briskin, L., & McPhail, M. (1988). *Feminists organizing for change: The contemporary women's movement in Canada* (p. 9). Toronto: Oxford University Press.
123. Reich, supra footnote 108, p. 814.
124. Ibid.
125. Sherwin, supra footnote 105, p. 49.
126. Ibid., p. 54.
127. Ibid.
128. Gilligan, supra footnote 16.
129. Reich, supra footnote 108, p. 810
130. Sherwin, supra footnote 105, p. 46.
131. Lind, A., Wilburn, S., & Pate, E. (1986, Spring). Power from within: Feminism and the ethical decision-making process in nursing. *Nursing Administration Quarterly, 10*(3), 50–57.
132. Reich, supra footnote 108, p. 810
133. Wolf, supra footnote 111, p. 15.
134. Ibid.

135. Ibid., p. 8.
136. http://www.utm.edu/research/iep/f/femethic.htm
137. Crowley, M.A. (1989, April). Feminist pedagogy: Nurturing the ethical ideal. *Advances in Nursing Science, 11*(3), 53–61.
138. Baker, C., Diekelmann, N. (1994). Connecting conversations of caring: Recalling the narrative to clinical practice. *Nursing Outlook, 42,* 65–70.
139. Reich, supra footnote 108, p. 811.
140. Sherwin, supra footnote 105, p. 50.
141. Ibid., p. 52.
142. Ibid.
143. Crowley, supra footnote 137.
144. Sherwin, supra footnote 105, p. 46.
145. Condon, E.H. (1992). Nursing and the caring metaphor: Gender and political influences on an ethic of care. *Nursing Outlook, 40*(1), 14–19.
146. Tschudin, V., & Marks-Maran, D. (1993). *Ethics: A primer for nurses.* London: Balliere Tindal. See also Niebuhr, R. (1963), *The responsible self.* New York: Harper & Row.
147. Jean, A., Pare, S., & Parizeau, M. (1991). Hospital ethics committees in Quebec: An overview. *HEC Forum, 3*(6), 339–346.
148. Storch, J.L., Griener, G.G., Marshall, A., & Olineck, B.A. (1990, Winter). Ethics committees in Canadian hospitals: Report of the 1989 survey. *Healthcare Management Forum, 3*(4), 3–8.
149. Ibid.
150. Ibid.
151. Jean et al., supra footnote 147.
152. Storch et al., supra footnote 148.
153. Storch, J.L., & Griener, G.G. (1992, Spring). Ethics committees in Canadian hospitals: Report of the 1990 pilot study. *Healthcare Management Forum, 5*(1).

The Canadian Legal System

LEARNING OBJECTIVES

The purpose of this chapter is to enable you to:
- distinguish between the two primary legal systems in Canada—French civil law and English common law—and appreciate their sources
- understand the legislative process
- distinguish between tort law and criminal law
- understand battery and negligence as they relate to nursing practice
- describe the federal structure of Canada, its Constitution and the *Charter of Rights and Freedoms*
- understand the basic structure and functions of the court system.

Introduction

The legal system is seen by most lay people as an obscure, complicated institution with its own language and rituals, shrouded in mystery. However, a good understanding of its basic machinery is indispensable for nurses. The legal and social interrelationships between individuals and institutions is becoming more complex in Canadian society. Thus, nurses with a working knowledge of the legal system are better able to deal with the myriad rules and regulations that govern their profession, their relationships with physicians and other health practitioners, and the health care system.

Foundations of Canada's Legal System

With the exception of the Province of Quebec, the Canadian legal system is derived from English common law. Historically, Canada is a confederation of former British colonies and colonial territories settled largely by French settlers first, and later by English, Scottish, Welsh, and Irish settlers in the 17th, 18th, and 19th centuries. These settlers brought with them not only their language and culture, but also the legal structures and principles of the mother country. The Province of Quebec was initially settled by French settlers and, for a large part of its history, was ruled by the kings of France under French civil law.

French Civil Law

What is today Quebec was governed exclusively under French **civil law** until the French colonies in North America were ceded by France to Great Britain in 1763 under the Treaty of Paris, which concluded the Seven Years' War. French civil law was based upon the Roman civil law system, which is still prevalent in most Western European countries. This is one of the legacies of the ancient Roman Empire, which controlled much of Europe until its collapse in the sixth century A.D.

In Roman civil law systems, legal rules and principles that establish the rights and responsibilities of individuals are formally written—or, as lawyers say, codified—in a single document known as a **civil code.** Lawyers and judges view this code as the chief source of all rules and principles necessary to resolve disputes or legal issues.

English Common Law

Unlike civil law systems, the majority of the **common law** is not written down or codified as statute law. Statute law is a formal written set of rules passed by a parliament or other legislative body to regulate a particular area, such as Ontario's *Highway Traffic Act,*[1] which regulates motor vehicles, drivers, and the rules of the road.

In the common law system, many of the essential rules and principles that govern day-to-day life, such as the laws of negligence and of contract, are informally contained in a massive and ancient body of precedent developed through centuries of adjudication. **Precedents** are individual sets of judges' written reasons for deciding a particular case. They usually contain the facts of the case, the legal issues to be decided, the legal principles to be applied, and a reasoned discussion of how those principles apply to the case at hand.

Precedents are usually published in volume form by category such as the jurisdiction (provincial or federal), subject matter (e.g., criminal law, family law, tort law, civil procedure) or the level of court that rendered the decisions (e.g., B.C. Court of Appeal, Federal Court of Appeal, Supreme Court of Canada).

Legal principles and rules are distilled and developed from these precedents, then applied to relevant cases by judges. These principles and legal rules are said to be pre-existing, culled from ancient customs and the unwritten common law of England. This body of precedent is called **case law.**

Sources of the Common Law

The two primary sources of law in the common law legal system are case law and statute law. A secondary source of law is found in textbooks and journals written by legal scholars and experts. These writers may address specific topics such as contracts or property law, and the scope may be narrow or broad. Such writings are called doctrine in civil law systems. Though invaluable to common law scholarship and legal education, doctrine is not as authoritative or persuasive to common law courts as it is to their civil law counterparts, and it is subordinate to statute and case law.

Custom constitutes another, less prominent source of law in common law systems. As its name suggests, custom means that in the absence of specific and applicable legal principles in either case law, statutes, or doctrine, the courts will be guided by the long-standing practices of a particular industry, trade, or other activity.

Table 3.1 on page 54 lists the four major sources of common law.

Case Law (Precedent)

Case law is a collection or body of judges' decisions rendered over centuries of judicial consideration and refinement. This feature is found in many nations, Canada among them, that have embraced the English common law. Each case expresses a legal principle which is applied by judges to resolve a legal issue arising in a given situation.

For example, there is a legal principle stating that a party (person) suing or claiming negligence against another person must prove that he or she has suffered **damages,** that the other party owed him or her a duty of care, and that the damages were caused by the other's breach or failure to perform that duty. This rule evolved from early cases in which someone was harmed as a result of another person's carelessness. The courts sought to protect people generally from carelessness, yet they did not wish to impose unreasonable restrictions on people. Therefore, they developed the requirement to prove the existence of three elements: duty of care; harm or damages; and cause and

TABLE 3.1
Sources of common law (in decreasing order of authority)

SOURCE AND DEGREE OF AUTHORITY	DEFINITION AND CHARACTERISTICS
Statute law and regulations Most authoritative in a common law court; override case law in a court of law.	Formal written laws and regulations passed by legislature or cabinet that set forth rules and principles governing a particular subject.
Case law (precedent) Very authoritative; depends on the level of court that rendered the particular decision and its relationship to the court considering the precedent.	Individual court decisions constitute body of precedent in which rules, definitions of legal concepts, and legal principles fashioned by judges over centuries are found; for application in future similar-fact situations.
Doctrine Seldom seen as authoritative by common law judges; depends on the stature of, and respect accorded to, the author of the work within the legal community.	Articles, studies, texts, treatises and other materials by leading legal scholars and academics that elucidate a particular area of law. These usually comment on statute and case law and attempt to elaborate upon, and further interpret, legal principles found in these sources.
Custom Least authoritative; there must be a complete absence of guidance from the other sources before the courts will resort to custom.	Principles and rules of a particular trade, upon which courts will draw when statutes and the common law are silent on a particular issue. The courts elevate accepted practice in a particular trade to a rule of law.

effect between the damages and the actions of the person who has the duty of care.

The use of precedent and case law is best illustrated in the example of a lawsuit. Here, each party to the suit, called a **litigant,** cites case law to the court containing facts similar to the case at hand. Each litigant relies on cases containing a principle or rule of law which, if applied in this case, will yield a result favourable to him or her. In our example in the previous paragraph, if the person bringing the suit cannot prove any damages, the case would, following precedent, be dismissed. Case law might be used to establish the amount of the damages, if they are proved.

The court must select from among these precedents those that are most relevant and most authoritative or binding. It applies the principle stated in the precedent to the facts of the case then before it. The court may elaborate or expand upon the principles derived from previous cases, thus further developing the law. In this sense, common law is fashioned by judges, who have to observe established legal rules in doing so. The decision itself then becomes a further precedent, which serves to bolster or destroy a future litigant's case in similar circumstances.

In English common law, unlike Roman civil law systems, **inferior courts** are bound to decide cases in a fashion similar to any applicable existing precedent of a superior court. This is called the doctrine of **stare decisis.** An inferior court (usually a trial court) is judicially subordinate to an appellate (appeal) court in the hierarchical court structure. We say that the lower court is subordinate in that it is bound to follow the decisions and precedents of the higher one. Stare decisis, which, translated from Latin, roughly means "to abide by the decision,"[2] dictates that a court presented with a prior decision containing facts similar to the case then before it, must decide the present case using the same legal principles and rules pronounced in the prior decision. (Jurisprudence is often used in similar ways by lawyers in Quebec; however, the bulk of legal argument that takes place in court usually relies heavily on the many articles and sections of the *Civil Code* itself.)

The application of precedent in the English common law is designed to achieve two primary objectives. First, the law must be consistent. Review of relevant case law is necessary to determine which judicial pronouncements have the force of law and which have been overruled by subsequent higher court decisions. Consistency is achieved by judges and the legal profession applying the same legal principles in the same circumstances in a similar manner over time. Consequently, a degree of certainty is a characteristic of the common law system.

Second, the common law strives to be predictable. Common law philosophy holds that if lower courts were not bound to follow the decisions and precedents of higher ones, then the outcome of a given case would be unpredictable. A court would be free to decide the case on the basis of any principle of its own choosing, regardless of existing legal principles and rules enshrined in case law. This would defeat the requirement of consistency, as we would never know which principles would be applied in a given situation.

In the common law tradition, predictability and consistency of the law are seen as conducive to a well-ordered society in which people know their rights and obligations towards one another. For example, they allow A. to enter into a **contract** with B., because A. knows that the law will enforce the contract in favour of A. if B. attempts to break it. This certainty follows from a primary legal principle established in case law that people who freely enter into contracts should and will be bound to perform their obligations, unless the contract is contrary to existing law or public policy. Within such a legal framework, a society flourishes both socially and economically, as people can predict the likely legal consequences of their activities. This lends greater stability to their social and economic endeavours.

This body of precedent spans roughly nine centuries and has become quite large and comprehensive. Over time, case law has developed and adapted, albeit slowly, to changing social, moral, and economic conditions and situations.

Statutes and Regulations

Case law is a slow means of altering and fashioning the law to meet changing social and economic conditions. Yet, the impact of court decisions on society is significant and far-reaching.

Courts are by nature conservative institutions. They define their main role as that of interpreting and applying an existing body of laws and regulations rather than creating law from abstract principles. The court, as the impartial arbiter of societal conflicts, is usually loath to infringe upon Parliament's power to make the nation's laws.

Perhaps the best example of this is found in the recent judicial treatment of **abortion** laws and laws dealing with **assisted suicide.** Until recently, the courts upheld laws that prohibit abortions except in special cases. The *Criminal Code of Canada* made it an offence for anyone to perform such a procedure unless it was intended to preserve the life of the mother and was deemed necessary by a hospital committee. In a legal challenge of the provision within the *Criminal Code,* the Supreme Court of Canada in *R v. Morgentaler* ruled the law unconstitutional as violating a woman's right to life and personal security.[3] Abortion is therefore regulated by provincial health legislation, not by the federal criminal power.

With respect to the controversial issue of assisted suicide, the *Criminal Code of Canada* makes it an offence for anyone to assist or counsel a person to take his or her own life.[4] The decision of the Supreme Court of Canada in the case of Sue Rodriguez illustrates the court's reluctance to strike down statutory provisions respecting assisted suicide. But in *R v. Latimer,*[5] the court, after the end of a new trial ordered by the Supreme Court of Canada, concluded that, while the accused was guilty of the second-degree murder of his daughter, who suffered from a severe form of muscular dystrophy, sentencing him to the maximum prison term prescribed by law would have violated his Charter right to be free from cruel and unusual punishment. Instead, he was sentenced to time served, with eligibility for parole after two years. This sentence was reversed on appeal to the Saskatchewan Court of Appeal, and a 10-year sentence was substituted. Mr. Latimer has appealed the matter further to the Supreme Court of Canada.

The Legislative Process

The slower pace of pre-industrial life may have been well suited to the gradual and incremental approach of common law courts. However, a modern and rapidly changing society demands more rapid response, which our legal institutions are ill suited to provide. For example, euthanasia has been a long-standing concern. Here, the legislative branch of government is called upon to enact new laws in response to such needs.

Canada is a constitutional monarchy with a **responsible government.** This means that government ministers sit in **Parliament** and are accountable to it for the exercise of governmental power. Its government comprises three branches: the judicial branch, or the courts that apply the law impartially to resolve disputes between individuals or an individual and the State; the executive branch, or the Queen and her ministers who enforce the law; and the legislative branch, which consists of Parliament and the provincial legislatures. Figure 3.1 illustrates the three branches of government in Canada.

In Canada the power to make law rests with Parliament or, in the case of a province, the legislative assembly. Parliament consists of the Queen, the Senate, and the House of Commons. Provincial legislatures in Canada have only one house, usually called the **Legislative Assembly.** Parliament and the provincial legislatures make statute laws which are also called "Acts" or statutes. These take priority over the common law and may confirm, clarify, alter, limit, or rescind the common law as determined by the courts. Further, Parliament and the legislatures can adopt urgently needed laws more quickly and comprehensively than can the courts if sufficient political will exists and is brought to bear. This may not always happen, however, and the courts will be left with this task. The legislatures may also legislate in new areas upon which the courts have not yet pronounced, thereby pre-empting judicial "lawmaking" that might steer the law in a direction other than that desired by elected lawmakers.

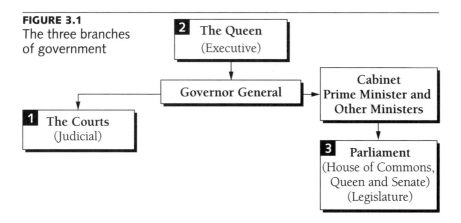

FIGURE 3.1
The three branches of government

2 The Queen (Executive)

Governor General

Cabinet Prime Minister and Other Ministers

1 The Courts (Judicial)

3 Parliament (House of Commons, Queen and Senate) (Legislature)

Cabinet ministers, including the prime minister, who is the head of the government, are usually elected members of the House of Commons belonging to a political party holding the majority of the seats in that House. Ministers can also be chosen from the Senate, but this is a rare occurrence. By unwritten **constitutional convention** (a practice that is not a part of the legal written **Constitution,** yet is followed by tradition), such members are entitled to form a government, since with their majority in Parliament, they are said to command the confidence of the House.

Government ministers and the Prime Minister are formally appointed and chosen to form a government by the Governor General, who is the Queen's representative. Provincial governments are formed in the same way; however, the provincial lieutenant-governor, the Queen's representative in that province, makes the formal appointment.

Before it can become law, a statute must pass the scrutiny of Parliament or, in the case of a provincial law, the legislative assembly. The draft version of a proposed law, called a **bill,** is usually prepared by a legislative committee made up of members of Parliament in order to address a specific area of concern to the government, special interest groups, constituents of a particular geographic region, or the general public. It can deal with any subject within the jurisdiction of the assembly in which it is to be proposed, such as criminal law, taxation and government spending, agricultural policy, health care, education, foreign policy, defence, and a host of other areas of concern to various sectors of society. The subject matter of the proposed legislation will depend on whether it comes within an area of federal or provincial jurisdiction according to the Constitution. (The federal structure of Canada's Constitution is discussed later in this chapter.)

The procedure followed in Parliament[6] and in the provincial legislatures when passing a bill into law is essentially the same, with a few variations across provincial boundaries.

The bill is first introduced in the legislature and given a formal reading. At this stage, the bill is read out in Parliament in summary form and may be taken to a vote without any further debate. The bill is then put through a second reading for lengthy debate on its merits. At this stage, no amendments may be introduced to the bill.

If approved in principle, the bill is then taken to a committee of the legislature for detailed study. Public hearings may be held at which witnesses, private individuals, special interest groups, and others may provide information, make submissions suggesting changes or deletions, or advocate for the addition of further provisions. The bill is discussed, refined, and amended, taking into account the recommendations of the participants and the members of the committee studying it. Upon completion, the committee usually prepares a report to the legislature recommending changes to the draft.

The hearings of the Ontario legislature's Standing Committee on Administration of Justice on the repeal of that province's *Advocacy Act,* and amendments to its *Substitute Decisions Act* and *Consent to Treatment Act,* provide an illustration of this process. During these hearings, held in February

1996, the Committee received presentations from hospital officials, lawyers practising in the area of mental incompetency, guardianships and estates, and advocates for the poor, among others. There were concerns with respect to the workings of those three statutes. It was generally agreed that the requirement that all witnesses to a signing of a power of attorney for personal care be satisfied that the person signing is competent was unworkable and should be eliminated. This was subsequently done in the final bill that was passed. Further, much controversy had resulted from the original legislation's requirement that mentally incapable patients have their rights explained to them by "rights advisers" before any substitute decision maker could act on a power of attorney for personal care. This was also eliminated in the amendments. *The Advocacy Act,* which had provided for advocates to intervene on behalf of mentally incapable patients, was entirely repealed in the end. This illustrates the many processes and considerations that affect the passage of a bill from the time it is first proposed, and the many hands that shape its final form.

On second reading, a bill is again taken to a vote, where the legislature may approve it in principle. After further debate and refinement, the bill is then put to a third reading in which the legislature considers the committee's report. Usually, each of the bill's provisions is debated until it is put to a third and final vote.

If passed, the bill is then submitted to the lieutenant-governor for Royal Assent in the case of provincial legislation; if it is a bill of the House of Commons of Canada, it is laid before the Senate, where it proceeds in the same fashion. If passed by the Senate, the bill is then submitted to the governor general for the Royal Assent. Royal Assent is given as a matter of course since, again by convention, the Queen's representative must defer to the wishes of the government of the day; otherwise, refusing such assent would prompt a constitutional crisis. This procedure is reversed if the bill originates in the Senate.

Figure 3.2 on page 60 illustrates the process by which a bill becomes law in Canada.

A bill becomes law on proclamation or on a specific date after it receives Royal Assent and becomes an Act of Parliament or of the provincial legislature. In many cases, an Act has the force of law upon proclamation and publication in an official government publication called a gazette.

At this point, all citizens are deemed to know the law and to be governed by it. As unreasonable as this may seem, the purpose of this rule is to ensure the efficient and impartial enforcement of the law. Otherwise, anyone could argue ignorance of the law as a defence. The law would then be unenforceable, and chaos would ensue. Thus, the rule that "ignorance of the law is no excuse" is fundamental to any society's ability to govern itself and maintain order.

In fact, most governments in Canada do much more to promulgate new laws than merely print them in gazettes. They usually send detailed press releases and communiqués to the media in an effort to make new laws known

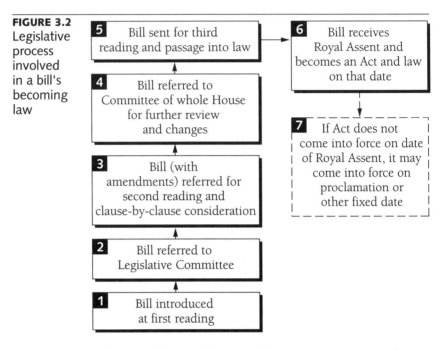

FIGURE 3.2
Legislative process involved in a bill's becoming law

to as many people as possible. Furthermore, the gazettes, statutes, and regulations themselves are available in law libraries and through government bookstores. Though it may not always be easy, it is always possible to find legislation in these sources.

Parliamentary and provincial statutes usually contain a short title, for example, the *Highway Traffic Act*.[7] They may have a preamble that briefly states why the Act was passed and its purpose. The Act will also contain one or more numbered and detailed sections or clauses setting forth definitions, conditions, prohibitions, and **remedies** that are sought to be regulated by the Act.

As comprehensive as these provisions may seem, they cannot provide for every situation that the government desires to regulate. Additional legislative details may be set forth in regulations passed by **Order-in-Council** by the cabinet under the specific authority of a particular statute. Details that must be amended from time to time are often governed by way of regulations. It is also significant that regulations are much easier to enact, since they are passed in cabinet away from the scrutiny of the full legislature.

Regulations, also known as subordinate legislation, have the same force of law as statutes, but are inferior to the Act from which they flow. The statute takes priority. In the event that a regulation goes beyond the authority granted in the statute, a court may strike down such a regulation and refuse to enforce it. The government of the day, therefore, must always ensure that any regulations it passes are consistent with the particular Act that gives it the authority to make these regulations.

Since the legislative branch of government has the ultimate power to make law (subject, of course, to any restrictions contained in the

Constitution), it follows that statute law will take precedence over the common (i.e., judge-made) law. If there is a conflict or contradiction between a principle of common law and a provision found in a statute of Parliament or of a provincial legislature, then a court is bound to apply the statute. The court presumes that it was the intent of the legislature to alter the common law by enacting the statutory provision.

For example, before the passage of the **negligence** statutes of the various common law provinces, the common law held that a person suing another for negligence could not recover any damages whatsoever regardless of fault if the person claiming the damages (the **plaintiff**) had in any way, however slight, contributed to the accident or occurrence that caused his or her injury or damage. Thus, even if the **defendant** (the person being sued) was 99% to blame for the plaintiff's injuries, the claim would fail if the plaintiff was just 1% at fault. This was found to be manifestly unjust, yet the courts continued to uphold the common law rule. It took the passage of various negligence statutes in the provinces early in this century to change it.

Today, a plaintiff who is, say, 20% responsible for his or her own injuries is still entitled to recover 80% of the damages from the defendant (provided the defendant has been found liable to that extent). If there is more than one defendant, the court will apportion **liability** among the various defendants to the extent to which each is to blame for the occurrence as well as the plaintiff (if he or she is in any way liable).

The Quebec *Civil Code*

Despite its many similarities with common law, Quebec civil law deserves a separate discussion. It has many features and characteristics that are unique to civil law countries. While Quebec's legal system is principally derived from the French one, for historical, social, and geographical reasons, it has also been influenced (to some degree) by English common law.

In the Quebec system, the primary source of law is the *Civil Code:* a lengthy, detailed, and comprehensive statute that sets out a variety of legal rules and principles dealing with such matters as contracts, civil wrongs (e.g., trespassing, slander, assault), negligence, family relations, children's rights, marriage, property rights, wills and the laws of inheritance, corporate law, and insurance law. (This list is not exhaustive.)

Quebec's legal system, as in the common law provinces, also has a body of precedents called **jurisprudence.** In the Quebec legal system, jurisprudence takes a back seat to the Code. Jurisprudence is merely persuasive evidence of how previous courts have treated a particular provision of the Code.

As well, Quebec has a body of statute law, but the *Civil Code* takes precedence unless the statute expressly states otherwise. Ultimately, the court consults the Code as its primary source of law to resolve civil disputes.

Doctrine, that is, the scholarly writings of experts in the law, is another guide that has the force of law for the civilian court. It takes precedence even over the jurisprudence of a higher court in helping a judge to interpret a provision of the *Civil Code* and to apply it in a particular situation. Doctrine may take the form of law review articles, textbooks on a particular topic, or frequently, multi-volumed treatises on various areas of the civil law. The more respected the author, the more respected, relevant, and authoritative that author's works will be in the eyes of the court. By contrast, doctrine in the common law is seldom seen as authoritative, and it is never treated as binding.

While a civilist court is not strictly bound by decisions of a higher court, this does not mean that it can ignore such jurisprudence. A court in Quebec is still required to treat such decisions with utmost respect and must have a sound reason, either in the Code itself, in accepted doctrine, or in subsequent decisions, for departing from a precedent. This is more so in Quebec compared to other civil law countries because of the influence of English common law on Quebec's judicial traditions. An added consequence of the non-binding nature of civil law jurisprudence is that the courts have somewhat greater leeway in applying the Code's various provisions to new situations. Because of this characteristic, civil law has often been said to have greater flexibility and adaptability than the common law.

Table 3.2 lists the three major sources of civil law.

An interesting illustration of the court's deliberative process is found in the controversial decision of the Quebec Superior Court in the case of *Nancy B. v. Hôtel-Dieu de Québec.*[8] This case involved a young woman of 25 stricken with Guillain-Barré syndrome, a rare and sometimes incurable neurological disease which, in its final stages, leaves a person completely paralyzed and dependent on a respirator. A patient such as Nancy B. can survive for years; however, he or she is incapable of physical activity. Nancy B.'s life was limited to lying in bed and watching television. Her mental faculties were keen, yet she felt trapped in a useless body, an existence that she found unbearable. She expressed a wish to die a natural death, and requested that her intravenous feedings be discontinued and her respirator turned off. The physician and hospital involved in her care had difficulty complying with her request and took the matter to a higher authority.

Nancy retained a lawyer and brought an application in the Quebec Superior Court for an **injunction** (a court order) directing the hospital and physician to cease all treatment, nourishment, and use of the respirator, so that she might die. The Court considered a provision of the *Civil Code*[9] then in effect which stipulated that no one could be made to undergo medical treatment of any kind without that person's consent. It held that this provision applied to this case, and thus Nancy had the right to refuse further treatment. The court also considered certain doctrine holding that, absent a threat to the rights of others or a threat to public order, the right was effectively absolute. To supplement the Code, the court relied on further doctrine stating that the act of placing a person on a respirator constituted medical treatment and thus fell within the meaning of the provision of the Code.

TABLE 3.2
Sources of civil law (in decreasing order of authority)

SOURCE AND DEGREE OF AUTHORITY	DEFINITION AND CHARACTERISTICS
Civil Code of Quebec, statutes and regulations Code is binding on all courts, as are statutes and regulations; Code is often used as an aid in interpreting a statute and usually takes precedence, unless the statute says otherwise.	The Code embodies rules, definitions, and legal principles regulating many areas of provincial law. Other statutes and regulations supplement the Code and usually regulate a specific area (e.g., highways).
Doctrine Usually given wide deference and seen as very persuasive and authoritative in a civil law court.	Articles, books, treatises, and other written materials by leading legal scholars. These are used by the courts as an aid to interpreting ambiguous provisions of the Code or statutes.
Jurisprudence Persuasive but not binding; accorded less authority in some cases than doctrine. It is seen as evidence of how other courts have interpreted and applied the law in past cases.	Resembles common law case law (see Table 3.1, page 54), but is not strictly binding on civil law courts.

In dealing with the argument that to remove Nancy from the respirator would entail a violation of the *Criminal Code of Canada* (insofar as the physician and hospital would be assisting her in committing suicide, or could be committing murder), the court stated that the discontinuation of treatment would merely allow a natural death to occur. It noted, referring as well to U.S. case law, that neither murder nor suicide is the consequence of a natural death. Thus, the removal of the respirator could not be classified as assisted suicide or murder.

The court further reasoned that these particular provisions of the *Criminal Code* could not reasonably be interpreted in such a way as to make removal of the respirator an offence. To do so would hamper the medical profession in that any course of treatment, no matter how ineffective, could never be discontinued once undertaken. This, the court held, could not have been the intent of Parliament in enacting these provisions. It thus ruled that Nancy had the right to withhold consent to this treatment, and accordingly granted her the injunction. After the time for an appeal of the decision had lapsed, the respirator was disconnected, and Nancy died shortly after.

This example demonstrates the civil court's use of doctrine and case law from another jurisdiction in interpreting a crucial provision of the *Civil Code,* and illustrates how the courts of Quebec tend to value doctrine to a far greater extent than do their common law counterparts.

The *Civil Code of Lower Canada* (as Quebec was called before Confederation) was originally enacted in 1866. Since that time, it has undergone numerous changes and additions, yet it remains essentially a 19th-century document. In response to massive changes and advances in technology and society since Confederation, the Quebec government commissioned a comprehensive study and review of the existing Code in 1955, with a view to preparing a completely new and revised Code ready to meet the needs of 20th-century Quebec.

The result of this lengthy undertaking was the passing in 1992 of a completely new Quebec *Civil Code,* which came into force on January 1, 1994. The new Code has added provisions dealing with areas of law unforeseen in the 19th century. It makes provision for consent to medical treatment, enshrines the right to refuse treatment, expands children's rights to have a say in their treatment, and enacts a host of other new provisions dealing with mentally incompetent or terminally ill persons, organ donation, substitute decision making, and other areas.

Due Process and Rule of Law

A common theme runs through both common law and civil law in Canada. As in other countries with highly developed legal systems, the concepts of due process and rule of law permeate them and give them legitimacy. **Due process** encompasses the concept that all people are equal before the law and are entitled to the same rights and benefits of it. In past times, many societies had separate rules and laws determined by a person's social status, ancestry, religion, race, or wealth. A basic tenet of the modern Canadian legal system is that any person, no matter how rich, poor, powerful, famous, or unknown, is entitled to be treated by the law in exactly the same manner as another. For example, if the son of a cabinet minister were arrested for drunk driving, he would receive no special treatment by the criminal justice system.

The rule of law means that those who are charged with administering and enforcing laws will behave in accordance with them, and that their decisions will be respected and complied with by members of society and persons in positions of authority. This gives a court order or judgement its finality and authority, or the decision of a government official its force. Rule of law ensures, for example, that conflicts between individuals (e.g., lawsuits) are resolved in accordance with set, predictable procedures and laws and are given finality and certainty. If it were otherwise, while a society might have the best written law, chaos and disorder would ensue if the rule of law were not observed. Rule of law ensures that contracts are enforceable, for example, and encourages a prosperous economy.

Civil Law as Distinct from Criminal Law

The term "civil law" has several distinct meanings to lawyers and judges. In one sense, it describes a legal system based on Roman law, such as Quebec's, in which legal principles and rules are codified and form the primary source of law.

In another sense, civil law refers to a body of rules and legal principles that govern relations, respective rights, and obligations among individuals, corporations, or other institutions. It is separate and distinct from **criminal law,** which is chiefly concerned with relations between the individual and the state and the breach of criminal statutes. Civil law includes law related to contracts, property, family, marriage and divorce, tort and negligence, wills and inheritance, the creation and administration of business and non-profit corporations or partnerships, insurance, copyright, trademarks and patents, employment and labour.

To give a simple example of a civil law relationship in a nursing setting, suppose that a nurse is called upon one night to administer an antibiotic to a patient suffering acute appendicitis. In error, the nurse administers the wrong antibiotic. Furthermore, it is noted in the chart that this patient is allergic to that particular antibiotic. The patient consequently suffers an anaphylactic reaction resulting in brain damage. He emerges from a coma two weeks later, at which time it is determined that he has suffered partial paralysis of his left side. The brain damage is later shown to be permanent and irreversible. In such a case, the patient and his family would have the right to sue the nurse, and even the hospital, for professional negligence.

This case is essentially a private dispute between two sets of individuals seeking redress in the courts. Here, the State (or more specifically, society) is not directly interested in the outcome of the case. It is a mainly private dispute which the court will resolve by drawing upon relevant legal principles and rules. The court's decision may later be applied in similar cases. In this broader context, society is indeed interested in the outcome, which may form the impetus for amending or creating legislation to regulate the particular nursing practice that gave rise to the negligence.

Another distinction within both civil law and criminal law is that between substantive and procedural laws. **Substantive** laws create rights and obligations between individuals—for example, laws governing the creation of a contract, the rights of a spouse within marriage, an employee's rights against an employer's, or the creation and governance of a corporation. **Procedural** laws, on the other hand, regulate how those rights are preserved and enforced in the courts. These would include the rules of court governing how a lawsuit is started, when it may be started, what documents must be filed, and in which court. They may also govern the application of substantive laws in other situations.

Torts

The nursing example discussed above illustrates a situation in tort law. A **tort** is a civil wrong committed by one person against another such as to cause that other some injury or damage, either to person or property. Torts may be *intentional* or *non-intentional*. An assault is an example of an intentional tort, in that the person who commits it intends the action that causes harm to the victim. Non-intentional torts generally constitute negligence. In our previous example, the nurse did not intend to cause harm to the patient, but was negligent in giving the wrong medication and in failing to notice that the patient was allergic to it. In acting, she may have breached a number of standards of nursing practice.

In civil law torts (and contractual matters), **duties** correspond with obligations. Specific provisions of the *Civil Code* define and govern the concept and the elements that must be proved in court for the plaintiff to recover damages. Under civil law, anyone under a duty not to cause harm to another is at fault if he or she fails in that duty by not acting according to the expected standard of care.

Intentional Torts

Battery and Assault

Of particular importance to the nursing profession is the concept of battery and assault. Since much of a nurse's work involves the physical touching of patients for the administration of injections, sutures, intravenous lines, and other such invasive measures, a nurse must understand that such procedures may be instituted only upon a consenting patient. Consent may be expressed and obtained in writing or may be implied and inferred from the patient's conduct.

Battery in the common law is defined as the intentional bringing about of a harmful or offensive and non-consensual contact with the person of another.[10] An example would be one person striking another. The harmful or offensive contact may be either direct, such as a slap in the face, or indirect, such as pulling away a person's chair, causing him to fall to the ground.[11] In either case, there has been an intentional interference with the bodily integrity and security of another. Moreover, these acts are seen as potential inducements to further violence, because the victim may be provoked into retaliation. The chief aim of tort law is to curb violence by making perpetrators of such acts civilly liable to their victims for damages. It is also concerned with the need to restore the victim of the tort, as much as is possible through the award of monetary damages, to the situation he or she was in prior to the battery or assault.

The offensive or intrusive conduct need not be violent, as even seemingly insignificant unwanted touching may amount to battery. The perpetrator need not intend any harmful result. Thus, even such conduct as a kiss on the cheek meant as a compliment may amount to battery if it is not consented to by the recipient.

However, certain common, everyday acts will not usually amount to battery. For instance, shaking hands is not considered battery, since it is a western custom in greeting acquaintances. Thus, one need not ask another's permission prior to shaking hands. Since it is a custom, the law would infer consent on the part of the recipient, especially where that person holds out his or her hand.

Assault is the "intentional creation of the apprehension of imminent harmful or offensive contact."[12] For example, if one person lunges threateningly at another who is close by, but does not actually strike, that person is still liable to damages for assault. A court would likely conclude that the victim was reasonably apprehensive of being harmed in this situation and that the threat was imminent. However, there will be no assault if the victim could not reasonably conclude from the circumstances that the perpetrator was actually able to carry out the threat. The reasonableness of the victim's state of mind is key here. There is no requirement that the perpetrator actually be able to carry out the threat. It is sufficient that the evidence of the circumstances in which the threat was made led to a reasonable conclusion that the defendant was able to carry it out.

Consent

In cases where the aggrieved person has consented to the conduct being visited upon him or her, the perpetrator may escape liability for such conduct in some cases. **Consent,** which can be defined as permission given by a person to someone else to perform an act upon the person giving such permission, can be *explicit* (expressed) or *implied* by the circumstances or the conduct of the aggrieved person. Expressed consent may be given orally or in writing. The written consent is not consent in and of itself, but rather is evidence that the party giving it has consented to an act.

Implied consent is agreement to an act inferred from the actions of the recipient. An example of implied consent in a medical setting might be a patient's holding out an arm to a nurse to have blood pressure checked. The patient cannot then say that he did not consent to the touching, since a reasonable person would imply from his conduct that he consented. This illustrates another aspect of implied consent, that is, the existence of consent is measured against an **objective standard.** Such consent is found to exist where the plaintiff's conduct is such that a reasonable person viewing all the surrounding circumstances would conclude that consent had been given.

For consent to be valid in law, the person giving it must be capable of giving consent. In the case of a mentally ill patient, consent to treatment may or may not be valid, depending on whether the mental illness makes that patient unable to appreciate the nature, quality, and consequences of the proposed treatment. Children under the age of majority (or under 16, in some provinces) usually cannot consent to medical treatment, in which case their parents or legal guardians would be called upon to give consent. However, if the child is old enough to understand the nature and risks of the proposed treatment, the caregiver or institution may rely upon that consent.

Consent will be **vitiated** (invalidated) if it was obtained by force or fraud. Duress or the use of force invalidates any consent, because the recipient is obviously not making a decision of his or her own free will. Only a freely given and voluntary consent is valid in law.

In the context of health care, it is important to remember that no medical treatment, no matter how crucial to the health or survival of the patient, may be administered without that patient's consent, unless the situation is life-threatening and the patient is unconscious or mentally incompetent.[13] Furthermore, only that specific treatment which is consented to may be administered, and in most cases, only those health professionals specified in the patient's consent may administer the consented-to treatment. The patient must give an **informed consent.** This means that the nature of the treatment to be administered, its benefits and attendant risks, and any and all material information must be given to the patient for the consent to be valid.

The issue of consent, and its many ethical and legal pitfalls, is as relevant to the nursing profession as it is to physicians. Many fine lines are drawn, and it is not always easy to determine the extent and scope of the consent. Chapters Six and Eight will elaborate upon this issue.

Non-intentional Torts

Negligence

As previously suggested, in the common law, negligence falls under the non-intentional category of torts. A defendant may still be liable for a tort while not having intended any harm or injury. For a defendant to be liable for negligence, three elements must be present.[14] First, the defendant must owe a duty of care in law towards the plaintiff. Second, the defendant must have breached that duty and failed to discharge the standard of care required by the law in the particular situation. Third, the plaintiff must have suffered damage or harm caused by the defendant's breach of the duty of care. Another related legal principle is that if the plaintiff was in any way partly responsible for his or her injuries as a result of negligence, the defendant will be absolved of liability to the extent of the plaintiff's own negligence. This principle is called **contributory negligence.**

To return to our nursing example, it is clear that the nurse owed a duty of care to her patient. In reading the medication labelling incorrectly and failing to notice that the patient was allergic to the medication he subsequently received, the nurse breached the duty she owed to that patient. As a direct result of that breach, the patient received a harmful substance and suffered a severe allergic reaction. His ensuing brain damage was a direct and foreseeable result of that breach.

Duty of care, standards of care, proximate cause, and contributory negligence are factors that help determine whether or not a defendant will be held liable (responsible) in a case of negligence. We will now discuss each of these factors in detail.

Duty of Care

To be liable in tort, a defendant must owe a duty of care to the plaintiff, either personally or as a member of a class. The law imposes a duty of care in many but not all situations. If there is no duty of care in law, the defendant will not be liable to the plaintiff, even if the defendant's conduct was the immediate cause of the plaintiff's injuries.

The common law holds that one owes a duty of care to those people who are close to, or closely connected with, one's conduct or activities such that a reasonable person could foresee harm or injury occurring to such persons as a result of negligent acts or conduct. Professionals such as nurses owe a duty of care to those who retain their services to act in a competent and diligent manner according to the standard of the reasonably competent nurse. This includes a responsibility for the nurse, as with any other professional, to keep abreast of current developments and techniques within the profession and to undertake retraining as necessary.

The classic definition of the duty of care can be found in an old case that originated in Scotland in the early 1930s: a person has a duty to avoid any acts or omissions that one could reasonably foresee would be likely to injure his or her neighbour. In the decision in *Donoghue v. Stevenson,* Lord Atkin, one of the Lord Justices of the House of Lords to which the case had been appealed, spoke of the duty thus:

> The rule that you are to love your neighbour becomes in law, you must not injure your neighbour; and the lawyer's question, Who is my neighbour? receives a restricted reply. You must take reasonable care to avoid acts or omissions which you can reasonably foresee would be likely to injure your neighbour. Who, then, in law is my neighbour? The answer seems to be persons who are so closely and directly affected by my act that I ought reasonably to have them in contemplation as being so affected when I am directing my mind to the acts or omissions which are called in question.[15]

A case from Alberta that arose in the mid-1980s will illustrate these concepts. In *Bergen v. Sturgeon General Hospital et al.,*[16] a young woman was admitted to a hospital complaining of abdominal pains. The hospital was modern and well equipped, and included general practitioners, surgeons, gynaecologists, and a radiologist, with appropriate nursing staff. Among other procedures, appendectomies and laparotomies were routinely performed.

The woman was admitted on Sunday afternoon by her personal physician, who advised three colleagues (who were subsequently involved in her treatment) that he wished to rule out the possibility of life-threatening appendicitis. It was accepted practice for a laparotomy to be performed so that the abdomen could be viewed and appendicitis confirmed or ruled out.

By Friday evening, having been confined to hospital since her admission, the patient was rushed to another hospital in Edmonton where she underwent an emergency operation by a gynaecologist and general surgeon. The woman died 13 h later from septic shock as a result of a ruptured appendix. Her husband and children brought a lawsuit against the hospital, attending nurses, and four physicians who treated her.

At trial, a judge ruled that three of the defendant doctors had failed to act upon the suspected appendicitis despite the fact that they had four and a half days in which to confirm such ailment. The admitting doctor was found to have acted with the skill, care, and knowledge expected of him under the circumstances. He admitted the patient promptly, diagnosed her, and noted the need for surgical confirmation.

A gynaecologist who examined the woman the day after her admission diagnosed pelvic inflammatory disease (PID); this diagnosis was accepted by the attending physician and the surgeon. No one had ruled out appendicitis. The attending physician was found to bear the ultimate responsibility for the patient's care and treatment. Although he noted fairly severe pain, he acknowledged under cross-examination at trial that he carried out no rectal, vaginal, or x-ray examination. He did note that the pain was in the right lower quadrant, typical of a ruptured appendix.

The patient's pain was treated with increasing doses of meperidine over the next few days, although the nurses' notes indicate that she was "not improving." The court ruled that ignoring the signs of appendicitis "showed a want of due care and diligence amounting to negligence."[17] It found two of the other physicians also liable, and similarly reviewed their conduct against the standard of care.

With respect to the nurses and nursing assistants, the hospital had a clear policy that complete and accurate notes, records, and charts be kept for all its patients. Prior to the woman's transfer to the second hospital, a registered nursing assistant cleaned her room and inadvertently threw out the vital signs record kept by the bed. The RNA considered that, as the patient had left, these documents were no longer needed. She also destroyed the sheet recording urine and stools output, among other records. In this case, the hospital policy on record keeping had not been followed in practice. In fact, evidence showed that vital signs sheets were not normally kept, but that only pertinent data from these would go into a patient's chart.

Of particular significance during the patient's hospital stay was a notation in the nurses' notes that the woman had experienced a "snap" in her abdomen and was found lying across her bed in pain. This was a most unusual occurrence in PID, and the nurse could not account for it. The other nurses testified similarly. A new shift was coming in at this time, and the outgoing charge nurse never told the incoming charge nurse what should be done with respect to this patient.

The outgoing charge nurse was found negligent; the incoming charge nurse was found to have acted promptly and reasonably under the circumstances in trying to secure the services of a physician when she began her shift. Another defendant nurse on duty in the earlier shift was found to have taken upon herself an assessment of a patient she had never seen before and never nursed, and to have dealt with a situation with which she was unfamiliar. According to the appropriate standard of skill and knowledge, she should have called a physician there and then. This nurse, too, was found negligent. These nurses clearly owed the patient a duty of care that her condition would be watched and monitored closely, as well as a duty to seek the assistance of a physician when the situation became serious.

A duty of care will be found to exist where one person has placed others in peril as a result of his or her conduct. Furthermore, a person who creates a hazard, even unwittingly and through no negligence of his or her own, may still be held liable if he or she fails to warn others of the hazard and they are injured.

It is both interesting and disturbing to note that under the common law (unlike Quebec[18] and the civil law countries of Europe), there is no general duty to aid someone in peril.[19] This is one illustration of the divergence that can occur between law and ethics. What may clearly be a moral or ethical imperative may not necessarily be a legal requirement.

For example, in common law provinces, a passer-by may observe a man in cardiac arrest without rendering assistance. There is no positive duty to act in such cases.[20] However, most people, acting morally, would likely intervene to save a person in obvious danger. Where someone does act, the law imposes a duty of care upon him or her not to conduct such rescue negligently. A person who fails in a rescue bid may be civilly liable for any injury or death resulting to the person being rescued.[21] Usually, however, to be found liable, the rescuer's conduct must amount to gross negligence—that is, a substantial and marked departure from the standard of the reasonably competent and skilled rescuer.

As we saw in the Bergen case, nurses have a special relationship to those whom they serve, and it is thus desirable to impose on them a duty of care.[22] They have special training and expertise, and are required to exercise a very high degree of care in carrying out their tasks.

Breach of the Standard of Care

How do courts determine whether or not a defendant's conduct has been negligent? The common law has developed the concept of the **standard of care** as an objective measure of such conduct. If a defendant's conduct is seen as having fallen below the standard of what a competent person, acting reasonably and responsibly in similar circumstances, would have done, a court may find that defendant's conduct to be negligent.

The particular standard against which any given conduct is judged will vary depending on the circumstances and people involved. For example, a doctor will be judged by the standard of the reasonably competent physician. Similarly, a nurse's conduct in the treatment of a patient who has suffered harm as a result of his or her acts or omissions will be judged by the standard of the reasonably competent nurse.

The nurses in our example would not be judged by the standard of the most highly qualified expert in the field of nursing, but rather by the average standards of the reasonable nurse possessed of reasonable knowledge, skill, and ability. These would include minimal standards of competence and knowledge set by the governing body for nurses in the various provinces, and any applicable standards prescribed by the health facility in which that nurse is employed. A paediatric nurse, however, might be judged by the standard of that specialized nursing practice. Similarly, an operating room nurse would be judged by the standard of the reasonably competent surgical nurse.

Such standards also include the requirement to keep up to date with the latest professional and technological developments. Additional training should be taken as required to maintain expertise to the appropriate standard. A professional who fails to keep up to date runs the risk of employing methods that have been discredited or proved harmful by the latest studies and thinking in that field. If that professional's conduct were ever called into question, such failure would be evidence of negligence.

Proximate Cause and Remoteness

The third element of negligence is that a defendant will be liable for harm to a plaintiff if that harm was caused by the defendant's negligent conduct. This seems straightforward and logical. However, can a plaintiff be compensated for all possible harm that may occur as a result of the defendant's negligent act?

To illustrate, suppose A. ignites fireworks in her yard, and that during the display, a live cinder from a descending rocket is carried by the wind into a nearby industrial park. Among the many enterprises in this park is a chemical factory that produces highly flammable cleaning solvents. In its yard are stored finished solvents, chemicals used in their manufacture, and several railway tank cars containing hazardous waste chemicals. An employee of this manufacturer has carelessly punctured one of the solvent containers, and highly flammable solvent has leaked out in and about the yard. The live cinder lands in a pool of solvent and immediately ignites it. The ensuing blaze destroys the facility and causes the toxic waste chemicals to burn. Hazardous fumes and heavy black smoke billow into the air, necessitating the evacuation of much of A.'s suburban neighbourhood. Furthermore, several firefighters are seriously injured by the fumes while dealing with the conflagration. Can A. possibly be held liable for all this damage? Some courts may hold A. liable only for the immediate damage to the yard, while others may extend the scope of A.'s liability to include the fire and injury to the firefighters. Of course, the chemical company will also be held partially responsible for the condition of its yard and hazardous storage methods.

Such a train of events is often referred to as a **chain of causation.** A chain of causation can easily be found in a health care setting, where many health professionals may be involved in treating a patient with numerous medical problems and complications. There are many situations in which a patient may suffer harm as the result of a combination of negligent acts by a number of health professionals. The actions of each member of the health care team in treating such a patient would have to be examined to determine how those particular actions influenced the course of the patient's condition and how reasonably foreseeable this could have been. Such a chain might start out with a nurse inaccurately recording one of the patient's vital signs. A second health practitioner may then not question the reading in light of his or her own physical observations of the patient and assume the reading is correct. An inappropriate course of treatment might be embarked upon as a result of this, leading to a further aggravation, rather than amelioration of the patient's condition, as we saw in the Bergen case. There, the court remarked upon the "tunnel-vision" that trapped the attending physicians into zeroing in on one diagnosis (PID) to the exclusion of all others.[23] The court noted that it was the duty of physicians to reassess their patients constantly and not to fall into this trap.

Negligence law holds that a defendant should be held liable only when his or her acts of negligence are the proximate cause of the ensuing harm. A defendant should not be held accountable to the plaintiff for all possible results of negligent conduct, no matter how remote or unforeseeable. The court will ask whether the resulting harm or damage was a reasonably foreseeable consequence of the defendant's act or omission.[24] If it was, the defendant will be held liable for any resulting loss. The exact manner in which the loss occurs, however, need not be foreseen.[25]

Contributory Negligence

In earlier times under the common law, if a plaintiff was found to be partly at fault for the harm he or she suffered, the law would deny him or her the right to recover damages from the defendant.[26] Today, in all common law provinces, a plaintiff may still recover even if partly at fault, but the damages awarded will be reduced by the percentage to which he or she was to blame or contributed to the loss.[27] Lawyers say in such situations that the plaintiff was contributarily negligent. Of course, if the evidence shows that the plaintiff was completely to blame for the harm that befell him or her, the defendant would escape liability entirely.

Returning to our fireworks example, suppose that the solvent manufacturer sued A. for damages resulting from the fire. A. can raise the fact that one of the manufacturer's employees carelessly punctured the solvent drum, and that this caused the solvent to leak and ignite more readily. A. might also argue that the manufacturer was partly to blame for the damage and harm because of the negligent way in which the various materials in the yard were stored.

The court will apportion the liability among the parties, that is, it will determine as best it can the percentage or proportion to which each party is to blame for the loss. In this respect, the law is basically the same in all common law provinces and the Province of Quebec, where it is known as the principle of common fault.[28]

Voluntary Assumption of Risk

A plaintiff may lose all rights of recovery against a negligent defendant if that plaintiff consented in some way to the defendant's conduct. The plaintiff may then be said to have **voluntarily assumed the risk** of harm that was likely to result from the defendant's conduct. This defence is known by the Latin maxim, *"Volenti non fit injuria."* ("He who consents cannot receive an injury."[29]) It is a defence insofar as the defendant must prove that the plaintiff voluntarily assumed the risk of injury.[30] There is no onus on the plaintiff in this regard. In most cases, the plaintiff's assumption of the risk is implied by the conduct of the plaintiff in the circumstances; it is rarely specifically expressed.

What Is a Lawsuit?

Thus far, we have dealt with the rights and duties of individuals, and with the mechanics and workings of tort law. This area has perhaps the greatest significance for the nursing profession. Tort law affects the nursing process directly insofar as nurses are professionals whose conduct must meet the appropriate standard of care. (Collective agreements and other employment matters that affect the daily working lives of nurses will be discussed in detail in Chapter Ten.) Individual rights are adjudicated and enforced by means of the court **action.**

In Canada, a **lawsuit** is not usually the first step in an attempt to resolve a contractual, tort, or other legal dispute. Informal attempts to resolve the problem may include discussions between the parties, mediation or arbitration, or other complaint mechanism. Lawyers should be engaged in the early stages to resolve the dispute without resort to the courts. If this fails, a court action must be started by the aggrieved party.

The Action (Lawsuit) and Pleadings

The process for starting a lawsuit is broadly similar in all provinces. It is controlled by a code usually referred to as the **rules of civil procedure,** or the rules of court, which are detailed regulations setting out how a court action is conducted, which documents must be filed in which court and by whom, other detailed provisions governing examinations of parties, summonses to witnesses (subpoenas), the manner of serving notice, the actual trial, and other such matters. It is initiated by filing a **statement of claim**[31] or writ of summons in the appropriate court.[32]

This document, which is usually filed on behalf of the plaintiff by his or her lawyer, is also referred to as an **originating process** because it starts the action. It sets out, in concise numbered paragraphs, the plaintiff's version of the facts relied on to support the claim made against the defendant(s),[33] but it may not set out any of the evidence by which the plaintiff intends to prove his or her case.

The statement of claim is issued by the court in which it is filed, and a court file is opened at the court office for that action. This file will contain all court documents relevant to this action. Once the claim is issued, the lawsuit officially commences. A copy of the statement of claim must then be served on (given to) the defendant(s) personally within a specified period of time.[34]

In turn, the defendant has the right to file a **statement of defence** to the plaintiff's claim within a specified time. Failure to file a statement of defence will prevent the defendant from participating in the action. Further, a defendant who fails to file a defence to the action may be deemed (considered) by the rules of court of the particular province to have admitted the truth of the allegations contained in the statement of claim.[35]

The statement of defence, like the statement of claim, sets forth in concise, numbered paragraphs those facts upon which the defendant relies in his or her defence to the claim. This statement of defence must, in turn, be served on the plaintiff and filed in the court office where the action was commenced within a specified time. Failure to file in time may mean the defendant will lose all opportunity to defend the action. The statements of claim and defence are collectively known as **pleadings.**

The Examination for Discovery

Assuming the defendant has filed a defence, the next step requires all parties to exchange all relevant documents upon which they intend to rely at the trial in order to help prove their respective cases. The intent of the rules of civil procedure of all provinces is that each party to a lawsuit make full disclosure to the others of all relevant evidence, both oral (i.e., from witnesses) and documentary, in that party's possession or control. This policy is designed to eliminate the element of surprise in litigation. It is felt by policy makers that avoiding surprise is less costly in the long run and promotes settlement of cases without the need for expensive trials. If both parties to a lawsuit are fully aware of the strength of the other's case, each can assess the chance of success more realistically.

Thus, a party who realizes that his opponent has the evidence necessary to prove her case will be more willing to settle the matter than risk a loss for a higher sum of damages at the conclusion of the trial. A key provision of the law of **costs** is a further incentive: the unsuccessful party must not only pay his or her own legal fees, but will usually be ordered to pay those of the victorious opponent at the end of the trial.[36]

Disclosure is achieved through two mechanisms: documentary discovery and the oral examination for discovery.[37] In **documentary discovery**, the party shows that he or she has disclosed all relevant documents by swearing an **affidavit** which lists all these documents. Failure to disclose the existence of a document relating to the action means that the party cannot rely upon it at trial.

In an **examination for discovery,** each party, in the presence of his or her own lawyer, is asked a series of questions relevant to any matter raised in the pleadings by the opposing party's lawyer. The questions and answers are recorded either by means of audio tape or by a stenographer at an official examiner's office. The party being examined answers under oath as if giving testimony in open court; however, no judge is present at this stage. An examination for discovery is not a trial.

The answers given at the examination enable each party to know the other's position and the kind of testimony that the other is likely to give at trial. They can also be used to test the credibility of a party whose answer at discovery differs from that given at trial. If the parties are unable to settle the action at this stage, then the matter proceeds to trial. Each party summons all necessary witnesses and documents to prove his or her case. Meanwhile, a trial date is set.

Before the trial, however, one last effort will be made to encourage the parties to settle by means of the **pre-trial conference.** Here the parties' lawyers, in the presence of a judge, advance (put forth) their clients' respective positions on liability, the amount of the damages, and the prospects of settling the case. With limited evidence, the judge then indicates how the matter might be decided at trial. To prevent bias, the pre-trial judge is not the one who will try the case. If a settlement is still not achieved, the parties prepare for trial held before a different judge.

The Trial

A civil action may be tried by judge alone or by a court consisting of judge and **jury,** according to the wishes of any one of the parties. However, certain types of actions, because of their nature or complexity, may only be tried by a judge alone.[38] The number of **jurors** varies from province to province. A civil trial jury is composed of fewer jurors than the 12 required in a criminal trial. For example, Ontario requires no more than six persons,[39] while Newfoundland requires nine. Civil jury trials were abolished a number of years ago in Quebec. Lawsuits in that province are now tried only by a judge.

During the trial, the **burden of proof** is upon the plaintiff. This means that the plaintiff must prove his or her case. It is not for the defendant to prove he or she is not liable. A plaintiff must present enough evidence to show that the injury or harm was caused, on a balance of probabilities, by the defendant. If at the end of the trial the plaintiff has failed to prove his or her case, or the evidence is at best inconclusive, the defendant will be found not liable, and the action will be dismissed.

If the plaintiff wins, judgement is granted, which is a court order stating that the defendant is to pay to the plaintiff a certain sum of money as damages. Damages, or monetary compensation for the harm incurred by a plaintiff as a result of the defendant's negligence, willful tort, or breach of contract, are one remedy the court may award. Damages compensate for losses due to pain and suffering, medical expenses incurred in the case of a personal injury suit, loss of earnings, and loss of future income.

Enforcing Judgement

Once having obtained judgement, the plaintiff will then have to enforce it. Many defendants do not pay a judgement once it is obtained. A plaintiff must now expend further sums to recover on the judgement by means of a **judgement debtor examination,** during which a defendant debtor (called a **judgement debtor** because he or she owes money according to a court order) is asked questions about his or her financial resources, property, and ability to pay the judgement.

The plaintiff can have any of the defendant's assets (e.g., the defendant's home, land, bank accounts, securities, automobiles, jewellery, or other such property) seized and sold by the sheriff (a court official) at an auction in order to realize the necessary funds to satisfy the judgement. The defendant's wages can also be subjected to **garnishment** procedures, meaning that the defendant's employer (or any other debtor of the defendant) will be required to pay a portion of the defendant's weekly or monthly wages (or the debt itself, in the case of a debt owed to the defendant) to the sheriff for the benefit of the plaintiff and any other creditors of the defendant. Through these mechanisms, the law permits a successful plaintiff to bring considerable pressure to bear on a delinquent judgement debtor.

Criminal Law

Thus far we have been discussing court actions involving one or more individuals asserting private claims. These are classed as civil law. Other cases concern society collectively when they involve a breach of fundamental values and rules that threatens the peace, stability, order, and well-being of all its citizens. This concern is the focus and province of criminal law.

The federal government is charged constitutionally with making criminal law in Canada.[40] This ensures one uniform set of criminal laws for the whole country. The provinces cannot make criminal law, though they may impose fines and short prison terms for breach of provincial laws, such as highway traffic laws, municipal by-laws, certain environmental offences, and health laws, for example.[41]

Most criminal law is contained in the **Criminal Code of Canada,**[42] which was originally passed by Parliament in 1892.[43] It is a lengthy statute containing a comprehensive and detailed list of criminal offences as well as a code of criminal procedure governing arrests, laying of charges, release on bail, preliminary hearings, trials, and sentencing. It also contains provisions dealing with appeals from verdicts and sentences, and release pending appeal. The most comprehensive revision in the Code's history took place in 1955;[44] however, it has since been amended many times.

As comprehensive as it is, the Code is not an exhaustive repository of all criminal offences in Canada. Other federal statutes, such as the *Controlled Drugs and Substances Act,*[45] the *Food and Drugs Act,*[46] the *Income Tax Act,*[47] the *Competition Act,*[48] the *Fisheries Act,*[49] and the *Canada Shipping Act,*[50] to name a few, create further criminal offences.

Classes of Criminal Offences

There are three classes of criminal offences under the *Criminal Code:*

- indictable offences,
- summary conviction offences, and
- dual procedure (or hybrid) offences.

Summary conviction offences are generally of a minor or less serious nature. They include such offences as causing a disturbance,[51] discharging a firearm in a public place,[52] loitering,[53] trespassing at night,[54] vagrancy,[55] and so forth.[56] Such offences are tried before a provincial court judge. No jury is employed in such a trial. If the accused is convicted, he or she is liable to a prison term of up to six months, a fine of up to $2000, or both, unless the Code or other statutory provision creating the offence specifies another punishment.[57]

Indictable offences are generally more serious. These include murder (both first- and second-degree),[58] manslaughter,[59] attempted murder,[60] **criminal negligence** causing death,[61] robbery,[62] theft of property having a value of over $1000,[63] treason,[64] and conspiracy to commit an indictable offence,[65] among others.[66]

Given their more serious nature, the procedure for trying indictable offences is more complex than that for summary conviction offences. After being arrested and charged, an accused person is first brought before a justice of the peace or a provincial court judge. Depending on the type of offence, the accused will be tried by a provincial court judge alone,[67] or may elect (choose) a mode of trial as allowed under the Code for certain indictable offences.[68] If the indictable offence is one that allows the accused to elect, the choices include:

- trial by a provincial court judge without a jury and without a **preliminary inquiry;**
- a preliminary inquiry and trial by a judge (other than a provincial court judge) without a jury; or
- a preliminary inquiry and trial by a court composed of a judge and jury.

If the accused fails to make an election, the third option is automatically assigned.[69] For those indictable offences listed in section 469 of the Code (treason, etc.), the accused is automatically tried by a court composed of a judge and jury, having first had a preliminary inquiry. The accused is given no choice, although he or she may, if the Crown prosecutor agrees, be tried by a judge without a jury.[70] The jury is composed of 12 Canadian citizens over 18 years of age.

The purpose of the preliminary inquiry is to determine whether the Crown has sufficient evidence such that a reasonable jury, reasonably instructed in the law could (not would) convict the accused of the offence.[71] It is not a trial. If the provincial court judge, after conducting the hearing, concludes that the evidence is deficient, the accused will be discharged. This does not mean, however, that the accused has been found not guilty, since there has been no trial. It means only that there is insufficient evidence to satisfy the standard (test) described above, and that the accused should not be made to stand trial.

Generally, an accused person cannot be charged and tried for the same criminal offence more than once. Since the preliminary inquiry is not a trial, the accused can, if the Crown obtains additional evidence, be charged again with the offence or a new offence, if the new evidence suggests that a separate and different offence was committed. If an accused is discharged following a preliminary inquiry, the Crown must adduce (present) new and more probative evidence in order to justify laying a new charge against the accused. If the new evidence is insufficient, the charge may be dismissed as an abuse of the court's process. Or, the charge may be dismissed because laying it violates the accused's rights under the *Charter of Rights and Freedoms* (discussed on pages 84–86).

Indictable offences carry much greater penalties, ranging from over two years to life imprisonment, as well as substantial fines. Such sentences are served in penitentiaries administered by the Government of Canada. If the sentence is less than two years' imprisonment, as in the case of summary conviction offences or provincial offences, it is served in a provincially administered correctional institution.

The third class of offence under the Code is that of **dual procedure** or **hybrid offences.** These are sometimes referred to as "offences triable either way."[72] They are hybrid in that the Crown, in whose name an accused person is prosecuted, may choose to try the accused summarily or indictably.[73] Until the Crown attorney prosecuting the case makes the choice, the offence will be deemed to be indictable.[74] If the Crown elects to proceed summarily, the accused will be tried by a provincial court judge alone. Should the Crown choose to proceed by indictment, the accused will be called upon to elect the mode of trial in accordance with the procedure outlined above.

The Presumption of Innocence

In Canada, as in most western democracies, an accused person is considered innocent until proven guilty. Not only is this principle enshrined in the *Criminal Code*,[75] but more significantly, it is also a fundamental right guaranteed in the Canadian *Charter of Rights and Freedoms*.[76] Section 11(d) of the Charter reads:

> 11. Any person charged with an offence has the right: ... (d) to be presumed innocent until proven guilty according to law in a fair and public hearing by an independent and impartial tribunal.

The *Charter of Rights and Freedoms* has been an integral part of the Canadian Constitution since 1982. It sets forth the basic legal and democratic rights of citizens, rights which the State cannot abridge or infringe upon without breaching the Constitution. (The Constitution and the *Charter of Rights and Freedoms* are discussed more fully later in this chapter.)

There are two consequences flowing from the presumption of innocence for both the Crown and the accused. First, the Crown must prove all the essential elements of a case. It is for the Crown to prove the offence and not for the accused person to disprove the charge against him or her. The burden of proof refers to the degree of proof that the Crown must attain in order to secure a conviction. In Canada, this burden of proof is proof beyond a reasonable doubt. Second, while the accused may refuse to lead (present) any evidence, more frequently the focus of the defence is to establish a reasonable doubt in the mind of either the judge or the jury, depending upon the mode of trial.

Rules of Evidence

Evidence is the material with which the Crown builds and proves its case against the accused. Only evidence that is relevant to an issue in the trial and is probative (proves something) may be admitted. **Hearsay evidence,** that is, testimony by a witness that he or she heard a third party make a factual statement regarding an issue in the trial, generally cannot be offered as proof of the truth of such facts, although there is a trend to allow some hearsay evidence provided it does not gravely damage the accused's case (i.e., it is not prejudicial) and proves something at issue.

For example, suppose A., a witness to a murder trial, testifies that he overheard B. (who is not a witness and is not present in court) say that C., the accused in this trial, had committed the murder. Such a statement would be ruled inadmissible as hearsay evidence, although it could be allowed for the sole purpose of proving that the statement was made.

Evidence usually takes the form of oral testimony from witnesses. It may also consist of written documents, photographs, video or audio tape, or other physical form, such as finger prints, DNA samples, blood samples, or ballistics (gunshot evidence, as in murder cases). This evidence must be sufficiently probative, that is, it must have sufficient weight and value to convince the judge or jury beyond a reasonable doubt that the accused committed the offence with which he or she stands charged. If the Crown's evidence leaves at least a reasonable doubt in the mind of the judge or jury, the law requires that the accused be acquitted (found not guilty).[77]

The accused need not present any evidence at the trial, since he or she cannot be compelled to give evidence against himself or herself.[78] This means that the accused may choose not to testify. If the Crown has presented enough evidence to secure a conviction, the accused, in turn, should present enough evidence to raise a reasonable doubt in the mind of the judge or jury. If the defence's evidence is enough to raise such a doubt, the accused must be acquitted.

Elements of a Criminal Offence

Most[79] criminal offences have two main elements: a physical element and a mental element. The physical element is known in law by the Latin term **actus reus.** Thus, for example, in the offence of assault, the actual physical conduct of striking the victim constitutes the actus reus. The mental component, known by the Latin term **mens rea,** is the element of intent. In most cases, a person must intend to commit the act with which he or she is charged. Thus, in an assault, the mens rea is the perpetrator's intention to strike the victim. The perpetrator's wilful direction of his or her body to commit the physical act is the actus reus.

The link between these two elements, insofar as proving the offence is concerned, is that a conscious rational person, thinking rationally, always intends the consequences of his or her physical conduct. This means that a sane person, acting voluntarily and rationally, who is seen physically striking another, is presumed to have intended that result. In other words, such conduct is the product of a conscious mind acting voluntarily. The two elements of the offence must therefore both be present.[80]

For example, suppose a woman suffers a head injury in an automobile accident. She is released from the hospital a few weeks later, seemingly recovered from her injuries. One night she gets out of bed, proceeds to the kitchen, and obtains a carving knife which she uses to stab her sleeping husband repeatedly. The husband dies. The woman discovers the murder the next day and to her horror, concludes from the physical evidence at the scene that she committed the deed.

She has no recollection of having done this. She and her husband loved each other. She had no motive nor any wish to see her husband dead, and cannot fathom how she could have done such a thing. Perhaps her head injury caused her to act involuntarily: that is, her actions were not the product of her conscious mind, but merely the automatic movement of her body resulting from the injury to her brain. In such a case, the accused could not be found guilty of murder, as she clearly was not aware of the circumstances, she was not conscious, and she was not acting voluntarily. This defence is known in law as the defence of non-insane automatism.[81] Strange though it may sound, it has been accepted in Canadian courts as a legitimate defence since the Supreme Court of Canada's decision in *R v. Rabey*.[82] However, it seems less strange when one considers the basic principle that persons should be held responsible only for intentional acts that are the product of a rational mind acting voluntarily.

One must not conclude that an accused in such a state is necessarily insane. She may or may not be. If the accused were conscious, she would not have committed the act voluntarily and would be fully capable of knowing the consequences of her actions and of discerning right from wrong. A truly insane person is afflicted with a disease of the mind and is not legally capable of appreciating the nature and quality of his or her actions and their consequences. Such a person, therefore, is incapable of formulating the necessary intent or mens rea. Since one of the elements necessary to prove guilt is absent, such a person would be acquitted (found not guilty). Specifically, this situation would attract a verdict of not guilty by reason of insanity, as provided in sections 16(1) and (2) of the *Criminal Code*:

16. (1) No person shall be convicted of an offence in respect of an act or omission on his part while that person was insane.

(2) For the purposes of this section, a person is insane when the person is in a state of natural imbecility or has disease of the mind to an extent that renders the person incapable of appreciating the nature and quality of an act or omission or of knowing that an act or omission is wrong.

We have said that a person's intent can often be discerned or inferred from the circumstances surrounding his or her actions or words. It is through this means that the Crown usually proves intent in an offence. This is known as the objective approach to evidence.[83] That is, the court or jury can draw reasonable inferences from the evidence of the accused's conduct or words or the circumstances surrounding the commission of the offence.

The accused who seeks to prove that his or her conduct was not the product of a conscious and voluntary mind bears the burden of presenting psychiatric and other such evidence to prove his or her defence.

Breach of a criminal law through **malfeasance** (doing something that is one's duty to do, but doing it badly) or **non-feasance** (failure to act altogether where a duty to do so exists, such as criminal negligence causing death)[84] is also punishable. Here, the accused clearly has not intended to cause death by his or her conduct, but has behaved in a way that departs from the standard of reasonable behaviour expected by society. That departure or negligence has resulted in injury to a third party. The injury is so severe (e.g., death) that it ought to be punished, yet the accused did not intend for such injury to result. Can he or she still be convicted?

For example, suppose an accused was driving his car at excessive speed on a residential street, thereby striking and killing a child. The accused's behaviour is clearly out of step with the standard of the reasonable driver. His negligent departure from that standard is the mental element required to prove the offence. In other words, he was aware that he was driving at excessive speed, and he knew or ought to have known that injury could result from his carelessness. The law would punish such reckless behaviour in the interest of protecting the public from gross carelessness.

The Canadian Constitution

History of the Constitution

Canada's Constitution was originally passed by the British Parliament in 1867 as the *British North America Act*[85] (now known as the *Constitution Act, 1867*). At that time, and up until well into the 20th century,[86] Canada was a self-governing colony of the United Kingdom. Unlike the United States and several other countries with colonial histories, Canada became an independent and sovereign nation by evolution, not revolution.

Since Britain possessed ultimate legislative power over Canada, it alone could provide supreme legislation to which all colonial parliaments in British North America, and later the Parliament of Canada, would be subject. Canada has had the power to amend its Constitution since 1982 with the enactment of the *Canada Act, 1982*[87] by the Parliament of the United Kingdom.

Supremacy of the Constitution

It is a fundamental requirement of any democracy that its government and its institutions must act legally according to a higher law. The constitution of a country is such a higher law. It is essentially a set of supreme laws that define and regulate the various branches of government, their powers, and restrictions on those powers. Canada's Constitution includes a *Charter of Rights and Freedoms*,[88] which sets forth the basic legal and democratic rights of Canadians. These are rights the government cannot infringe upon unless it has a justifiable reason. Any governmental action or law that breaches the Constitution or a person's constitutional rights is itself illegal and invalid. A government is neither above the law, nor is it immune from the law's reach. It must always act legally. This is an adjunct to the principle of the rule of law and of due process, discussed above.

The *Charter of Rights and Freedoms*

Fundamental Rights

Canada's *Charter of Rights and Freedoms*[89] is an entrenched (integral) part of its Constitution. It codifies as constitutional law many of the **fundamental rights** and freedoms enjoyed in Canadian society, including freedom of religion and conscience,[90] freedom of thought and expression,[91] freedom of the press,[92] freedom of peaceful assembly,[93] and freedom of association.[94]

Democratic Rights

The Charter also protects **democratic rights,** such as the right of citizens to vote,[95] the provision that no Parliament or provincial legislature may continue for more than five years from the date of the last election,[96] and the requirement that Parliament or a legislature must sit at least once every 12 months.[97] These particular rights are meant to ensure that governments remain responsible and accountable to the electors and do not become tyrannical.

Mobility Rights

As well, Canadian citizens have the right to enter, remain in, and leave Canada, as well as to move and to take up residence in any province to pursue a livelihood (subject to laws providing for reasonable residency requirements in that province).[98] These are called **mobility rights.** Thus, neither level of government can erect barriers or systems of internal passports, for example, to control the flow of citizens across provincial boundaries or to prevent citizens from moving about the country freely, as is the case in many totalitarian countries.

Legal Rights

Perhaps the most important rights enshrined in the Charter are **legal rights.** These include the right to life, liberty, and security of the person;[99] the right to be secure against unreasonable search and seizure;[100] and the right not to be arbitrarily detained or imprisoned.[101] Thus, for example, the police in Canada do not have the right to arrest a person because they do not agree with that person's political views or fear that such person may engage in behaviour that is not illegal but which the police, other governmental officials, or politicians might find objectionable or offensive. Likewise, the authorities do not have the right (as they do in many totalitarian countries) to apprehend a person and hold him or her in prison for an indefinite period of time without a trial or specific criminal charges being laid.

Any resident who has been arrested or **detained** (held in police custody) has the right to be informed of the reasons for the arrest;[102] to speak with a lawyer without delay, and to be informed of that right;[103] to have the validity of the detention determined by a court, and to be released if the detention is unlawful.[104]

Rights accorded to all accused persons in a criminal trial or other proceeding include the right to be informed without delay of the specific offence;[105] to be tried within a reasonable time;[106] not to be forced to give testimony against himself or herself;[107] to be presumed innocent until and unless proven guilty;[108] to reasonable bail;[109] and to be tried by a jury where the punishment for the offence is imprisonment for five years or more.[110]

If tried and acquitted of an offence, a resident of Canada has the right not to be tried for it again. If found guilty and punished, he or she has the right not to be punished a second time for the same offence;[111] not to be subjected to cruel and unusual punishment;[112] not to have evidence given as a witness in a proceeding subsequently used against him or her in another proceeding;[113] and the right to an interpreter if he or she does not understand or speak the language in which the proceedings are being conducted, or is deaf.[114]

Equality Rights

Finally, all persons in Canada are equal before the law regardless of race, sex, national or ethnic origin, colour, religion, age, and mental or physical disability.[115] This provision is subject to the enactment of laws implementing affirmative action programs for the benefit of disadvantaged groups in society.[116] It is important to note that the absence of any right from those specifically enshrined as **equality rights** in the Charter does not mean that such unwritten right does not exist and is not otherwise enforceable.

The "Notwithstanding" Clause

While any statute law enacted in Canada is subject to the Charter, it is possible for Parliament or a legislature to forestall this result by invoking the **"notwithstanding" clause** of the Constitution. This clause provides that a law may continue to apply for up to five years, even if it contravenes a provision of the Charter. The five-year limit is designed to ensure that rights are not permanently infringed (violated) by a law. After five years, the "notwithstanding" clause expires insofar as it applies to that particular law, unless it is invoked again.

Language Rights

The Charter also contains minority language education rights, and makes French and English the official languages of Canada.[117]

Supremacy of the Charter

Since the Charter is part of the Canadian Constitution,[118] and the Constitution is the supreme law of Canada,[119] any law that is inconsistent with that supreme law has no force or effect. This means that any such law has the same status as if it had never been passed, and any action taken pursuant to it may be declared illegal by the court that rules upon its constitutionality. However, all laws are presumed to be constitutionally valid until the law is determined to be invalid by a court.

Division of Legislative Powers

Canada is a federal state modelled somewhat after the United States' federal system. There are two basic levels of government: federal and provincial. There is also, arguably, a third level of government at the municipal level. However, municipalities (cities and towns) are created by provincial law and not by the Constitution.[120]

The Constitution assigns power to make law to both levels of government. Thus, the federal Parliament can make law in those areas listed in section 91 of the *Constitution Act, 1867*. These categories include (but are not limited to)[121] the public debt and property, regulation of trade and commerce, unemployment insurance;[122] raising money by any mode or system of taxation; borrowing money on the public credit; the postal service; the census and statistics; national defence; salaries for the civil service; navigation and shipping; marine hospitals and quarantine; coastal and inland fisheries; weights and measures; currency and coinage; the incorporation of banks, banking law, and issue of paper money; cheques and negotiable instruments; interest; bankruptcy and insolvency; patents and copyrights; Indians and Indian reserves; immigration and citizenship; marriage and divorce; criminal law (except establishment and administration of the courts), including criminal procedure and penitentiaries; and any subject excepted from those reserved for the provinces.

Similarly, each province may make laws for itself exclusively within those areas listed in section 92 of the *Constitution Act, 1867*. Some of these include: direct taxation to raise revenue; borrowing money on the credit of the province; salaries and establishment of the provincial civil service; provincial prisons, hospitals, and charities; municipal institutions; licences to raise revenue for the province or municipality; local works and undertakings (except certain types reserved for the federal government); the incorporation of companies with provincial objects; solemnization of marriage; property and civil rights; administration of justice, including establishment of courts and civil procedure; power to levy fines or punishment by imprisonment for breach of any provincial law; and matters of a local or private nature.

It is apparent from this **division of powers** that there is overlap between the two levels of government. However, in the 131 years since the enactment of our Constitution, the courts have fleshed out these provisions and have built up a detailed body of case law to deal with conflicts between these two levels. These rules ensure that each level knows what areas these categories encompass, and whether its legislation is valid under the powers granted to it by the Constitution.

If there is a conflict between a provincial law and a federal enactment, the courts have determined that the federal law takes precedence. The provincial law will be suspended to the extent that it conflicts with the federal law, even if the provincial law is valid under section 92 of the *Constitution Act, 1867*. Furthermore, any power or area not assigned or mentioned in the Constitution is reserved for the federal Parliament.[123]

Municipalities are created by provincial law. Each province gives its municipalities the power to regulate such matters as garbage collection, road maintenance, maintenance of municipal parks and recreational facilities, licensing of local businesses and activities, land use planning and zoning, traffic by-laws, public health facilities and programs, libraries, and the raising of municipal taxes to fund these activities. The provinces cannot grant municipalities powers that they themselves do not possess under the Constitution.

Of particular significance to nurses is the fact that health care is largely an area of provincial responsibility.[124] (Specific provincial legislation regulating the nursing profession is discussed in Chapter Four.) Hence the provinces, through their ministries of health, administer and regulate health care systems within their boundaries. This includes such matters as the establishment, administration, and funding of hospitals and clinics; regulations governing public hospitals and private health care institutions such as nursing homes, long-term care facilities, and the like; and public health insurance. Regulation of the nursing profession (and other health professions) including professional self-governing bodies comes under the province's powers to make laws governing property and civil rights and hospitals.

In cases where one level of government has overstepped its constitutional authority and enacted legislation that infringes on another level's powers, the courts are called upon to resolve the dispute. Since Confederation, the courts (in particular, the Judicial Committee of the Privy Council, and since 1949, the Supreme Court of Canada) have gradually defined the extent and distribution of powers under the *Constitution Act, 1867*.

For example, the Constitution decrees that the federal Parliament has authority over telegraph lines connecting the provinces.[125] When the Fathers of Confederation drafted the Constitution, telegraphy constituted the state of the art in communications technology. Future developments in telephone, wireless telegraphy, radio, television, fibre optics, digital and satellite communications technology could not have been foreseen at that time. Over the years, the courts have interpreted this particular provision to include such technologies as a logical extension of federal authority over telegraph lines.

The thinking behind such interpretations is that the Constitution is a living document, capable of growth and interpretive development, that should be construed in light of current social, economic, and technological conditions, rather than according to the standards and conditions that existed at the time it was enacted. This is a logical extension of the principle that Parliament, which always expresses its will and intent through its legislation, is deemed to be "speaking" in the present at all times. Since the Constitution is a product of Parliament (in our case the British Parliament), that legislative body is said to be expressing its will in the present. Therefore, the Constitution should be interpreted as if it had just been written.

The Canadian Court System

The Canadian Constitution also provides for the establishment of a court system to adjudicate upon criminal and civil matters and to interpret the laws.[126] Our court system is organized primarily at the provincial level, where the bulk of litigation occurs. The Constitution gives the provinces the power to establish and maintain provincial civil and criminal courts and to set the rules of civil procedure in these courts. (Recall that criminal procedure is set out in the federal *Criminal Code of Canada*.) The specific court structure varies somewhat from province to province; however, there are fundamental similarities.

Provincial and Superior Courts

Each province has two basic levels of court: a trial level and an appellate (appeals) level. The **trial courts** vary from province to province in organizational structure and number, but their jurisdiction (i.e., the types of matters they can hear and the orders and judgements they can make) is much the same. Trial courts are further split into two types: a provincial court and a superior court.

For example, in British Columbia,[127] the provincial court hears summary offence criminal matters and preliminary hearings under the *Criminal Code,* and it operates as a youth court to hear cases involving young persons under 18 years of age charged with a criminal offence pursuant to the *Young Offenders Act.*[128] It also hears civil matters as a small claims court for claims under $10 000.[129] The superior trial court is known as the Supreme Court of British Columbia.[130] The appellate court is a separate court, the British Columbia Court of Appeal.[131]

The difference between the superior courts and provincial courts in the various provinces is that the former are higher in rank and have generally broader powers than the latter. The judges in the superior courts are appointed by the federal government, whereas provincial court judges are appointed by the provinces. Provincial court judges are more restricted in their powers and in the types of matters they may hear.

Alternatively, the superior court of a province may be further divided into a trial division and an appeals division, as in Nova Scotia. Sometimes the superior trial court and the appellate court are completely separate, as in Ontario, where trials occur in Ontario Court (General Division) and appeals in the Court of Appeal of Ontario.

In some provinces, some family law matters (except divorce proceedings) are heard in family courts. These may be set up as a division of the provincial court, as in Manitoba,[132] or as a separate court set up by the province, as in Nova Scotia.[133] Either way, family court judges are appointed provincially. Family law matters include custody applications, paternity disputes (the question of whether a named male is the biological father of a particular child), maintenance and support, and criminal matters involving young offenders, that is, children under 18 who are charged with criminal offences.

Administrative Tribunals

The provinces have also established boards and commissions which, although not courts in the strict sense, nevertheless **adjudicate** upon the respective rights and obligations of the parties who come before them. Examples of such boards or commissions, known as **administrative tribunals,** include the various provincial human rights commissions, labour boards, energy boards, provincial securities commissions, municipal boards, assessment review boards, and health disciplines boards (which regulate and govern nurses and other health professionals). The federal government has also created administrative tribunals, such as the National Transportation Agency, the Canadian Radio-television and Telecommunications Commission (CRTC), the Canada Labour Board, the National Energy Board, the Competition Tribunal, and others.

Administrative tribunals are established to administer and adjudicate under laws that govern a particular area or sector of the economy. Such boards may given power to grant licences, rule on complaints, set rates or tariffs, and hear grievances against persons or parties coming within their jurisdiction.

For example, the health disciplines boards established by the various provinces establish minimum standards of competence and enforce these standards among various health professionals. They may have the power to grant permission to practise a given profession or use a professional title (such as RN) within the province, and to discipline members who breach the standards or ethical rules of that profession. Thus, they operate like a court in that they have a duty to decide on such matters fairly and impartially and to give the parties before them a full opportunity to be heard and to present their case.

In the event that the board in question has failed to live up to the duty of fairness, its decisions are reviewable by a court. Otherwise, the operations and decisions of these boards are final and cannot be appealed to the courts. In this way, the government seeks to avoid overburdening the courts with highly complex matters best left to a board whose members have the necessary experience and expertise to decide on them.

Figure 3.3 illustrates the structure of the provincial court system.

Roles of Trial Courts and Appellate Courts

A trial court hears matters as a court of **original jurisdiction** or a **court of first instance.** This means that it is the first court to hear a case. Once a trial court makes a decision or renders a verdict, that decision or verdict may be appealed to an appellate court, which reviews the proceedings of the lower trial court to ensure that no procedural, evidentiary, or other rules of law were breached or misapplied, that the trial court acted within its powers or jurisdiction, and that the accused's constitutional rights were not violated (especially in the case of a criminal trial).

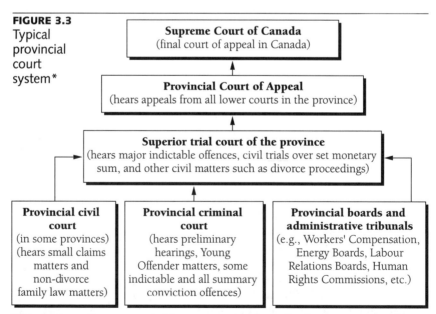

FIGURE 3.3
Typical provincial court system*

Supreme Court of Canada
(final court of appeal in Canada)

Provincial Court of Appeal
(hears appeals from all lower courts in the province)

Superior trial court of the province
(hears major indictable offences, civil trials over set monetary sum, and other civil matters such as divorce proceedings)

Provincial civil court	**Provincial criminal court**	**Provincial boards and administrative tribunals**
(in some provinces) (hears small claims matters and non-divorce family law matters)	(hears preliminary hearings, Young Offender matters, some indictable and all summary conviction offences)	(e.g., Workers' Compensation, Energy Boards, Labour Relations Boards, Human Rights Commissions, etc.)

*This structure will vary somewhat from one province to another. In some provinces, the Superior trial court and Court of Appeal are combined to form one supreme court for the province. In Ontario, the Superior trial court has a second branch called the Divisional Court which itself hears appeals from that province's administrative tribunals. In Quebec, on the other hand, municipal courts also exist to hear certain by-law offence and local matters.

An appeal is not a new trial. There are no witnesses, and new evidence is seldom heard. It is simply a review of the trial proceedings to ensure that no errors of law were made and that **findings of fact** are based on properly admitted evidence. Appeals courts review the decisions of trial courts if a party to the case appeals the decision because he or she believes the decision is unsound in law or unsupported by the evidence at trial. At an appeal hearing, lawyers for the parties argue (depending on whether they are the **appellants'** or **respondents'** counsel) that the trial court made a mistake in its interpretation or application of a point of law in some way material to the verdict or finding of liability, or that it erred in the way it assessed the plaintiff's damages, for example. The appellate court then has the power to substitute its own verdict or decision for that made by the trial court, or, if there were sufficient and serious errors made at the trial, it may order that a new trial take place. In such case, the matter is treated as if the first trial never took place, and the whole procedure is repeated anew.

The Federal Court and Supreme Court of Canada

Under the Constitution, the Parliament of Canada may also establish courts for the administration of the laws of Canada. This essentially means laws made specifically by Parliament, or matters over which the federal government has constitutional authority (except matters governed by the *Criminal Code*), and not provincial laws. Under this provision, the federal government has established the Federal Court of Canada,[134] which is divided into a trial and an appellate division.

The Federal Court of Canada

The trial division of the Federal Court hears a more restricted class of subjects, since most matters are heard in the provincial courts. It hears matters involving lawsuits against the Queen in right of Canada (i.e., the federal government) and federal employees in their capacity as employees of the government; taxation matters; suits involving First Nations people or land claims and bands; matters relating to members of the Canadian Armed Forces serving outside Canada; claims made against any federal board, commission, or administrative tribunal; suits between a province and the federal government or between two provinces, where the provinces have agreed by legislation that such matter should be heard in the Federal Court; matters involving patents, trademarks, copyrights, and industrial designs; matters involving suits under federal legislation; immigration and citizenship appeals; matters arising out of maritime (shipping) law or admiralty law; aeronautics; bills of exchange and promissory notes where the federal government is a party; and matters involving works or undertakings connecting one province with another.

The Federal Court of Appeal may hear appeals from a decision or judgement of the trial division, or of a federal board, commission, or tribunal, and any appeal which by law may be taken to the Federal Court. By leave of the Supreme Court of Canada, the Federal Court of Appeal decision may be further appealed to the Supreme Court.

The Supreme Court of Canada

The Supreme Court, established in 1875, is today Canada's highest court. Prior to 1949, any case heard by the Supreme Court could be further appealed to the Judicial Committee of the Privy Council in the United Kingdom. This step reflected Canada's slow evolution to a fully independent nation. Because Canada was still legally a colony of Britain, Canadian citizens (who were also British subjects) could appeal to the Privy Council (i.e., His Majesty in Council). Privy Council appeals in criminal cases were abolished in 1931 and in civil cases in 1949. Since that time the Supreme Court has been the final court of appeal for all cases arising out of Canadian courts. The Supreme Court[135] hears appeals from all provincial appellate courts in Canada and from the Federal Court of Canada. It also is the final interpreter of the Constitution. Its decisions are final until and unless the law is changed by Parliament or the Constitution is amended to reverse the Court's interpretation of one of its provisions. Furthermore, all decisions of the Supreme Court are binding on all lower courts. This is in accordance with the principle of stare decisis, discussed earlier.

The Supreme Court is made up of nine judges who serve until age 75 and are appointed by the Governor General on the advice of the Prime Minister. They, like all other federally appointed judges, may be removed from office only by resolution of Parliament. In this way, their independence is assured. They need not fear removal if they do not rule upon matters as the government of the day might wish. However, they may be removed if they have broken the law. No federally appointed judge has ever been removed in this fashion since Confederation, though a few judges have resigned following controversy impugning their integrity or impartiality.

Figure 3.4 illustrates the structure of the federal court system.

Summary

In this chapter we have gained a basic understanding of the workings of the Canadian legal system. We have discussed the sources of the law in Canada's two basic legal systems: the English common law and French civil law. We have examined the elements of negligence in the common law and reviewed the concepts of causation, foreseeability and remoteness. A good knowledge of these is an invaluable asset to any nurse today.

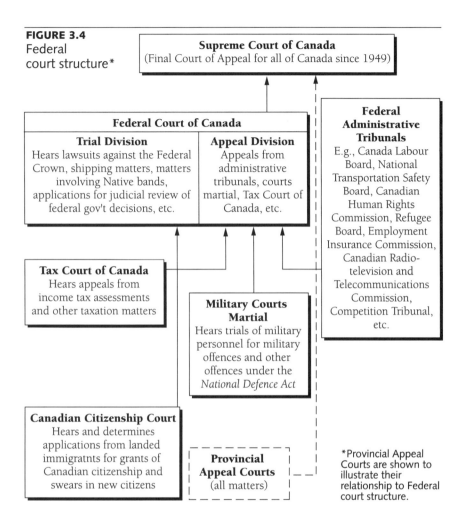

FIGURE 3.4
Federal
court structure*

Supreme Court of Canada
(Final Court of Appeal for all of Canada since 1949)

Federal Court of Canada

Trial Division
Hears lawsuits against the Federal Crown, shipping matters, matters involving Native bands, applications for judicial review of federal gov't decisions, etc.

Appeal Division
Appeals from administrative tribunals, courts martial, Tax Court of Canada, etc.

Federal Administrative Tribunals
E.g., Canada Labour Board, National Transportation Safety Board, Canadian Human Rights Commission, Refugee Board, Employment Insurance Commission, Canadian Radio-television and Telecommunications Commission, Competition Tribunal, etc.

Tax Court of Canada
Hears appeals from income tax assessments and other taxation matters

Military Courts Martial
Hears trials of military personnel for military offences and other offences under the *National Defence Act*

Canadian Citizenship Court
Hears and determines applications from landed immigratnts for grants of Canadian citizenship and swears in new citizens

Provincial Appeal Courts
(all matters)

*Provincial Appeal Courts are shown to illustrate their relationship to Federal court structure.

The chapter has also reviewed the structure of the provincial and federal court system and described how laws are passed. Finally, the workings of the Canadian Constitution, *Charter of Rights and Freedoms,* and criminal law have rounded off our overview of the legal system.

The key points introduced in this chapter include:

- the two primary legal systems in Canada—French civil law and English common law—and their sources
- the legislative process
- the distinction between tort law and criminal law
- battery and negligence as they relate to nursing practice
- an overview of the federal structure of Canada, its Constitution and the *Charter of Rights and Freedoms*
- the basic structure and functions of the Canadian court system.

Critical Thinking

QUESTIONS FOR DISCUSSION

1. Compare and contrast the key elements of English common law and French civil law.
2. Describe the concept of due process and the rule of law in Canada. Discuss the benefits and advantages of due process and rule of law in modern society.
3. What is negligence? How does it compare with, and relate to, tort law? Discuss how concepts of negligence might apply in a nursing practice setting.
4. What is a lawsuit, and how does an action typically progress through the court system?
5. What is Canada's Constitution, and what is its function?
6. What is the purpose of the Canadian *Charter of Rights and Freedoms?* Apply your discussion to a nursing setting.

References

1. RSO 1990, c. H.8, as amended.
2. This translation is from D. Stuart (1982), *Canadian criminal law* (p. 7). Toronto: Carswells.
3. *R v. Morgentaler,* [1988] 1 SCR 30; (1988) 63 or (2d) 281 (note); 82 NR 1; 26 OAC 1; 62 CR (3d) 1; 44 DLR (4th) 385; 31 CRR 1 (sub. nom *Morgentaler v. R*), 37 CCC (3d) 449, rev'g. in part (1985), 52 or (2d) 353; 22 DLR (4th) 641; 22 CCC (3d) 353; 48 CR (3d) 1; 17 CRR 223 (ca), rev'g. (1984), 47 or (2d) 353; 12 DLR (4th) 502; 14 CCC (3d) 258; 41 CR (3d) 193; 11 CRR 116 (HCJ).
4. *Criminal Code of Canada,* RSC 1985, c. C-46, section 241, as amended.
5. *Rodriguez v. British Columbia* (AG), [1993] BCWLD 347; (1992), 18 WCB (2d) 279 (SC), aff'd. (1993), 76 BCLR (2d) 145; 22 BCAC 266; 38 WAC 266; 14 CRR (2d) 34; 79 CCC (3d) 1; [1993] 3 WWR 553, aff'd. [1993] 3 SCR 519; *R v. Latimer* (1997), 121 CCC (3d) 226 (Sask. QB).
6. The procedure is well described in R. Dawson (1970), *The government of Canada* (5th ed.; N. Ward, Ed.) (pp. 356–357). Toronto: University of Toronto Press.
7. Supra footnote 1.
8. *Nancy B. v. Hôtel-Dieu de Québec et al.,* [1992] RJQ 361; (1992), 86 DLR (4th) 385; (1992), 69 CCC (3d) 450 (SC).
9. Article 19.1, *Civil Code of Lower Canada.* This legislation is no longer in effect, having been replaced by the Quebec *Civil Code* in January 1994.
10. Fleming, J. (1983). *The law of torts* (6th ed.)(p. 23). Sydney: The Law Book Co. See also Linden, A. (1993), *Canadian tort law* (5th ed.)(p. 40). Toronto: Butterworths.
11. Linden, ibid., pp. 40–41.
12. Ibid. p. 42.
13. E.g., see Saskatchewan's *Emergency Medical Aid Act,* RSS 1978, c. E-8, sections 2(b) and 3. This statute permits a registered nurse to administer emergency medical treatment to an unconscious person involved in an accident without incurring liability for negligence as a result of an act or omission on his or her part. It does not, however, excuse the nurse from

gross negligence, that is, conduct that drastically departs from the standard of the reasonably competent nurse. At time of writing (July 1998), other provinces were in the process of considering similar legislation.

14. Linden, supra footnote 10, p. 92.
15. *Donoghue v. Stevenson,* [1932] AC 562, at p. 580; 101 LJPC 119, at p. 127; 147 LT 281 (HL); see also Linden, supra footnote 10, p. 258; see also *Heaven v. Pender* (1883), 11 QBD 503.
16. (1984), 28 CCLT 155 (Alta. QB).
17. Ibid., p. 165.
18. See, e.g., *Gaudreault v. Drapeau* (1987), 45 CCLT 202 (Que. SC) and Quebec's *Charter of Human Rights and Freedoms,* RSQ 1977, c. C-12, articles 1, 2, 4, 5, 7, 8, and 49. Article 2 of the Quebec *Charter of Rights* creates a duty to rescue any person in peril. Such a person has the right, under article 2 of this statute, to aid and rescue and may bring an action for damages against anyone who fails to aid the plaintiff where the defendant's life or that of others is not imperiled by such rescue.
19. Linden, supra footnote 10, p. 266.
20. There are a few exceptions found in criminal legislation as well that require persons to act; see, e.g., *Criminal Code of Canada,* RSC 1985, c. C-46, section 215 (failing to provide necessaries of life to a child), section 218 (abandoning a child), section 216 (duty of persons undertaking acts dangerous to life to use reasonable skill and care in so doing), and section 217, which reads: "Every one who undertakes to do an act is under a legal duty to do so if an omission to do the act is or may be dangerous to life."
21. Linden, supra footnote 10, pp. 279–281.
22. Ibid., pp. 270–272.
23. Supra footnote 16, pp. 174–175.
24. *Overseas Tankship (UK) Ltd. v. Mort's Dock Engineering Co. Ltd., The Wagon Mound (No. 1),* [1961] AC 388; [1961] 1 All ER 404 (PC); see also *R v. Coté* (1974), 51 DLR (3d) 244 (SCC); *Abbott et al. v. Kasza,* [1975] 3 WWR 163 (Alta. DC), varied [1976] 4 WWR 20 (Alta. CA); and see Linden, supra footnote 10, pp. 308–309.
25. *Hughes v. Lord Advocate,* [1963] AC 837; [1963] 1 All ER 705 (HL).
26. See *Butterfield v. Forrester* (1809), 11 East. 60; 103 ER 926.
27. See Alberta: *Contributory Negligence Act,* RSA 1980, c. C-23, as amended; British Columbia: *Negligence Act,* RSBC 1996, c. 333, as amended; Manitoba: *Tortfeasor's and Contributory Negligence Act,* RSM 1987, c. T90, as amended; New Brunswick: *Contributory Negligence Act,* RSNB 1973, c. C-19, as amended; Newfoundland: *Contributory Negligence Act,* RSN 1990, c. C-33, as amended; Northwest Territories: *Contributory Negligence Act,* RSNWT 1988, c. C-18, as amended; Nova Scotia: *Contributory Negligence Act,* RSNS 1989, c. 95, as amended; Ontario: *Negligence Act,* RSO 1990, c. N.1, as amended; Prince Edward Island: *Contributory Negligence Act,* RSPEI 1988, c. C-21, as amended; Saskatchewan: *Contributory Negligence Act,* RSS 1978, c. C-31, as amended; and Yukon Territory: *Contributory Negligence Act,* RSYT 1986, c.31, as amended.
28. Quebec *Civil Code,* article 1478; and see Linden, supra footnote 10, pp. 440–441.
29. *Black's law dictionary* (1968) (4th ed.), p. 1746. St. Paul: West.
30. Linden, supra footnote 10, p. 457.
31. The document that starts the action is usually referred to as a statement of claim in Ontario and several other provinces. In some provinces, it may instead be referred to as a writ of summons.
32. The appropriate court will be the court that has jurisdiction (i.e., is authorized by law) to hear the particular matter. This is discussed in greater detail below.
33. See, e.g., rule 25.06(1) of the Ontario Rules of Civil Procedure (herein referred to as ORCP).
34. This time limit varies from province to province, depending on the provincial rules of civil procedure. In Ontario, for example, the statement of claim must be served within six months of its issue; see rule 14.08(1), ORCP. In British Columbia, a writ of summons must be served within 12 months; see rule 9(1), British Columbia Supreme Court Rules.
35. E.g., rule 19.02(1)(a), ORCP.

36. See, e.g., Ontario's *Courts of Justice Act,* RSO 1990, c. C.43, section 131(1) re: court's general discretion to award costs in a proceeding.
37. E.g., rule 30.02(1), ORCP
38. These matters include actions where the plaintiff asks for an injunction, the sale of land, a children's or family law matter, the dissolution of a partnership, foreclosure on a mortgage, and other such matters; see, e.g., Ontario *Courts of Justice Act,* supra footnote 37.
39. E.g., Ontario *Courts of Justice Act,* ibid., subsection 108(4).
40. *Constitution Act, 1867,* UK 30 & 31 Vict., c. 3, subsection 91(27).
41. For example, the highway traffic legislation of each province provides for fines and, in some cases, prison terms for breach of its provisions. The provinces have constitutional authority to make laws governing roads and use of motor vehicles. They need to be able to enforce these laws; therefore, they are permitted by subsection 92(15) of the *Constitution Act, 1867* to enact penalties for breach of such legislation.
42. *Criminal Code of Canada,* RSC 1985, c. C-46, as amended.
43. SC 1892, c. 29.
44. *Criminal Code,* SC 1953–54, c. 51. This revision came into force on April 1, 1955. See, generally, Mewett, A. (1993), *The Canadian Criminal Code, 1892–1992, 72 Can. Bar Rev.* 1.
45. SC 1996, c. 19.
46. RSC 1985, c. F-27, as amended.
47. RSC 1985, c. 1 (5th Supp.) as amended.
48. RSC 1985, c. C-32.
49. RSC 1985, c. F-14, as amended.
50. RSC 1985, c. S-9, as amended.
51. *Criminal Code,* section 175(1)(a).
52. Ibid., section 175(1)(d).
53. Ibid., section 175(1)(c).
54. Ibid., section 177.
55. Ibid., section 179.
56. This list is not exhaustive.
57. *Criminal Code,* section 787(1).
58. Ibid., section 235(1). Murder is first-degree murder if the accused has deliberately planned the act. Murder that is not planned and deliberate but, for example, committed in the heat of passion, is second-degree murder. Murder is first-degree murder regardless of planning and deliberation when the victim is a police officer, prison guard, or prison employee, or where the murder occurred as a result of a kidnapping, sexual assault, aircraft hijacking, or hostage taking. See section 231.
59. *Criminal Code,* section 236.
60. Ibid., section 239.
61. Ibid., section 221.
62. Ibid., section 344.
63. Ibid., section 334(a).
64. Ibid., section 47.
65. Ibid., section 465(1)(c).
66. This list is not exhaustive.
67. I.e., for offences such as theft or possession of stolen property of a value under $1000, counselling such an offence, keeping a gaming or betting house, betting, bookmaking, placing bets, lotteries and games of chance (unless held under a government licence), keeping a common bawdy house, cheating at play, fraud in relation to fares, and driving while disqualified (see section 553).
68. I.e., those not listed in *Criminal Code* section 553 and those not contained in section 469. Section 469 offences include treason, alarming Her Majesty, intimidating Parliament or a legislature, inciting to mutiny, seditious offences, piracy, piratical acts, murder, being an accessory after the fact to high treason, treason, or murder, bribery of a judicial office holder, attempting to commit any of these offences, or conspiring to commit any of these offences (see section 554).

69. *Criminal Code,* section 536(2).

70. Ibid., section 473(1).

71. *United States of America v. Sheppard,* [1977] 2 SCR 1067; (1976), 30 CCC (2d) 424; 34 CRNS 207; 9 NR 215; 70 DLR (3d) 136.

72. Marrocco, F. (1989–90). "The classification of offences and trial jurisdiction." Law Society of Upper Canada Bar Admission Course lecture notes, pp. 1–3.

73. An example is found in section 266, which reads: "every one who commits an assault is guilty of (a) an indictable offence and liable to imprisonment for a term not exceeding five years; or (b) an offence punishable on summary conviction."

74. This is so by virtue of section 34(1)(a) of the *Interpretation Act,* RSC 1985, c. I-21.

75. *Criminal Code,* section 6(1)(a).

76. Section 11(d) of the Canadian *Charter of Rights and Freedoms,* Part I of the *Constitution Act, 1982,* being Schedule b of the *Canada Act 1982* (UK), 1982, c. 11 (herein referred to as "the Charter").

77. This principle has been affirmed in the seminal English decision in *Woolmington v. Director of Public Prosecutions,* [1935] AC 462, at p. 481; (1936) 25 Cr. App. R. 72 (HL); for further discussion of the principle, see Stuart, supra footnote 2, at pp. 32–39. Woolmington has been adopted by the Supreme Court of Canada in *R v. Manchuk,* [1938] SCR 341, at p. 349.

78. *Charter of Rights,* section 11(c).

79. Some offences, known as absolute liability offences, merely require proof that the prohibited conduct took place without the requirement that the accused actually intended to commit the offence. For a fuller and leading discussion of absolute liability, strict liability, and mens rea offences, see *R v. Sault Ste. Marie,* [1978] 2 SCR 1299; (1978), 3 CR (3d) 30; 40 CCC (2d) 353; 85 DLR (3d) 161; 21 NR 292.

80. *Fowler v. Padget* (1798), 7 TR 509; 4 RR 511; 101 ER 1103 (KB); but see *R v. Bernard* (1961), 130 CCC 165; 47 MPR 10 (NBCA).

81. See Stuart, supra footnote 2, pp. 77–91.

82. [1980] 2 SCR 513; (1981) 54 CCC (2d) 1; 15 CR (3d) 225; 114 DLR (3d) 193; 32 NR 451. In *R v. Rabey,* the accused was convicted at trial of assaulting a woman with whom he was infatuated and who had rebuffed him. He had no recollection of having done so. The Supreme Court of Canada recognized (in a split decision) that a person might suffer a psychological blow that could cause him to act unconsciously.

83. Stuart, supra footnote 2, pp. 120–123.

84. *Criminal Code,* section 220.

85. UK, 30 & 31 Vict., c. 3.

86. It can be argued that Canada did not legally become fully independent from Britain until April 17, 1982, when the *Canada Act, 1982* was proclaimed by Queen Elizabeth II.

87. UK (1982), c. 11.

88. *Charter of Rights,* supra footnote 76.

89. Ibid.

90. Ibid., section 2(a).

91. Ibid., section 2(b).

92. Ibid.

93. Ibid., section 2(c).

94. Ibid., section 2(d).

95. Ibid., section 3.

96. Ibid., section 4(1).

97. Ibid., section 5.

98. Ibid., section 6.

99. Ibid., section 7.

100. Ibid., section 8.

101. Ibid., section 9.

102. Ibid., section 10(a).

103. Ibid., section 10(b).

104. Ibid., section 10(c). This is known as the right to a writ of habeas corpus, which is an

ancient type of court order dating back to medieval England. It was granted to those who were detained by the authorities without charge and for no lawful reason, and it is designed to protect citizens against arbitrary detention without charge or trial.

105. Ibid., section 11(a).
106. Ibid., section 11(b).
107. Ibid., section 11(c).
108. Ibid., section 11(d).
109. Ibid., section 11(e).
110. Ibid., section 11(f).
111. Ibid., section 11(h).
112. Ibid., section 12.
113. Ibid., section 13.
114. Ibid., section 14.
115. Ibid., section 15(1).
116. Ibid., section 15(2).
117. Ibid., section 16(1).
118. Ibid., section 52(2).
119. Ibid., section 52(1).
120. *Constitution Act, 1867*, supra footnote 85, section 92(8).
121. This list is not exhaustive.
122. This provision was added in 1940. There was no such scheme in Canada before that time and it was felt that the Parliament of Canada should expressly be given the power in the Constitution to legislate such a scheme.
123. *Constitution Act, 1867*, supra footnote 85, section 91(29).
124. Ibid., section 92(7). The federal government does play an active role in health care, however, through its funding activities, transfer payments to the provinces, and federal/provincial arrangements. In this way, it can influence health care policy in Canada. A major federal law in this area is the *Canada Health Act*.
125. *Constitution Act, 1867*, supra footnote 87, sections 91(29) and 92(10)(a).
126. Ibid., sections 92(14) and 96 through 101.
127. *Provincial Court Act*, RSBC 1996, c. 379, as amended.
128. RSC 1985, c. Y-1, as amended.
129. *Small Claims Act*, SBC 1989, c. 38.
130. *Supreme Court Act*, RSBC 1996, c. 443.
131. *Court of Appeal Act*, SBC 1982, c. 7, Index c. 74.1.
132. *Provincial Court Act*, CCSM c. 275.
133. *Family Court Act*, RSNS 1989, c. 159,
134. *Federal Court Act*, RSC 1985, c. F-7.
135. *Supreme Court Act*, RSC 1985, c. S-26, as amended.

Regulation of the Nursing Profession in Canada

LEARNING OBJECTIVES

The purpose of this chapter is to enable you to:
- understand the scope of laws regulating the nursing profession across Canada
- clarify the role, function, and responsibility of nursing governing bodies
- clarify some of the rules and standards regulating the nursing profession
- articulate the processes and procedures used by governing bodies relating to registration, complaints, discipline, and quality assurance
- understand the role of regulatory bodies in defining standards of professional practice
- utilize the *Code of Ethics for Registered Nurses* of the Canadian Nurses Association as a guide to ethical nursing practice.

Introduction

Like other health professionals today, Canadian nurses are held to an ever-increasing standard of accountability. In the last few years, new structures and mechanisms have arisen to make professional regulatory bodies such as provincial nursing colleges more responsive to their duties to ensure competent and safe nursing standards. Nurses need to be aware of the basic organization of the regulatory bodies charged with the self-governance of the nursing profession throughout Canada. While these vary in structure from province to province, the main objective is to make them accountable, responsible, flexible, and adaptable to rapid changes in nursing standards and ethics, while remaining responsive to the professional needs of their members.

As with all self-governing professions in Canada, nursing is regulated provincially. Each province has passed statutes and regulations respecting the profession's governance and its governing body. Such legislation sets out the body's powers to establish educational requirements, prerequisites for entry into the practice of nursing, fees, complaints and disciplinary procedures, and professional practice standards, to name but a few.

These regulatory bodies must be distinguished from nurses' unions such as, for example, the Ontario Nurses Association. The latter exist as collective bargaining agents and act solely in the interests of members as employees of various health facilities. (Labour issues, as they relate to nurses, are discussed more fully in Chapter Ten.)

As Canadians become increasingly aware of their legal rights, they are also questioning the efficacy of health professionals to regulate themselves for the public interest. Thus, the nursing governing bodies and health disciplines must set practice standards and codes of ethics that protect the public and provide the benchmarks against which professional practice may be measured. This is of prime importance, as all such bodies are given a mandate to protect the public from incompetent, unskilled, unqualified, or unethical practitioners. Thus, the primary purpose of each governing body is to serve as a watchdog and to promote the welfare of the public in relation to its profession.

This chapter will outline the laws governing the nursing profession in the various provinces and territories of Canada, including organizational structures, methods of regulation, licensing systems, establishment of educational standards, evaluation of the qualifications and skills of nurses, and management of complaints and disciplinary procedures.

Legal and Organizational Structure of Nursing Bodies in the Provinces and Territories (Other Than Quebec and Ontario)

The laws regulating nursing in the provinces and territories of Canada (other than Ontario and Quebec) are fairly uniform. They are essentially single-tiered systems, excluding the ultimate governmental authority of their respective ministers of health. In none of these jurisdictions is there an all-encompassing regulatory body for all health professions, although both

Alberta[1] and British Columbia[2] have health disciplines boards[3] that regulate a number of health professions. Each provincial nursing regulatory body is responsible directly to the provincial or territorial government and, ultimately, to the public.

Regulatory Bodies

In British Columbia, there are three professional nursing groups: registered nurses, licensed practical nurses, and registered psychiatric nurses. Registered nurses are governed by the Registered Nurses Association of British Columbia, which is incorporated by the *Nurses (Registered) Act*.[4] Licensed practical nurses do not have their own association per se, but are governed by the Council of Licensed Practical Nurses, whose members are appointed by the provincial cabinet and are now governed by the *Health Professions Act*.[5] Registered psychiatric nurses are governed by their own professional body, called the Psychiatric Nurses Association of British Columbia, which is created under the *Nurses (Registered Psychiatric) Act*.[6] The Registered Nurses Association of British Columbia is administered and governed by a board of directors. There are four categories of membership in the B.C. Association: registered nurses, licensed graduate nurses, student members, and honorary members.[7] Further classes of members may be established by the by-laws of the Association as required.

Similarly, in Alberta, registered nurses are self-governed by the Alberta Association of Registered Nurses, which is incorporated under the *Nursing Profession Act*.[8] Licensed practical nurses, psychiatric nurses, and mental deficiency nurses are governed and licensed separately under Alberta's *Health Disciplines Act*.[9] The remaining provinces and both territories also have provincially (or territorially) incorporated associations that self-govern and regulate nursing in their respective jurisdictions.[10] Alberta, however, is presently considering a health professions statute with a structure somewhat similar to those presently existing in Ontario and Quebec.[11] It would create separate colleges for various health professions and vest the powers of the present director of health professions in those colleges.

Objectives of the Associations

The objectives of the various associations are to regulate education, entry into the profession, and standards of practice of members of the profession in the public interest, as well as providing for discipline of members not in compliance.[12] The British Columbia Association's objectives also include the establishment and enforcement of standards of professional ethics among members, as well as the establishment of a patient relations program to prevent professional misconduct of a sexual nature. This provision appears to have been enacted in response to recent findings of widespread sexual abuse of patients by physicians in Canada.[13] In each province, it is the duty of the professional association, as a servant and protector of the public, to regulate the nursing profession and to discharge its responsibilities consistent with the public interest, while balancing the need for autonomy in the functioning of its professionals.

Board's or Council's Role

Each association is headed by a board of directors or a council (depending on the province) which governs the day-to-day affairs of the association, as well as providing the mechanism to establish entry criteria and standards of practice. As the primary rule-making body, the council or board enacts rules and by-laws respecting nursing practice standards; standards for admission to nursing schools; the curricula and teaching standards of such schools, although the provinces also have a say in this; student membership; continuing education; reinstatement and renewal of membership; licensing, membership, and other fees; rules governing types of duties and activities that may be carried out by licensed graduate nurses, and so forth. In British Columbia,[14] Alberta,[15] the Yukon,[16] Saskatchewan,[17] Manitoba,[18] New Brunswick,[19] Nova Scotia,[20] and Prince Edward Island,[21] the provincial association's board or council also hears appeals from decisions of its disciplinary or professional conduct committees.

The councils or boards may also, in some cases, hear appeals from decisions of the registration committees, or the association's Registrar (as the case may be). In the case of British Columbia,[22] its Council also hears appeals from decisions of the Association's Board of Examiners. The British Columbia, Prince Edward Island, and Newfoundland nursing associations each have a Board of Examiners whose duty is to arrange, set, and mark examinations administered to applicants for registration as registered nurses.[23] The exam administered to applicants is the Canadian Nurses Association Test Standards exam. It is a national exam designed to enable registration of students from one province into the nursing body of another. An appeal from the Board might, for example, involve the Board's decision to refuse an applicant permission to write the registration examination on the grounds that he or she had not met pre-examination requirements.

Registration and Licensing of Nurses

The registration and licensing schemes of the remaining provinces and territories are similar but more traditional. All provincial and territorial laws require applicants for membership in their respective provincial or territorial association to have graduated from an approved school of nursing, and to have passed the requisite nursing registration examination, before they may be admitted as members of the association.

Where applicants have received their training in a province other than the one in which they are applying, the education and training received must be either equivalent to that association's educational standards, or it must have been obtained from a Board-approved institution.[24]

In some provinces, applicants who are already registered and licensed to practise nursing in another province, who demonstrate that they are competent, and who are not currently the subject of disciplinary or competency proceedings in any other jurisdiction, will be entitled to registration in the province in which they are then applying.

Some provinces, notably British Columbia, Alberta, Saskatchewan, and Nova Scotia, have instituted licensed (or certified) graduate nursing categories. In British Columbia, Alberta, and Saskatchewan,[25] this is a temporary provision for applicants who have graduated from an approved school or course of nursing and have been employed for a period of time, but have not yet passed the national nursing registration examinations required by the association. This authorizes such nurses to continue to practise under certain terms and conditions pending their passing such examinations. Other provinces and both territories achieve the same result by granting temporary permits to such applicants.

In many provinces and territories, special classes of membership have been established, such as associate membership or (in the case of the Newfoundland Association) honorary membership. The purpose of these separate classes is to provide for those who do not practise in the particular province. The association will want to ensure that the member is still competent, keeping in mind the obligation to the public to ensure that members are subject to its discipline and competency requirements.

Unauthorized Practice and Use of Titles

All provinces and both territories restrict the practice of nursing and the use of the title "registered nurse," and the initials "RN" or "RegN," to members of the particular provincial or territorial nursing association who hold a registration certificate or licence, and are members in good standing (i.e., they have paid all membership fees, have not been suspended, nor had their membership or licence revoked). Moreover, the provinces of British Columbia, Saskatchewan, New Brunswick, and Prince Edward Island have gone as far as restricting the use of the title "nurse."[26] Any person who represents himself or herself as a registered nurse, provides or offers to provide nursing services, or engages in the practice of nursing, or who uses the term "nurse," or the initials "RN," or any variation thereof, without being a member in good standing of a provincial or territorial association and holding a valid registration certificate, commits an offence. Penalties vary from a $1000 fine up to one month in jail (or both) in Newfoundland to as much as several thousand dollars and up to six months' imprisonment in Alberta.[27]

Similarly, a member of an association who is under suspension or whose certificate of registration has been revoked or suspended may be deemed, for the duration of such suspension or revocation, not to be a member of the provincial or territorial association. Such a person then ceases to be a registered nurse and is not entitled to practise nursing, or to represent that he or she is licensed to practise nursing, in the province or territory. If the nurse nevertheless continues to practise, he or she may be charged with unauthorized practice and may be subject to the penalties mentioned above. In addition, continuing practice while under suspension constitutes **professional misconduct** under some provincial laws.[28]

It is thus important for the registered nurse to make sure that all membership fees are paid on time, as many provincial laws provide that a member's privileges and right to practise are suspended on failure to pay such fees when due. Most (if not all) provinces send notice advising the member that fees are due,[29] but this is not necessarily the case in all jurisdictions.

Exemptions

Certain health professionals are exempted from registration and licensing requirements under many of the nursing laws across the country. For example, physicians and surgeons, dentists and dental surgeons, registered nursing assistants or licensed practical nurses (who are regulated under another law specifically dealing with RNAs or LPNs), and nursing students need not apply for registration and licensing before they may practise in their field. Because these health professionals are already authorized or licensed by their own regulatory bodies to perform such treatments, it would be redundant to require dual registration. As well, persons rendering emergency first aid to people involved in an accident are exempt from registration and licensing.

In the case of those administering first aid, the law's policy is to encourage "good Samaritans." It is felt that there should be no regulatory prohibitions preventing one person from giving first aid to another in desperate need of it. People should be free to render first aid without fear of prosecution because they are not licensed health professionals. The acts undertaken, however, should be reasonable and fall reasonably within the competence of the person who undertakes them.

There is an interesting provision respecting registered nurses in the Northwest Territories. In that jurisdiction, a nurse who does anything for which a licence would normally be required under the *Dental Profession Act,* the *Medical Profession Act,* the *Pharmacy Act,* or the *Veterinary Profession Act* in the course of rendering emergency first aid or treatment or alleviating the pain or suffering of a person or animal, is not restricted from acting by any of those statutes. Thus, for example, if a nurse is required, in an emergency, to perform a surgical procedure, and no competent or qualified surgeon is available, he or she may proceed without fear of committing an offence. If the treatment is provided to an animal to relieve its suffering, the nurse is permitted to continue without requiring a veterinarian's licence.[30]

Temporary in Another Jurisdiction

The laws of some provinces and the Yukon Territory do not restrict the right to practise of nurses who are duly licensed and qualified to practise in another province, territory, state, or country. For example, suppose Nurse A. is a registered nurse qualified to practise in Alberta. She is accompanying an ill patient from that province on a two-week trip to visit the patient's relatives in Newfoundland, and she is not a member of the Newfoundland Association. Nurse A. will nevertheless be permitted to continue providing nursing services to her patient while they are in Newfoundland, provided the stay is temporary and she does not represent to others that she is licensed or authorized to practise nursing in Newfoundland.[31]

Disciplinary and Competency Matters

Disciplinary and competency matters are investigated by an investigator. If criteria are met, the matter is referred to the professional conduct or disciplinary committee of the provincial or territorial association. Committee members are usually appointed by the board of directors or council of that association, and include lay persons. The procedures for disciplinary hearings and the findings and penalties that can be assessed by the committee are similar to those in Ontario and Quebec.

Step 1: Complaint in Writing

In most cases, a complaint relating to alleged professional misconduct will be filed by the person making the complaint with the Registrar or executive director of the provincial or territorial association to which the member belongs. The complaint must be in writing, must be signed and dated by the person making the complaint, and should name the health professional who is alleged to have acted in an unprofessional manner. (However, failure to name him or her will not necessarily invalidate the complaint.) Further, it must outline the facts and particulars of the alleged misconduct. A complaint that is not in writing and that is made anonymously is usually ignored.

It is the ethical (and, in Alberta and New Brunswick, the legal) duty of each nurse to report any other nurse who has acted in an unprofessional manner or whose lack of skill, knowledge, or judgement poses a threat to the safety of patients in the nurse's care or who is, by reason of addiction to alcohol or drugs, or mental or physical illness, unable to discharge his or her nursing duties competently or safely. In Alberta, New Brunswick, and many other provinces, failure to report such conduct or situation will constitute professional misconduct on the part of the nurse whose duty it was to disclose it.

The duty to disclose unprofessional conduct or incompetence is accompanied by a potentially conflicting duty to observe the nurse–patient/client relationship and to keep confidential any information disclosed by the patient to the nurse in the course of treatment and the provision of nursing care. If, in the course of providing treatment to a patient, a nurse gained knowledge from that patient that another nurse was acting in an unskilled manner, that nurse may not be entirely free to disclose such information, if to do so would in any way compromise the confidentiality of the conversation.

It will usually be possible to disclose the information without divulging the identity of the patient, or other details that would readily identify him or her. The patient who feels strongly about the professional's conduct may choose to waive privacy rights and authorize full disclosure. For example, Ontario's legislation allows (and indeed requires) nurses and other health professionals to report knowledge of such allegations obtained in the course of practising nursing without naming the patient involved, unless the patient consents in writing to having his or her name disclosed in the report.[32] Nevertheless, this seems to apply only to situations involving sexual abuse, and may not necessarily protect the reporting nurse if the allegations relate to incompetence or other non-sexual misconduct. Manitoba's legislation, on the other hand, exempts the disclosure of information obtained, which is confidential by reason of the nurse–client relationship.[33] Yet even in Manitoba, a nurse, with the patient's written and freely given consent, could disclose such information to the Manitoba Association's investigators and disciplinary committee.

Step 2: Investigation

Usually, a complaint will be investigated in a preliminary way by a complaints committee, an investigator, or the Registrar of the association in order to ascertain whether it is well founded or merely frivolous or malicious (e.g., where it is brought deliberately to injure a person's reputation).[34] In Newfoundland, complaints may be investigated and reviewed either by the Council of the Association itself or by a special committee appointed by the Council for that purpose. One member of each such committee is required not to be a member of the Association.[35] This ensures lay representation and, in small measure, gives the public some input into disciplinary matters. The growth in public participation in professional disciplinary matters is an increasing trend in Canada in many professions. While some have welcomed this trend, others have seen it as a threat to the self-governing nature of the professions and to their independence.

By statute, members whose conduct or competency is the subject of an investigation must be notified immediately upon receipt of a written complaint by their provincial or territorial association. They may also[36] be entitled to make submissions to the committee or individual conducting a preliminary investigation. At this stage the complaint may be dismissed if it is unwarranted or unsupported by the results of the investigation.

In the Yukon and Manitoba, in a preliminary investigation, inspectors appointed by the board of directors or the committee investigating the complaint have wide powers to attend, inspect, observe, or inquire into a member's records, place of practice, equipment, and the supervision of the practice, without a court order. This inspection must comply with the provincial statute in this regard.[37] Such inspector may copy any records required in the investigation and must report any findings to the committee. In British Columbia, if authorized by the committee, such investigator may apply for a court order allowing him or her (or another so delegated) to enter the premises or land of anyone named in the order for the purpose of conducting an inspection, examination, or analysis, or to require the production of any record, property, or other items. The order may authorize such a person to inspect or analyze anything seized and to remove any such items for further inspection or analysis. A court order is generally required in British Columbia when a search is to be conducted outside regular business hours.[38] An investigator appointed by the Professional Conduct Committee must be authorized to apply for such an order. It is essential, for the purposes of fairness and natural justice, that an investigator be independent of the disciplinary committee or other tribunal hearing the matter. Otherwise, it may be alleged by the professional under investigation that the committee was biassed and directed the investigation against that professional.

Nurses must recognize that they are under a legal duty to co-operate with an inspector and to allow him or her to make examinations without interference. But patient confidentiality must be protected. A lawyer's advice and assistance should always be sought without delay. Legal counsel will be able to apply to an appropriate court for a ruling on whether such a search or seizure is lawful and made according to the procedural safeguards contained in the legislation.

Step 3: Interim Investigation

If well founded, the complaint may be referred to a disciplinary committee or a professional conduct committee (depending on the province or territory) for further investigation and then to a hearing, if necessary. If the allegations show that the nurse being investigated poses a threat to the safety or security of patients, the committee usually has the power to order that the nurse's right to practise be suspended or restricted pending the conclusion of the disciplinary proceedings. This effectively halts the nurse's practice for the duration of the matter, and may be a source of financial or other hardship to the nurse.

A nurse, when faced with an interim suspension or restriction, will in most cases appeal the decision to a court. The nurse may ask that the court lift the disciplinary committee's order on the grounds that the suspension was harsh, unreasonable, or excessive, or that the circumstances do not warrant suspension from practice in that no threat is posed to the public's safety. The granting of such an order is in the court's sole discretion and is not an automatic right.

Step 4: Disciplinary Committee

Before a hearing is scheduled to consider the matter, the committee must first notify the nurse against whom the complaint was brought. The date and time of the hearing will usually be coordinated with the nurse's legal counsel, if any. The notice usually specifies the nature of the conduct being reviewed, and the date, place, and time of the hearing by the committee.

The committee will usually hear evidence under oath and record it for the purpose of preparing a transcript for use at a possible appeal. Both the committee or board of directors (as the case may be), and the member whose conduct is being investigated, are entitled to have lawyers present and to submit evidence.

In cases where physical, sexual, or other abuse of a patient by the nurse is alleged, the patient may also be present and be represented by a lawyer. The patient may be the complainant, and if so, will be given an opportunity to relate the facts and basis for the complaint. The complainant may also give a **victim impact statement,** in which he or she explains the personal consequences of the complained-of behaviour.

The committee, after hearing the evidence, will consider its decision. Depending upon the provincial law, among the possible findings it may make are: that the nurse is innocent of any wrongdoing; or, that the nurse involved is incompetent, unskilled, or otherwise lacking in essential knowledge; or, that he or she is guilty of professional misconduct; or, that the nurse is habitually impaired by the use of alcohol or drugs such that he or she is unable to discharge nursing duties and obligations safely. Many of the provincial statutes specify acts that constitute professional misconduct. Such definitions are not meant to be exclusive, but serve to identify many common situations.

A nurse convicted of an indictable offence under the *Criminal Code,* or an offence under the *Narcotic Control Act* or the *Food and Drugs Act,* may, in British Columbia, Manitoba, Saskatchewan, New Brunswick, and the Northwest Territories, be liable to suspension from nursing practice in some cases, without any hearing. However, the *Charter of Rights and Freedoms,* as well as principles of natural justice, make it doubtful whether such legislation providing for permanent suspension without a hearing would pass constitutional scrutiny. It is likely that some form of hearing would have to be held, especially if the nurse runs the risk of permanent suspension and, hence, his or her livelihood. However, the particular legislation under which such a suspension would be initiated by a provincial association will require, in some cases, that the nature of the offence be such as would affect the member's nursing practice.

A 1990 British Columbia court decision involving a licensed practical nurse illustrates how provincial human rights laws may intervene to protect an applicant's right to membership despite that person's prior criminal record.[39] Although the case involved specific legislation applying to practical nurses, the principle is equally applicable to RNs. In this case, a woman had applied for a licence as an LPN after having worked unlicensed as such for a number of years. The Council of Licensed Practical Nurses of British Columbia refused her application on the grounds that she had a prior criminal record consisting of a conviction for shoplifting in the early 1970s. The B.C. *Human Rights Act*[40] then in force prohibited discrimination in employment based on a person's past criminal record unless such a record was related to the person's intended occupation. The practical nurse took her complaint to the B.C. Human Rights Council, claiming that the Licensed Practical Nurses' Council had illegally discriminated against her on this basis. The Human Rights Council found in the nurse's favour and ordered the LPN Council to grant the nurse a licence.

The LPN Council appealed, and the case ultimately found its way to the B.C. Court of Appeal, which upheld the Human Rights Council's decision and confirmed its view that the *Human Rights Act* superseded the statute granting the LPN authority to deny a licence to applicants who are not deemed fit to be licensed. The court further stated that the Human Rights Council was correct in asserting that the prior criminal record, in this case, was unrelated to the applicant's intended occupation as a licensed practical nurse, and that the discrimination was therefore unlawful.

It is arguable that such a ruling could apply to other provinces, since most provincial human rights laws contain similar provisions with respect to discrimination on the basis of a criminal record. Of course, other prohibited grounds of discrimination apply to bar refusal of a licence or registration on the basis of race, creed, ethnic origin, sex, religion, marital status, physical or mental disability, and, in some most provinces, sexual orientation.

Penalties

The penalties awarded to the nurse who has been found guilty of professional misconduct, or who has been found incompetent, include: censure or reprimand before the committee or in writing; conditions placed on the nurse's right to practise, including a requirement that he or she take additional courses or education and pass further examinations; suspension from practice for a specified period of time (e.g., for the completion of such additional training or education); or, in more serious cases, permanent revocation of the nurse's right to practise and expulsion from the nursing association. This, in some provinces, may be accompanied by a further order that the nurse pay the association's legal costs and fees incurred in conducting the investigation and hearing, or pay a fine, or repay to the patient any monies received from the patient for treatment services.

Criminal Record Checks (British Columbia)

In 1995, British Columbia passed the *Criminal Records Review Act*.[41] This law provides a scheme for initiating criminal record checks by a variety of persons (including governing bodies) from a number of professions such as social workers, health professionals including nurses, and teachers.[42] It requires governing bodies to initiate criminal record checks on all members applying for registration.[43] Those who wish to become registered nurses or licensed practical or psychiatric nurses in British Columbia must authorize the governing body to initiate a criminal record search.[44] If such authorization is not provided, the member cannot be cleared to work with children. Furthermore, if a nurse (or other professional) refuses to authorize a criminal record check, the board of directors of the governing body must take that refusal into account in deciding whether to register the nurse or to set conditions on his or her practice.[45] In this way, policy makers in British Columbia have provided the nursing (and other professional) bodies the means to ensure the health and safety of children and to stem the flood of cases involving the physical and sexual abuse of children by persons entrusted with their care and education.

Appeals

The decision of the professional conduct committee as to the finding of guilt, or the penalty awarded, or both, may be appealed to the board of directors or the council of the association by notifying it in writing within a specified time (usually within 15 or up to 30 days of the decision's being rendered).[46] If the decision on the appeal is still unfavourable, the nurse may appeal, in most provinces, to the provincial superior court (in Alberta, to the Alberta Court of Appeal, which may order a new hearing before the Alberta Court of Queen's Bench). Prince Edward Island, Nova Scotia, and the Yukon Territory do not allow further appeals to the courts, although an application for judicial review can always be brought to challenge the decision on the basis of the denial of natural justice, fraud, or the committee's having exceeded its jurisdiction. In the Northwest Territories and Newfoundland, the decision of the Trial Division of the Supreme Court on an appeal from a disciplinary committee's decision is final and may not be appealed further to their respective Courts of Appeal.

Many of the structures and procedures outlined above are equally applicable to registered nursing assistants (or licensed/registered practical nurses, as they are called in some provinces), as well as registered psychiatric nurses (specifically in British Columbia, Alberta, Saskatchewan, and Manitoba), pursuant to the statutes that regulate those professions.

Quebec and Ontario

Ontario and Quebec have somewhat different and more complex legislation regulating the nursing profession; however, the objectives and functions are basically similar to those of the other provinces and territories. Each province's laws, in particular Ontario's, is more highly detailed and structured compared with those of the remaining provinces and territories. Thus, the schemes of these two provinces will be looked at in more detail.

In both provinces, the nursing profession is regulated by a two-tiered system: at the higher level, a central administrative body established to govern all professions (as in Quebec) or all health professions (as in Ontario); and under this, the various professional organizations.

The Nursing Profession in Quebec

Office des professions du Québec

In Quebec, a central administrative agency, the Office des professions du Québec, has been established to regulate all professions including lawyers, notaries, chartered accountants, engineers, and architects, as well as physicians, dentists, chiropractors, nurses, and nursing assistants.[47] In short, all the professions that Quebec has decided should be regulated are included in the jurisdiction of the Office. The Office itself and its powers and functions are created and set forth in Quebec's **Professional Code**.[48] This statute also sets out the powers and procedures of the various Bureaus, that is, the rule- and policy-making councils of the various professional corporations that govern the members of each profession. These corporations are akin to the various colleges that regulate the health professions in Ontario.

The Office is primarily engaged in supervisory functions over the many professions under its jurisdiction. Its main task is to ensure that each self-governing profession acts with the protection of the public as its main priority.[49] It oversees the activities of the professional corporations, ensures that each corporation adopts a code of ethics, and further, that each adopts various regulations required by the Code. In particular, the Office must ensure that each professional corporation determines the composition, membership, and procedures of its professional inspection committee, and that each adopts regulations governing quorums at general meetings, dates and procedures for election of the president and directors of the corporation, standards for the equivalence of diplomas issued by educational institutions outside Quebec, and so forth.[50]

In addition, the Office has the power to suggest amendments to any of the regulations made by a corporation. In the event that a corporation fails to make a regulation required by the Code or suggested by the Office, the Office has the power to make the regulation for it, subject to government approval. Finally, the Office is required to make an annual report of its activities to the appropriate minister who, in turn, is required to present the report to that province's Legislative Assembly.[51] In this way, the legislature maintains a watchful eye over the Office, and policy matters that may arise out of the Office's activities are brought up for debate in a public forum.

Corporation professionnelle des infirmières et infirmiers du Québec

Like similar legislation in other provinces, Quebec's *Nurses Act*[52] defines the practice of nursing as an activity whose object is to identify the health needs of people, to contribute to the methods of diagnosing illness, to provide and control nursing care needed to promote health, to prevent illness, to treat and rehabilitate, and to provide care according to medical prescription. This definition is less detailed than that of other provinces, but is fairly succinct and allows greater flexibility of interpretation. It is worded broadly enough to encompass many daily activities and tasks undertaken by modern nursing professionals. Of course, it is not exhaustive of all aspects of nursing; in particular, it does not address ethical concerns directly or explicitly.[53]

The definition also serves a legal purpose: it helps in delimiting which acts constitute the practice of nursing for the purpose of identifying possible unauthorized practice. A legal definition of nursing thus assists a court or other administrative tribunal in determining whether a particular act by an individual constitutes nursing practice. In Quebec, the practice of nursing, as in other provinces and territories, is restricted. No one may practise nursing unless he or she is a registered nurse and a member of the Corporation professionnelle (or Ordre) des infirmières et infirmiers du Québec, or is otherwise permitted to do so by law. A breach of this provision leaves a person liable to the penalties set out in the *Professional Code.*

In Quebec, each professional corporation is governed by a Bureau whose size varies with the size of the membership in the particular profession. Most of the members of the Bureau are elected from among the membership. The nursing profession is governed by the Order and the *Professional Code* subject to the *Nurses Act.*[54] Its Bureau consists of a president and 28 directors, including a vice-president and a treasurer.[55] The elected directors are chosen at a general meeting by votes of delegates who represent the various sections of the corporation.[56] The Order of Nurses also has a secretary chosen from among the membership for an indefinite term who acts as secretary of the Order, the Bureau, and the Bureau's executive committee, and has custody and control of all records of the Order.[57]

Certain duties of the Bureau are established in the *Nurses Act.*[58] Specifically, the Bureau must establish the procedures for entry of members on the membership roll; advise the Minister of Health and Social Services on the state and quality of nursing care in the province and of ways to improve the quality of that care; determine the date and place of the annual meeting of the Order; maintain the register of nursing students, and procedures for entry in that register; require annual reports from the various sections; determine those sections that, because of their insolvency or poor use of funds, are to be dissolved or placed under trusteeship, or order inquiries into the affairs of such sections.

In addition, the Bureau must carry out those duties assigned to it by the *Professional Code.*[59] These include, among others, the obligation to appoint committees and determine their powers, issue specialist certificates, hold refresher courses or training periods for members, fix the amount of the annual assessment to be levied of members, strike members off the roll who fail to pay dues, and so forth.[60] The Bureau is also required to set the amounts required to defray the cost of a group professional liability insurance plan, and to designate a provisional custodian who temporarily holds and disposes of the professional records, books, equipment, etc. of a nurse who has ceased to practise. The Bureau has passed a regulation requiring that its members furnish proof of **professional liability coverage** of at least $500 000. A member must file a certificate that indicates, among other things, the period of insurance coverage and the dollar limits of the policy.[61]

The Bureau must also pass a code of ethics to govern its members, and the *Professional Code*[62] sets out the minimum requirements that must be contained in it. Pursuant to this, the Bureau of the Order of Nurses of Quebec passed its code of ethics in 1976.[63] A new draft code was published in 1992; however, it had not been passed into law as of the date of writing. The existing code defines the duties and obligations of the nurse towards the public and towards clients (i.e., persons who are receiving care from a nursing professional), as well as duties owed to the profession. In particular, it requires that the nurse be reasonably available and diligent, and that he or she subordinate personal interest to that of the client, respect the client's privacy, and refrain from disclosing confidential information.[64]

Although many nurses are employed in the public sector, some are employed as private nurses and, in some cases, render their accounts directly to their patients. Consequently, the Bureau must establish a conciliation and arbitration procedure for disputes arising between patients and private nurses in connection with nurses' accounts. These procedures provide a streamlined mechanism for settling disputes over accounts, thus avoiding the more costly process of litigation.

Nursing students must be registered with the Order and, once registered, are issued a certificate of registration by the secretary of the Order. Any person possessing a high school certificate or diploma recognized by the Bureau, and who has observed specific formalities set by it, is entitled to registration.[65]

Sections of the Corporation

The Order is further divided into sections based on geographical regions of the province. By law, there must be at least 11 such sections, although the exact number and precise boundaries of each are set by regulations passed by the Bureau.[66] There are currently 13 such sections in Quebec.[67] Each constitutes a separate corporation; thus, an attempt has been made to achieve a greater degree of decentralization and regionalization in the governance of the profession.

These sections are not altogether independent, however, since the *Nurses Act* gives the Bureau the power to dissolve or place a particular section under trusteeship if it is determined that the section is insolvent or has failed to make beneficial use of the funds at its disposal.[68] Each section is administered by a council made up of a president, a vice-president, and up to eight councillors.[69] To the extent that these regional sections are autonomous, they are free to determine the rules and procedures for elections of members of the council of the section, the length of their terms, and the exact number of councillors (not to exceed eight); set the date for the election; designate the returning officer for the election; and pass by-laws for the management of the council and administration of its property.[70] In this way, the regional regulation of the profession is encouraged, and each member is given more input into the running of his or her local section. Yet, the degree of autonomy actually enjoyed by these sections must not be overstated, as the Bureau also has the power to disallow any by-law passed by a section if such a by-law conflicts with its own regulations or is "inconsistent with à the general interest of the Order."[71] As well, each section is required to choose auditors at its annual general meeting and to have its books of account audited every year.[72]

The Professional Inspection Committee

The Bureau must have a professional inspection committee[73] to inspect the individual practices of the members of the Order. Its procedure and make-up are determined by regulations passed by the Bureau. The committee may inspect the records, books, registers, medications, poisons, products, substances, and equipment relating to a particular member's practice. It may also, at the Bureau's request, inquire into the professional competence of any member. Members must cooperate with any investigation conducted by the committee, as it is an offence under the *Professional Code* to hinder an investigator retained by the committee or any committee member in the performance of his or her duties.[74] Conviction for an offence under the Code carries with it a fine ranging from $600 to $6000.[75]

The Disciplinary Committee

Each Bureau also has a disciplinary committee responsible for investigating and conducting hearings on disciplinary matters involving members. The chair of such committee must be a lawyer with at least 10 years' experience, appointed by the Government of Quebec from among a list of names submitted by the Quebec Bar. This requirement is unique to Quebec. Although the majority of the members of such a disciplinary committee are themselves members of the professional corporation, it is felt that the complex procedural rules and regulations respecting the investigation and hearing of disciplinary matters require the expertise of a lawyer. Hence, the chair of the committee is entrusted to a lawyer skilled in civil procedure, the rules of evidence, and basic procedural requirements of such hearings.

The consequences of a hearing into a member's professional conduct carry potentially grave penalties, including permanent revocation of the member's licence, and hence the removal of that member's right to practise.

This provision warrants ensuring that all procedural rules and requirements are met, and that the member being investigated is given due process (i.e., a full opportunity to defend himself or herself), and a chance to make a complete answer to any allegations of professional misconduct.

Furthermore, a nurse who has had an adverse disciplinary decision made against him or her, such as a **reprimand,** or more seriously, temporary or permanent **revocation** of his or her right to practise, may appeal the decision of the disciplinary committee to the Professions Tribunal with permission (in most cases) of that tribunal.[76] The Tribunal itself resembles a court. It is made up of 11 judges of the Court of Quebec, chosen by the Chief Judge of that court.[77]

The Disciplinary Process

Disciplinary procedures under the *Professional Code* of Quebec, as in most other provinces and territories, are fairly straightforward. However, the nursing professional, no matter what province or territory in which he or she practices, is always well advised to obtain legal advice from a lawyer (preferably one who specializes in disciplinary matters involving professionals) immediately upon receiving notification that such proceedings have been brought against him or her. In virtually all cases, a professional facing disciplinary proceedings is entitled to be represented by a lawyer. The lawyer is best able to make sense of the procedures and rules of the disciplinary hearings and is well versed in the rules of evidence. He or she will likely have trial experience and will be skilled in the art of presenting a defence case and of cross-examining witnesses.

In a disciplinary matter in Quebec, a person wishing to make a complaint against a nurse must do so in writing under oath or solemn affirmation, stating the date, place, and nature of the offence that is alleged to have been committed.[78] The complaint is filed with the secretary of the disciplinary committee. Complaints may be lodged by an individual or by a syndic or assistant syndic chosen by the complainant (the person filing the complaint) or the Bureau.[79] (A syndic's role and duties are like those of complaints investigators in the other provinces.) The complaint may deal with the member's breach of, for example, the code of ethics, the *Professional Code* itself, the *Nurses Act,* or any regulations made under either of those statutes.[80] It may allege abuse of a patient by a nurse, or that a nurse abandoned or stole from a patient.

The Bureau must then appoint a syndic and assistant syndics, who investigate the complaint made against the member[81] and decide whether or not to lodge a formal complaint against him or her with the disciplinary committee. In either event, they must inform the complainant of their decision and, if a complaint is not lodged, of the reasons for that decision. Everything that is disclosed to the syndic or assistant syndics during an investigation is held in strict confidence, and these officials must take an oath not to divulge any such information without being legally authorized to do so.

If the facts of the offence with which a member is charged are such that the continuation of those acts would pose a serious threat to the public, the complainant can request that the committee strike the member off the roll provisionally (i.e., for the time being).[82] This suspends the member's right to practise. A copy of the complaint is served (given) to the member, who then has 10 days to file an appearance (a written notice that he or she will appear to answer the complaint).

If a request has been made to have the member struck off the roll provisionally, a hearing must be held on this question within 10 days of the complaint's being served on the member. If the committee deems it in the public interest to strike the member from the roll provisionally, it may do so at the conclusion of the hearing, and the order is effective from the time it is served on the member who is the subject of the complaint.[83]

This hearing determines only whether or not the professional's name should be provisionally removed from the Order's roll, and does not deal with the substance of the complaint itself. The question at this stage is whether the member's alleged conduct is of such nature that it poses a danger to the public and further, whether the protection of the public requires that the member be provisionally suspended. The suspension lasts until such time as it is overturned on appeal, or until the disciplinary hearing itself is resolved in favour of the member.

If the member chooses to appear, he or she, or the member's lawyer, must file an appearance with the Order, accompanied by a declaration in which the member either denies or acknowledges the act that is alleged to have been committed. Failure to file such a declaration is taken to mean that the nurse denies the allegations. A written contestation that sets out the member's own version of the facts may then be filed within 10 days of filing an appearance.

The hearing itself is conducted by a panel of the disciplinary committee, made up of three of its members including the chairman of the committee. A notice of the date, place, and time of the hearing must be served on the member and the member's lawyer (if any) at least three days before the date set for the hearing. Testimony given during the hearing (called a deposition) is recorded, unless the parties agree otherwise. These recorded proceedings will form the record in the event that the member wishes to contest the committee's decision.

During the hearing, the member must be given every opportunity to make a full and complete defence. The committee has the power to subpoena witnesses, and all parties and witnesses must answer all questions put to them. However, any evidence given by a witness (including the member) may not be used against the member in court.[84] All evidence is given under oath, as in a court trial. This means that anyone who lies or misleads the committee in giving testimony is subject to the same penalties for perjury as in a court case.

Only the committee has the power to determine guilt or innocence with respect to an offence under the Code. In the event that the member is found guilty, the reasons for the verdict must be recorded in writing and signed by the committee members. A penalty must be imposed within 30 days of a conviction. The committee also has the power to order the guilty member to pay the costs of the proceedings, other parties' costs, and the costs of recording the proceedings.[85] These penalties include any one or more of the following: a reprimand of the member; temporary or permanent striking of the member's name from the roll; a fine of at least $500 for each offence; the obligation to remit any money the nurse is holding to any person entitled to it; a revocation of the member's permit or specialist's certificate; or a restriction or suspension of the member's right to engage in professional activities. As well, the committee must publish its decision in a regular newspaper or professional publication in the place where the nurse principally practises. This ensures that notice of the disciplinary proceedings and their result is given to the nurse's clients and members of his or her community. The stigma of such publication alone should be enough to deter a breach of the Code and rules of professional conduct and ethics. Often, however, it is not.

In the event that the Bureau is required to pay a sum of money to the client of a member who was ordered to pay it, such payment is made from an **indemnity fund** set up for that purpose by the Bureau. This is to ensure that there is money available to compensate persons who have been injured or have suffered harm as a result of the member's breach of a provision of the Code or regulations. It is used in the event that the committee recommends that the Bureau make the payment. If the fund pays the injured client on the member's behalf, then the member is automatically struck from the rolls of the Order until such time as he or she repays the money to the professional corporation.[86]

As part of the penalty assessed against an offending nurse, the committee may order that he or she take a refresher course or refresher training, and it may suspend or restrict the member's right to practise until such time as that course or training has been completed.[87] A member whose name has been struck from the roll or whose right to practise has been suspended or restricted may request that he or she be reinstated. The disciplinary committee may make a recommendation to the Bureau as to whether that member should be so reinstated before the expiry of the penalty period originally assessed. The Bureau has the final say in the granting of such a reinstatement, but it is up to the committee whether or not a recommendation to reinstate is passed on to the Bureau.[88]

Appeals of any decision of the disciplinary committee must be made to the **Professions Tribunal** within 30 days of the date of service of the decision of the disciplinary committee on the member. Most decisions may be appealed only with leave (permission) of the Tribunal. Only a decision of the committee to strike a member from the rolls provisionally may be appealed as of right (i.e., automatically, without permission from the Tribunal). A petition for an appeal is filed by the member with the office of the Court of Quebec (because the Tribunal's members are judges from that court), and a copy is served on every party to the proceedings, as well as the secretary of the disciplinary committee. Other parties might include the person who filed the original complaint and any additional parties who may have had similar complaints arising from the member's conduct, plus any other parties who may have been given permission to participate in the disciplinary proceedings. A petition for leave to appeal (in cases where this is required) must also be filed within 30 days of the committee's decision being served on the member. Such petition must, in turn, be served on the parties to the proceedings and the secretary of the committee.[89]

The Tribunal also has certain investigatory powers. In addition, it may receive, in special circumstances, other evidence that was not presented at the hearing before the disciplinary committee. A date for hearing the appeal is then set and is held open to the public unless the Tribunal orders that it be held in camera (Latin, "in private"). It has the power to punish for **contempt of court** anyone who disobeys one of its orders or publishes evidence contrary to a publication ban. Finally, the Tribunal may confirm, alter, or quash (cancel) any decision submitted to it from a disciplinary committee and make the decision that it feels should have been made in the first place. It can also order the parties, or any among them, to pay the costs of the appeal.[90]

The *Professional Code* also imposes other duties upon the disciplinary committee and the Bureau, such as the obligation to publish notices of disciplinary action and decisions taken against specific members. The corporation must notify its members of the fact that a member has been disciplined, and of the penalty meted out, including the fact that the member's right to practise has been suspended or restricted, or that his or her name has been struck from the roll.

The Nursing Profession in Ontario

The Health Professions Board

The regulatory scheme for nursing in Ontario resembles that of Quebec in that it is a two-tiered system. The Health Professions Board, established under the *Regulated Health Professions Act, 1991*[91] (*RHPA*), is responsible for the overall supervision of health professions in the province and hears disciplinary appeals from the various professional colleges. This Board is roughly equivalent to the Office des professions du Québec. However, the Ontario statute limits the Board's jurisdiction to health professions only.

The Board is made up of 12 to 20 members appointed by the provincial cabinet, with a chair and one or more vice-chairs as designated by the chair. Each member of the Board serves for a maximum three-year term but each may be reappointed for further three-year terms.[92] As well, the Board is given the power to employ people to aid it in carrying out its many functions. It may hire investigators in disciplinary matters before it, and experts to provide the Board with professional advice and information in connection with registration hearings and reviews or reviews of complaints.[93]

The Health Professions Board is essentially a supervisory body. Its various functions and duties are set out and defined in the *Health Professions Procedural Code*,[94] which is enacted as a schedule to the *RHPA* and is deemed to be a part of each health profession Act. The *Nursing Act, 1991*[95] is such an Act; therefore, the *Procedural Code* is a part of that Act[96] and has the force of law.

The *Health Professions Procedural Code*

The *Health Professionals Procedural Code (HPPC)* is the core of Ontario's system for the regulation of health professions, and it is perhaps the most comprehensive such code in the country. It defines in greater detail the powers and responsibilities of not only the upper tier of the system, that is, the Health Professions Board, but also delimits the powers and authority of the professional colleges of all the health professions subsumed under the Act (including the College of Nurses of Ontario). It establishes procedures for hearing complaints against college members; reviews of registrations of members and appeals of those reviews; inquiries into the fitness or capacity of a member to practise the profession; judicial review of decisions of the Board and committees of the colleges; investigations conducted by the Registrar of a college; and the establishment of a quality assurance committee and a patient relations program. Finally, the *HPPC* establishes procedures for dealing with complaints of sexual misconduct of a member of a college. The Code strives to provide for more input from individual consumers of health services. It provides as well for more sensitive recognition of the rights and needs of those consumers.

The College of Nurses of Ontario

Each of the health professions is regulated and administered by its own professional college, such as the professional corporations in Quebec, and each college is set up under a specific Act of the legislature. Apart from the *RHPA*, nursing in Ontario is regulated under the *Nursing Act, 1991*.[97] This Act incorporates the College of Nurses of Ontario and defines its powers and responsibilities. In addition, the Act contains a legal definition of nursing, which codifies the scope of nursing practice in Ontario:

> The practice of nursing is the promotion of health and the assessment of, the provision of care for and the treatment of health conditions by supportive, preventative, therapeutic, palliative and rehabilitative means in order to attain or maintain optimal function.[98]

The purpose of this legal definition is to describe the nature and scope of nursing practice by delimiting those acts and procedures that constitute nursing practice. This provides a framework to determine whether certain actions constitute the practice of nursing and allows a distinction to be drawn between nursing and other professional practices. The definition also aids the courts in interpreting other sections of the Act.

Infrastructure

The College of Nurses of Ontario is led by an executive director who also acts as its Registrar.[99] All persons who are authorized to practise nursing or practical nursing in Ontario, are registered with the College, and have met the prerequisites (including fees) are its members. College membership is divided into two classes, namely, registered nurses and practical nurses (formerly known as registered nursing assistants or RNAs).[100] This feature of combining both registered and practical nurses under the jurisdiction of one professional college is unique to Ontario. In all other provinces and territories, licensed practical nurses, certified nursing assistants, and RNAs are governed by a separate body or other governmental agency.

The College's objectives are set out in the *HPPC* and include:

- regulation of nursing practice and governance of its members;
- development, establishment, and maintenance of criteria for persons to whom certificates of registration are issued;
- standards of practice to ensure quality professional practice;
- standards of knowledge and skill, and programs to promote continuing competence among members of the profession;
- standards of professional ethics for members;
- development of programs to assist individuals to exercise their rights under the *Procedural Code* and the *RHPA*;
- administration of the *Nursing Act, 1991,* and the *RHPA*; and
- any other objectives relating to human health care that the Council may consider desirable.[101]

Such a list assists the courts in interpreting the provisions granting the College specific powers and duties. Similarly, it provides legislative guidance to the courts when interpreting regulations made by the Council (see below). It also helps the College interpret the legislation for the purpose of making policy, creating regulations, and performing its duties under the Procedural Code, the *Nursing Act, 1991,* and the *RHPA*. When acting pursuant to these powers, the College must always have service and protection of the public interest foremost in mind.[102]

Council

The College's governing body is the Council or Board of Directors,[103] which is made up of 39 persons. Twenty-one of the Council are elected by the members of the College according to election procedures set by the Council.[104] Of these, 14 must be registered nurses, and seven practical nurses. The remaining 18 members are appointed by the provincial cabinet and must neither be members of the College, nor members of any other health profession's college or council. In this way, there is input from lay persons, which will potentially result in greater public input, scrutiny, and accountability not only of nursing, but also of other health professions.

As self-governing groups are generally regarded with suspicion, lay representatives may demystify professional regulation and make it more accessible and accountable to the public. The professions have expressed the concern that lay involvement will sacrifice self-governance and professional autonomy. The policy thinking behind such governing structure is that professionals retain the ability to govern and enforce professional standards while still allowing the public some influence on decision making. The drawback to this is that increased input from persons who are not sufficiently versed in the procedures and practices of a profession may unduly hamper the College's activities and independence. On the other hand, input from the consumer should greatly assist answering the question: What makes patients happy? The trend towards allowing non-professionals to sit on the governing bodies of professional organizations is desirable, but some would argue that it should not be permitted to suppress professional independence and self-regulation.

The Council has a president and two vice-presidents elected annually from among its members, one vice-president being a registered nurse and one a practical nurse.[105] It also has seven statutory committees: an executive committee, a registration committee, a complaints committee, a discipline committee, a fitness to practise committee, a quality assurance committee, and a patient relations committee.[106]

The Executive Committee

This committee is charged with exercising the powers of the full Council between meetings of Council. It has all the powers of Council (except the power to make or change regulations or by-laws) to deal with any matter that, in its opinion, requires immediate attention.[107] On the surface, this looks like a great deal of delegated power; however, it allows for greater flexibility in that the full Council need not be called to deal with every crisis or urgent matter. Thus, the committee acts as a caretaker between full meetings of the Council, deals with the day-to-day routine of administration, and screens complaints made against particular members respecting competency and fitness to practise.

The Registration Committee

This committee is responsible for processing applications for registration from prospective members.[108] When a registration application is filed with the Registrar of the College together with the registration fee, the applicant will be registered immediately if the Council's prerequisites have been met. If the application does not meet established prerequisites, it is referred by the Registrar to the registration committee.[109]

The College of Nurses of Ontario has five classes of registration certificates for registered nurses:

- General,
- Temporary,
- Special Assignment,
- Provisional, and
- Extended.

Identical classes exist for registration as a practical nurse.[110]

The Special Assignment class of certificate is intended for special programs such as, for example, exchange programs involving nurses from other provinces or countries. It is valid for up to a maximum of one year, as specified.

The Provisional class applies to those who have a number of criteria outstanding and are therefore not eligible for general registration (for example, graduate nurses who have completed their course of study but have not yet written their CNATs). It will be valid for a maximum of the earlier of three years or a lesser period stated in the certificate. A Provisional member also may not perform a delegated controlled act and may not self-initiate or delegate a controlled act (see Controlled Acts, below).

The General class applies to members fully qualified to practise within the full scope of nursing.

The Temporary class is reserved for those who will practise only for a specific period of time.

In order to permit nurse practitioners to practise in areas under-serviced by physicians and to add greater flexibility to the role of nurses in Ontario in primary and acute care, a new class of certificate was recently introduced with amendments to the *Nursing Act, 1991*.[111] The Extended certificate, when adopted by regulation passed by the College of Nurses of Ontario, permits nurses holding it to communicate to a patient, or to his or her representative, a diagnosis made by the nurse that identifies, as the cause of the patient's symptoms, a disease or disorder that can be identified from the patient's own health history, the findings of a comprehensive health examination, or the results of any laboratory tests, or other such tests and investigations that the nurse is authorized to perform. The Extended status also permits a nurse to order x-rays and radiation therapy, to prescribe certain specified drugs, and to administer, by injection or inhalation, such specified drugs. The ability to diagnose is limited by the necessity of the nurse to comply with a standard of practice that requires consultation with members of other health professions, where necessary.

It is the role of the registration committee to review those applications for membership that do not fully comply with the detailed registration requirements. Thus, the committee would, for example, review a foreign applicant's educational credentials to determine whether or not they are equivalent to those that an Ontario resident would obtain in an approved nursing program in that province. As part of its review, the committee might find that an aspect of the applicant's training was deficient, and may order him or her to take further courses or practical training. Alternatively, the committee may require the applicant to take and to pass further examinations set by the panel reviewing the particular case.[112] The Registrar or the committee may impose restrictions and conditions on the granting of a certificate of any class to the applicant. It may also recommend that the Registrar grant a certificate to a person who does not meet all the requirements, except where the requirements cannot be exempted. Any terms and conditions imposed on the certificate must be consented to by the applicant.

The *HPPC* sets out specific procedures for review of an application. Provisions for notice of the proceedings to the applicant, as well as for reasons why the application has not been automatically approved, are outlined.[113] The applicant is given the right to make written submissions to the committee within 30 days of being given such notice by the Registrar. The review is actually undertaken by a panel of at least three members of the committee. Once a certificate with conditions or limitations is issued, the applicant may later request the committee to vary those conditions and limitations. The committee would do so presumably in the event that the applicant has demonstrated that he or she has met the conditions originally imposed, such as, for example, passing an examination or taking further courses or training.

If the applicant is not satisfied with the committee's decision, he or she may appeal it to the Health Professions Board within 30 days of receiving written notice of the committee's decision.[114] The committee is also given notice of the applicant's appeal, and has 15 days to respond in writing to the Board. If such an appeal is launched, the committee's decision may not be carried out until and unless it is confirmed by the Board upon review or until the expiration of the time for launching an appeal (i.e., 30 days). The review is conducted by a panel of the Board consisting of at least three, but no more than five, of its members as selected by the chair. Applicants are given opportunity to make their case before the Board. It may confirm or vary the order of the registration committee or may send the decision, together with the Board's recommendations, back to the committee for further consideration.

The Registrar of the College is charged with keeping a complete and timely register of the names of all members. The register includes details of the class of certificate held by each member. In addition, terms and conditions (if any) imposed on a member's certificate, plus information required to be kept on a member by the committees on fitness and discipline, should be noted. Finally, the Registrar may suspend a member for failure to pay required fees upon giving the defaulting member two months' notice.

The Complaints Committee

This committee deals with complaints about a member's conduct or incompetence brought by such member's patients, colleagues, or other persons. A complaint filed with the Registrar of the College is investigated by a panel of three members of the committee selected by the chair.[115] A complaint must be in writing or recorded on tape, film, disk, or other such medium. If it alleges sexual abuse by a member, it may also be referred by the panel to the quality assurance committee after the panel has concluded its investigation.

The committee's role is to screen complaints involving specific allegations concerning a member's conduct or competence, which may then be referred to the discipline committee. However, the committee may choose to take no further action if it finds the complaint unsubstantiated or frivolous; or it may caution the member about his or her conduct; or it may refer the matter to the executive committee for incapacity proceedings if the conduct demonstrates that the member is incapable of safe or proper practice because of a mental or physical problem.

Before the investigation, the member complained of must be given a copy of the complaint. The committee investigates the complaint and, on completion, is required to give the complainant and the member a written notice of its decision within 120 days, otherwise the Health Professions Board may investigate the complaint itself. This is meant to ensure the timely disposition of complaints. If the panel decides to take no action, it must give to both the complainant and the member a copy of its reasons and a notice advising them of the right to request a review of the panel's decision by the Health Professions Board within 30 days.[116] A decision to refer the matter to the discipline committee or the executive committee cannot be appealed. In an appeal to the Health Professions Board, both the complainant and the member who is the subject of the complaint are parties to the appeal. Each is entitled to participate in the review.

The Discipline Committee

The discipline committee is responsible for investigating and adjudicating upon matters involving unethical or otherwise unprofessional conduct of members. This includes matters involving sexual misconduct. It is important to stress that the *Health Professions Procedural Code* applies to all health professions stipulated in statute in Ontario. Any member of any health profession who is alleged to have sexually harassed either a patient, a colleague, or a member of another health profession, including nursing, is subject to the same complaints and disciplinary procedures as nurses. Therefore, the procedures for initiating complaints, including those involving allegations of sexual misconduct, may be used by nurses in respect of improper conduct by other health professionals or fellow members of the College of Nurses.

If, as part of an investigation of a complaint against a member, a specific allegation of professional misconduct is found (since not all complaints against health professionals, no matter how justified, will necessarily involve professional misconduct), the executive committee may refer the matter to the discipline committee.[117] In the case of sexual misconduct, the executive committee, in deciding whether to refer the matter to the discipline committee, must consider the reports filed by other health professionals with respect to the member's conduct and, in particular, their opinions as to the likelihood of the member's abusing patients in the future.[118] In the meantime, the member's licence may be suspended or restrictions may be placed on the member's certificate of registration. However, the member must be notified in writing of the committee's intentions before such restrictions or suspension may be imposed.

Where the matter is referred to the discipline committee, a hearing will be held by a panel of at least three but no more than five members of that committee. The professional whose conduct is being investigated has the right to participate in the proceedings and to be represented by a lawyer.[119] The College and the professional against whom allegations have been made will be the parties to the hearing. If another person's conduct, competence, or good character is an issue in the proceedings against the professional, that other person may also be permitted to participate in the hearing to the extent permitted by the panel hearing the matter.

The professional complained of must be given at least 10 days' advance opportunity to examine any evidence and a copy of any expert's report to be given at the hearing. He or she must be advised of the identity of any witnesses who will be testifying. If these requirements are not met, the evidence will be inadmissible. However, the panel still has the power to allow the evidence if it ensures that the professional's interests in the case are not harmed thereby, that is, that he or she is not harmed by the lack of notice or opportunity to examine the evidence in advance of the hearing.

The hearing will normally be open to the public; however, where issues of personal privacy or safety or public security outweigh the policy of open proceedings, the hearing may be closed. As well, any evidence disclosed at an in camera (closed) hearing must not be disclosed to the public or anyone not involved in the hearing.[120] If a witness will be testifying as to the professional's sexual misconduct (including, but not limited to, sexual abuse), that person's identity must, at the person's request, be kept confidential. All evidence given at the hearing must be recorded, and a transcript made available to any party at that party's request and expense.

The panel is also bound by the rules of evidence. Any evidence that could not be admitted in a civil court cannot be admitted at the hearing. In making its findings, the panel must confine itself to considering the evidence properly before it.[121] In other words, the panel cannot consider anything that its members may have heard or read (e.g., in the news media or in discussions or conversations outside the hearing), nor may it consider any evidence that it has ruled to be inadmissible. As well, it would be ethically improper and illegal for any member of the panel to discuss the matter with other persons outside the confines of the hearing room.

If a member has been found guilty of an offence relevant to his or her suitability to practise, has sexually abused a patient, has been found guilty of professional misconduct in a jurisdiction outside Ontario, or has committed an act of professional misconduct as defined by regulations passed by the College, that panel must find the member guilty of professional misconduct.[122]

The College of Nurses of Ontario has passed extensive definitions of professional misconduct, including 37 specific acts. Examples include contravening a standard of practice of the profession or failing to meet the standard of practice of the profession;[123] improperly discontinuing professional services that are needed unless requested by the client to do so, or unless alternative services are arranged, or the client is given a reasonable opportunity to arrange alternative or replacement services;[124] abusing a client verbally, physically, or emotionally;[125] or failing to keep records as required.[126]

One interesting provision having important consequences for nurses states that it is professional misconduct to do anything to a client for a therapeutic, preventive, palliative, diagnostic, cosmetic, or other health-related purpose where consent is required by law, without first obtaining such consent.[127] This is significant in light of Ontario's *Consent to Treatment Act, 1992*,[128] which deals with a patient's consent to medical treatment. This statute, which contains provisions for informed consent and disclosure of material risks, will be discussed further in Chapter Six.

The penalties that may be levied against the guilty professional include revocation or suspension of the certificate of registration; imposition of terms, conditions, or limitations on the certificate for a specified period of time, including criteria that must be satisfied before the restrictions, terms, or conditions may be lifted; a reprimand by the panel; or a fine of up to $35 000.

Where the professional has been found guilty of sexual misconduct, he or she can be ordered to reimburse the College for expenses incurred in providing a program for therapy and counselling for patients who were sexually abused by professionals.[129] The guilty professional may also be reprimanded, or his or her licence may be revoked if the sexual abuse consisted of certain specified acts.[130] In such a case, the patient is allowed to make, and the panel must consider, a statement describing the impact that the abuse has had on him or her.

The panel may also, in an appropriate case, order the guilty professional to pay the College's legal costs, its costs of investigating the matter, and of participating in the hearing. A panel might make such an award where the case against the professional was clear and the evidence against him or her so compelling that the professional should have admitted responsibility, but instead chose to force the matter to a hearing.

The committee may find that the professional is incompetent. If his or her professional care demonstrated a lack of knowledge, skill, or judgement, or exhibited disregard for the welfare of a patient, this behaviour may be deemed incompetent. If the professional's conduct demonstrates that he or she is unfit to continue to practise, or that his or her practice should be restricted, the committee may also find that professional incompetent to practise. This is different from a finding of professional misconduct.

Regardless of the nature of the finding, the panel must render its decision in writing and give it to all parties. The College is required by the *HPPC* to publish its decisions and the reasons for these, including the member's name if he or she requests it, in its annual report and in any other of its publications. (A member might make such a request, for example, where he or she has been cleared of any wrongdoing and wishes to make this known to colleagues and patients.)

The Fitness to Practise Committee

Situations may arise concerning a member's fitness and capacity to practise. Investigation of such matters is the responsibility of the fitness to practise committee of the College of Nurses. Such an investigation will not necessarily raise questions of professional misconduct, but the member's behaviour may be such that there is doubt as to his or her physical or mental abilities.

Inquiries as to a professional's capacity will usually be commenced by the Registrar, using the extensive investigatory powers granted under the *HPPC*. If the Registrar has reason to believe that the member in question may be incapacitated, the Registrar must report these findings to the executive committee for further action.[131] If further action is warranted, and it has received the Registrar's report or a referral from a panel of the complaints committee, the fitness to practise committee may appoint a board of inquiry to determine whether the professional is incapacitated. A notice of the inquiry must be given to the professional. Some of the board must be drawn from among the College's general membership. In this way, the professional's fitness to practise is evaluated by his or her peers.

As part of its inquiry, the board may order the member to undergo any physical or psychological examinations conducted or ordered by a health professional (e.g., a physician or psychiatrist). Further, the member's licence may be suspended until he or she agrees to be examined.[132] Upon conclusion of the inquiry, the board is required to submit its report to the executive committee which, in turn, may refer it to the fitness to practise committee if it decides that further proceedings are necessary. The professional's licence may be suspended or restricted in the interim on such terms as that committee may order. In any such decision, however, the professional must be notified in writing of the committee's or the board's intention to suspend or place restrictions on his or her certificate. The professional has 14 days in which to make written submissions to the committee or board stating why such suspension or restrictions should not be imposed.

The fitness to practise committee then selects a panel of at least three of its members to hold a hearing into the fitness of the professional to practise nursing. Since a hearing will be held, the professional is again entitled to be represented by legal counsel, as are any witnesses who will testify, including any person who may have suffered harm or have been otherwise affected by the member's conduct. Evidence at the hearing will include testimony by medical or psychiatric experts. However, the professional who is the subject of the hearing must be given a copy of the expert's report or a summary of the evidence before it is presented at the hearing.

Unless the professional requests otherwise, the hearing must be closed. The professional's request for a public hearing may be refused if this would compromise public security, or any person's safety or privacy.[133] If the panel concludes that the professional is incapacitated, his or her certificate of registration may be revoked or suspended, or conditions, terms, or restrictions may be imposed on it. In cases where a certificate has been revoked, the professional may apply to the Registrar to have a new certificate issued, or the suspension removed, no earlier than one year after the suspension or revocation.[134]

If the application is turned down by the committee that originally ordered the suspension or revocation (e.g., discipline, fitness to practise), the professional may not bring another application for reinstatement until six months after the decision on the first application for reinstatement.[135] In an application for reinstatement, the committee may lift the suspension or revocation or order the Registrar to impose terms, conditions, and limitations on the certificate.

Any party to a proceeding before the Health Professions Board concerning a registration hearing or review, or before a panel of the discipline or fitness to practise committees (except a hearing for reinstatement), can appeal a decision of one of these bodies to the Divisional Court of Ontario. However, there is no suspension of the order revoking or suspending the member's certificate pending the outcome of such appeal.[136]

The Quality Assurance Committee

Every health profession's college is required under the *RHPA* to establish a quality assurance committee whose task is to review and examine individual members' practices to identify incompetency, incapacity, professional misconduct, and in particular, the sexual abuse of patients by health professionals. For example, if either the executive committee, the complaints committee, or the Health Professions Board receives a report from the Registrar following an investigation into a member's conduct involving sexual remarks or behaviour directed towards a patient, it may refer the matter to the quality assurance committee.

The *HPPC* defines sexual abuse of a patient as "sexual intercourse or other forms of sexual relations between the member and the patient, touching of a sexual nature of the patient by the member, or behaviour or remarks of a sexual nature by the member towards the patient"[137] unless it is touching, behaviour, or remarks of a clinical nature that are appropriate in the context of the treatment being provided by the member.

The quality assurance committee will conduct its own investigation into the professional's practice, not only to identify incompetency or incapacity, but also to pinpoint inadequacies in the professional's overall practice, including its operations and facilities. It may appoint an assessor to enter and inspect the professional's premises and records, obtain any other information on the professional concerning the care of patients, confer with the professional concerning the conduct, or require the professional to participate in a program designed to evaluate his or her skill, knowledge, and judgement. Anyone having control of such premises or records must allow an assessor to inspect them unless that person is a patient or a representative of a patient.

If the quality assurance committee believes that, based on its assessment, the professional may have committed an act of misconduct, or may be incompetent or incapacitated, it may disclose the professional's name to the executive committee and the allegations against him or her. On receipt of such information, the committee would refer the matter to the discipline committee or the fitness to practise committee, as required.[138]

The Patient Relations Program and Committee

In conjunction with the activities of the quality assurance committee with respect to sexual abuse of patients by professionals, the College was also required to establish and implement a patient relations program commencing December 31, 1994.[139] This program is intended to prevent and deal with the sexual abuse of patients by health professionals governed by the *RHPA*. It requires each college to adopt educational requirements for its members dealing with sexual abuse, guidelines for the conduct of members with their patients, training for college staff in this area, and the dissemination of information to the public regarding the program. The Council of the College will be required to submit a written report describing its program and any changes after the program is implemented. The role of the patient relations committee is to advise the Council as to the nature and content of such a program. Membership of this committee also consists of members of the College who are not members of its Council.

In addition, the *HPPC* requires any health professional to report a member of any health profession where the person has reasonable grounds, obtained in the course of practice, to believe that the other has sexually abused a patient.[140] The reporting member must file a complaint in writing with the other professional's college, stating the nature of the allegations, the offender's name, and the reporting member's name within 30 days of becoming aware of the sexual abuse. The patient's name may be disclosed in such report only with the patient's consent. Each college must set up and fund a therapy and counselling program for patients who have been sexually abused by its members. Such programs are administered by the patient relations committee.

Controlled Acts

One of the distinctive features of Ontario's system of regulation of the health professions is that the law specifically defines which medical actions and procedures may be performed, and who may perform and delegate them. The system no longer licenses areas of practice, but focuses on these specific acts. Thus, being a registered nurse does not grant a blanket authorization to perform controlled procedures that the nurse believes to be a part of the profession. A nurse may perform only those controlled acts that nurses are specifically authorized to perform. Needless to say, any act within the scope of nursing practice may be performed by a registered nurse or practical nurse unless it is specifically designated a **controlled act,** in which case that act may be performed by the nurse only if he or she is authorized by the *RHPA*, the *HPPC*, the *Nursing Act, 1991*, and nursing regulations to perform it.

The *RHPA* strictly regulates health care controlled acts,[141] and states who may perform or delegate them, to whom and by whom. In addition, the registration committee or the Registrar may impose restrictions or limitations upon a specific nurse's right to practise nursing.

The *RHPA* sets out 13 controlled acts, which may be performed only by members of a professional college authorized by the college's particular governing statute and regulations[142] to perform the controlled act.[143] If the particular act is to be delegated, it may be delegated only by a member so authorized and only in conformity with the regulations made under the statute governing the member's profession. For example, if a registered nurse is authorized to administer a particular substance by injection,[144] then he or she may delegate the act to a registered practical nurse, provided that the regulations under the *Nursing Act* allow such delegation, and all procedures for delegation set out in such regulations are followed.

The 13 controlled acts include:

(1) communicating a diagnosis or a disorder or disease to a person or that person's personal representative where it is reasonable to believe the person or the representative would rely on such diagnosis;

(2) performing a procedure below the dermis, surface of the mucous membrane, the cornea, or in or below the surface of the teeth (including scaling teeth);

(3) setting or casting a fracture of a bone or a dislocation of a joint;

(4) moving the joints of the spine beyond a person's normal range of motion using a fast, low-amplitude thrust;

(5) administering a substance by injection or inhalation;

(6) putting an instrument, hand, or finger beyond the external ear canal, the point in the nasal passages where they normally narrow, the larynx, the urethral opening, the labia majora, the anal verge, or into an artificial opening into the body;

(7) applying or ordering the application of a form of energy controlled and authorized by law (e.g., radiation);

(8) prescribing, dispensing, or selling drugs (e.g., controlled drugs);

(9) prescribing or dispensing contact lenses or eye glasses other than simple magnifiers;

(10) prescribing hearing aids;

(11) fitting or prescribing a dental prosthesis or periodontal appliance or device used inside the mouth to protect teeth from abnormal function;

(12) managing labour or delivery of a baby; and

(13) allergy testing.[145]

It is readily apparent that some of these acts would never, under normal circumstances, be performed by a registered nurse or registered practical nurse, although as we have seen above, Ontario has recently given primary

care nurse practitioners the ability to make and communicate diagnoses, prescribe certain drugs, and order x-rays and radiation therapy.

Currently, therefore, of these 13 controlled acts, registered nurses and
practical nurses (in certain circumstances) are authorized to perform items 1,
2 (only those specific procedures below the dermis or mucous membranes,
as allowed in the regulations made by the College), 5 (administering a substance by injection or inhalation and certain drugs as authorized by the
regulations), 6 (intrusions by finger, hand, or instrument, as outlined in the
regulations made by the College), 7 (ordering the application of a form of
energy prescribed by the regulations under the *Nursing Act, 1991*, and 8 (prescribing and dispensing certain drugs as designated in the regulations). As
noted earlier, items 1, 5, 7, and 8 can be performed only by nurses holding
an Extended certificate of registration.[146]

Interestingly enough, people falling into certain categories are authorized
to perform a great many of these acts regardless of whether or not they are
members of a health profession. The *RHPA* allows anyone to perform any
such act if it is done when rendering first aid or temporary assistance in an
emergency.[147] This is designed to encourage people to give aid and render
assistance in emergencies without fear of contravening the law.

A person is allowed to perform these acts if they are done to fulfil the
requirements to become a member of a health profession and the acts are
within the scope of practice of that profession and are supervised by a member of that profession,[148] or if the person performs such an act when treating
a member of the person's household.[149] In this latter case, however, only
those acts numbered 1, 5, or 6 in the above list may be performed.

Exemptions

A person may also perform the acts set out in items 5 and 6 if he or she is
assisting someone with routine activities of daily living. This would apply, for
example, in the case of a home care worker or friend who was assisting a
handicapped person in certain daily tasks which that person could not do
unassisted. There has been some concern with this particular exemption. It
is felt that persons involved in providing attendant care to the disabled will
fall outside the regulatory scheme of the *RHPA*, thereby defeating the purpose
of regulation. On the other hand, advocates for the disabled argued, prior to
passage of this legislation, that they did not wish for activities of daily life of
the disabled to be subject to governmental regulation and potential interference. This would have occurred had this exemption not been included.

If such an act is done in the context of treating a person by spiritual
means in accordance with the tenets of the religion of the person giving the
treatment, this is permitted.[150] It is difficult, however, to envisage a situation
in which some of these enumerated acts would be performed in a spiritual or
religious ceremony, especially procedures below the dermis, or the administration of substances by injection or inhalation. Certain specific acts, such as
religious circumcision, are expressly permitted.[151]

The *RHPA* also exempts certain communication when it is made in the course of counselling a person about emotional, social, educational, or spiritual matters, provided that the communication is not one that a health profession Act authorizes a member to make.[152] Equally significant, the RHPA does not apply to aboriginal healers or midwives when they are providing their services to members of an aboriginal community.[153] This would, for example, exempt aboriginal healers providing services to residents of an Indian reserve or members of an Indian band. However, if the aboriginal healer is a member of a college, he or she is still subject to its jurisdiction, regulations, and by-laws.

The fact that persons are permitted to perform acts 1, 5, or 6 in the context of treating a member of their household raises some interesting situations. For example, suppose a registered nurse in charge of and responsible for the care of a terminally ill patient is asked by a member of the family to permit a family member to administer morphine by injection to the patient to control pain. The *RHPA* would allow this provided that the nurse, having delegated a controlled act, ensured that the family member had been adequately instructed in the administration of injections, and that all necessary procedures had been followed.

Delegation

The Ontario *RHPA* also allows nurses to delegate the performance of specific controlled acts to non-qualified persons, provided the nurse has adequately instructed the person on how to perform such act properly and in accordance with professional standards, and that he or she adequately supervises performance of that act. This allows a greater degree of flexibility in the provision of health care services.

Use of Titles

Apart from regulating the performance and delegation of controlled acts, the *RHPA* also controls and restricts the use of certain professional titles such as "doctor,"[154] "nurse," "registered nurse," "registered practical nurse," or "registered nursing assistant."[155] In addition, no person may represent to anyone that he or she is qualified to practise nursing in Ontario as an RN or an RPN or as a specialist in nursing unless that person in a member of the College.[156] Anyone violating these provisions is guilty of an offence and is liable to a fine of up to $5000 for a first offence, and up to $10 000 for each subsequent offence.[157]

Other Offences

Both the *RHPA* and the *Nursing Act, 1991* set out other offences. These include obtaining employment for an individual knowing that that person is not competent to perform the duties of that position without contravening a provision of the *RHPA*.[158]

A distinction should be drawn here. "Competent" is used in the sense that the professional has the necessary skills, experience, and knowledge to carry out the duties of the particular provision. This is quite different from being "registered" or "authorized" to perform those duties. The latter expressions convey the idea that an official regulatory agency has assessed and passed judgement upon that person's skills and knowledge and has found these to meet the requirements of regulations. For example, suppose an employment agency found a position for a private nurse who was not a member or was not properly qualified in Ontario, knowing full well that that person was unable to perform any of the controlled acts that nurses are permitted to perform.

Other offences include: obtaining a registration certificate from any one of the colleges by false pretences or knowingly assisting a person to do this;[159] obstructing an investigator appointed by the Registrar of the College in an investigation into professional misconduct, incompetency, or incapacity of a member;[160] disclosing any information revealed at a hearing or inquiry that is closed to the public;[161] failing to permit an assessor of the quality assurance committee of a college to inspect a member's records or premises;[162] and failing to report a member (of the same or any other college) when there are reasonable grounds to believe that that member has sexually abused a patient.[163]

Finally, no professional may treat a person where it is reasonably foreseeable that serious physical harm may result from the treatment or advice, or from an omission from such treatment or advice.[164] Therefore, if serious physical harm is likely to result from a particular treatment or advice given to a patient, that treatment must not be undertaken, nor the advice given. Counselling about emotional, social, educational, or spiritual matters is excepted. These might result in psychological harm, but this is not prohibited by the *RHPA*. Despite this, it would certainly be unethical to counsel someone such that psychological harm might foreseeably result. Perhaps including "psychological" or "mental" harm in this prohibition would have placed too onerous a burden on health professionals, as the mind, its workings, and the genesis of mental disorders are still imperfectly understood. Others would argue that this gap in the law is a further example that what is legal is not necessarily ethical.

Standards of Practice

Nursing regulatory bodies and legislation establish standards of nursing practice and professional behaviours, which serve as yardsticks to measure the actions and competence of nurses in Canada. Nurses are accountable for meeting these standards, which clarify expectations for the delivery of safe, effective, and ethical nursing care. Standards make explicit nurses' accountability to the regulatory bodies, their employers, patients and clients, and the public.[165] These standards, which are considered minimum, are used to evaluate the actions of any nurse who is the subject of a complaint or disciplinary process within the regulatory body, or of a legal proceeding. Further, these standards are considered a component of the performance appraisal of nurses, and serve as a guide for ongoing professional development and education.

Nursing standards reflect the values of the nursing profession[166] and hold nurses accountable to the public with respect to the delivery of safe, competent nursing care. In general, most standards of practice:[167]

- provide a guide for safe practice;
- describe the responsibilities and accountabilities of the nurse;
- provide performance criteria;
- interpret nursing's scope of practice;
- provide direction for nursing education;
- facilitate peer review;
- provide a foundation for research-based practice;
- provide benchmarks for quality improvement.

For example, the College of Nurses of Ontario (CNO) defines "standards of practice" as "the provincial legislation, regulations, standards, policies and guidelines which establish CNO's expectations in relations to member practice and conduct." Examples of the standards produced by the College include CNO's *Guidelines for Professional Behaviour,* the professional misconduct regulations; *Nursing Documentation Standards;* and the *Professional Standards for Registered Nurses and Registered Practical Nurses in Ontario.*[168] Recently, this College produced more specific guidelines for nurses: the *Ethical Framework for Nurses in Ontario* and the *Standard for the Therapeutic Nurse–Client Relationship.* These address nurses' professional obligations to clients, colleagues and the profession, and explore how nurses develop and maintain relationships that benefit the client.

The professional standards document, similar to those produced in other provinces, reflects the philosophy of nursing practice and ethical standards and codes. Its standards focus on professional service to the public, knowledge, application of knowledge, ethics, continued competence, and professional behaviour. For each standard, the CNO has identified indicators, which assist in clarifying the standard's application. The indicators in this document reflect the concepts of "communication, leadership, critical thinking and legal professional requirements."[169] They are a guide to the evaluation of the nurse or nurses and serve as a benchmark with respect to the extent that standard is achieved.

To ensure these standards are met, and in order to meet the expectations of the *Regulated Health Professions Act,* the CNO has introduced a quality improvement program called the *CNO Quality Assurance Program.* All nurses who are registered with the College are expected to participate in this program, which has three parts: reflective practice, competence assessment, and practice setting consultation.[170] Each nurse must participate in one of these components.

The reflective practice component of this quality improvement program involves a self-assessment based on the standards and guidelines for practice, obtaining feedback from peers in order to identify strengths and improvement opportunities, development of a learning plan based on the self-assessment and feedback, implementation of the learning activities, and an evaluation.[171]

Approaches to competency assessment include volunteering for assessment, random selection by the College from the general pool of nurses or from an identified group to participate in an assessment, or referral from a statutory committee (e.g., as part of a complaint or disciplinary process).[172]

A practice setting consultation program was introduced by the CNO "to help nurses and agencies identify, and cultivate or maintain, characteristics in their workplace that support quality professional practice."[173] In this model, the College partners with employers to achieve quality care by "creating practice environments that support competent nurses to provide a quality outcome for the client."[174] The CNO has identified seven key attributes of a quality practice environment: care delivery processes, professional development system, leadership, organizational supports, response systems, facilities and equipment, and communication systems. The program is self-directed and allows an agency to examine its key attributes in order to build on its strengths and create opportunities for improvement.[175] The process embraces a quality improvement model which emphasizes organizations and systems, rather than individuals, and supports the notion that systems and performance can be improved even when high standards appear to have been met.[176] Success factors of this process include collaboration and partnership, the involvement of front-line staff, seeking staff input, integrating the changes into existing systems, and sustaining the improvements.[177]

Though legislation and regulatory bodies establish broad standards of professional practice, standards are developed in more specifically in particular organizations or institutions to represent nursing practice in that setting. Nurses are required to meet these standards, and their actions are evaluated accordingly. Standards of practice also exist for specialty areas within nursing. For example, standards of practice for a nurse in critical care will differ from those in a community or psychiatric setting. These standards lay out the specific competencies nurses in those settings must meet.

Professional Codes of Ethics

Standards of ethical practice are made explicit in professional *codes of ethics*. Professional groups have a duty to serve the public interest and the common good. Members of professional bodies have this obligation because their roles, missions, and ethical foundations focus not only on the individuals they serve, but also on society as a whole.[178]

Professional codes of ethics articulate the professional's ethical standards and obligations to clients and to society.[179] They define acceptable and unacceptable behaviour and rules of conduct, and articulate general principles that guide professionals' decisions and actions. The public trusts that professionals will use their knowledge and skill in the best interests of the individuals and the communities they serve. To maintain this trust, it is essential that professionals maintain scrupulous standards of conduct and be held accountable to the public.[180] When nurses accept their role, they commit to the profession's clearly articulated codes of practice and conduct.

As well, many health care organizations have their own codes of ethics. These include institutions such as hospitals, community agencies, professional associations, and registration bodies.

The Canadian Nurses Association

The Canadian Nurses Association (CNA) is a national nursing organization with links to 11 provincial and territorial nursing associations representing more than 110 000 registered nurses.[181] The CNA assists and supports the provinces in the development of standards of nursing practice, education, and ethical conduct. It initiates and influences legislation, government programs, and national and international health policy. It establishes and supports research priorities, facilitates information sharing, and represents the profession to health groups, government bodies, and the public.

The CNA *Code of Ethics for Registered Nurses*

The *Code of Ethics for Registered Nurses* of the Canadian Nurses Association (reprinted in Appendix A) offers a framework and guide for ethical practice for Canadian nurses.[182] It affirms that each nurse must recognize his or her responsibility not only to individual patients or clients but also to society, and must participate in activities that contribute to the community as a whole.

Since its first publication in 1980, the Code has been revised periodically (in 1985, 1991, and 1997) to respond to changing needs in Canadian nursing, including the consequences of economic constraint, expanded technological development, and new ways of delivering nursing services. The experience of nurses in all practice settings is considered, particularly in light of the current transition of care to the community.

Elements of the Code

The Code is organized around seven primary values:[183]

- health and well-being;
- choice;
- dignity;
- confidentiality;

- fairness;
- accountability; and
- practice environments that are conducive to safe, competent, and ethical care.

The values expressed in the Code provide a broad sense of the ideals of nursing. Specific direction is provided through statements of moral responsibilities, which have their basis in nursing values. The Code is prescriptive in cases where an ethical violation would result if the value is not followed. Otherwise, the Code is advisory, and is intended to guide ethical reflection and judgement.[184]

These standards provide direction for professional conduct and guidance for action within specific contexts or circumstances. The Code does not claim to provide rules of moral behaviour in all circumstances. It aims to provide guidance to the nurse in identifying areas of ethical violation, and in identifying and seeking some resolution to ethical dilemmas. In providing guidance for nurses in these areas, it is hoped that ethical distress can be minimized and a high standard of care can be achieved.[185]

In the following section, summaries of the values expressed in the code are listed in tables, followed by a brief summary of the responsibilities. Case studies provide a framework for discussion on how each specific value and its responsibilities guide the ethical practice of Canadian nurses.

Health and Well-being

In expressing this value, the Code makes explicit that the major focus of nursing is on the health and well-being of the patient or client. It acknowledges that health is more than the absence of disease or infirmity, and is influenced by a number of factors that fall within the domain of nursing. The Code acknowledges that nurses do not function in isolation. In collaboration with other health care providers, nurses are encouraged to advocate for a continuum of health services, beyond the treatment and cure of disease and injury.[186]

This value reinforces the important role that nurses play in health promotion, disease, and injury prevention, rehabilitation, and palliative care. Nurses are guided to alleviate suffering and to assist clients in a dignified and peaceful death. The value of health and well-being supports the principle of beneficence and the pledge that nurses accept to help others. Further, it clarifies that in order for nurses to achieve a consistently high quality of care, the nursing role must be promoted, and nurses' practice must be grounded in good science and research.

Consider this value when reflecting on the responsibilities of the nurse in the case study that follows on page 138.

TABLE 4.1
Health and well-being[187]

Nurses value health and well-being and assist persons to achieve their optimum level of health in situations of normal health, illness, injury, or in the process of dying.
- Nurses' major focus is on the health and well-being of their clients.
- Health is more than the absence of disease or infirmity.
- Health status is influenced by social, political, institutional, and other factors.
- Nurses support and advocate for a continuum of health services, including health promotion, disease prevention, rehabilitation, and palliation.
- Recognizing that maximal benefits to the client can be achieved through teamwork and collaboration, nurses respect the knowledge and skill of other health care providers.
- Nurses alleviate suffering and support a dignified and peaceful death.
- Nurses provide the best care they can in emergencies that arise outside the work environment.
- Nurses contribute to the ongoing development of the profession through participation, as able, in research and other related activities.

CASE STUDY

What outcome? What interventions?

Stephanie is a nurse case manager with an insurance company. Her role is to coordinate the resources needed by clients to ensure they achieve optimal recovery and return to health. There is usually a package of services aligned to each type of injury. Stephanie, as an employee of the insurer, is expected to utilize resources efficiently and to keep within prescribed guidelines.

Stephanie is assigned to manage the care of a client who sustained a fracture of his cervical spine in a motor vehicle accident. Mr. C. was taken to the closest hospital, 30 km from his home, which is located on the outskirts of a major city. When Stephanie first visits Mr. C. in hospital, she learns that he is recovering well from surgery and is now in halo traction. However, he is extremely depressed and withdrawn. He confides to Stephanie that he is worried, not only about his future employability, but about his ability to support his wife and child. Further, his wife is blind and must rely on friends to drive her to the hospital. Consequently, her visits are infrequent. As Mrs. C. is unable to care for their child on her own, their son is now staying with relatives.

In consultation with Mr. C.'s hospital team, Stephanie learns that there are no imminent plans to discharge him. The team plans to transfer him to a rehabilitation unit in the same hospital once he has sufficiently recovered from surgery.

Issues

1. Although Mr. C. is progressing well physically and plans are under way for his rehabilitation, is everything being done to ensure his well-being

and return to health? What factors would contribute to Mr. C.'s optimal health?

2. What is Stephanie's responsibility to Mr. C., his family, her employer, and the other members of the health care team?

3. How would the value of health and well-being guide Stephanie's practice?

Choice

Based on the principle of autonomy and respect for persons, this value stresses the significance of informed patient choice. Whether given in writing or verbally, or simply implied, a valid consent is one that must be: (a) based on the relevant information required to make that choice, (b) free from coercion, and (c) made by someone capable of this level of decision. For example, a client may be able to make decisions about her activities of daily living, yet may not be competent to decide whether surgery is in her best interest. The challenge for health professionals is to assess competence and to ensure that choices are made in a non-coercive environment.

TABLE 4.2
Choice[188]

Nurses respect and promote the autonomy of clients and help them to express their health needs and values, and to obtain appropriate information and services.

- Nurses attempt to involve clients in planning and decisions about their care.
- Nurses ensure that clients receive accurate and truthful information in order to be able to act on their own behalf.
- Nurses are sensitive to readiness of the patient/client to receive and understand information, and are respectful if that information is not wanted.
- Nurses are guided by the relevant legislation regarding consent, and ensure that their practice meets the established standards.
- Nurses respect an individual's right to refuse treatment, regardless of the consequences, when they are reassured that the person appreciates these risks. Nurses are not obliged to act on the wishes of a client when those actions fall outside the law or pose a serious moral conflict for the nurse. However, the nurse is obliged to ensure that other arrangements are available to a patient/client when the care required conflicts with the nurse's beliefs but is legally acceptable.
- Nurses are aware of their position of power with clients and how this may unduly influence clients' decisions.
- Nurses are clear about their own values and are alert to potential value conflicts.
- Nurses respect advance directives.
- Nurses recognize that individuals deemed incompetent may still be able, and should be encouraged, to make some decisions regarding their care.
- Nurses seek the input of a substitute decision maker when the client is unable to make decisions on his or her own behalf.

Even if it is not the nurse's responsibility to obtain informed consent, it is the ethical duty of the nurse to take action if this standard is not met. In acknowledging the role of substitute decision makers, the Code acknowledges recent legislation in this area, and the nurse's responsibility to ensure that the competent client's wishes are respected.[189] If a substitute decision maker has been designated, this person is best positioned to appreciate the values and beliefs of the patient who is no longer able to act on his or her own behalf. An important consideration is the role of beneficence in ensuring that the client's wishes are respected. Decisions about health care are not always easy. Nurses have the responsibility to ensure that their clients have the time and opportunity to reflect and consider their options, and to make the choice they think is best for them.

Consider this value when reflecting on the responsibilities of the nurse in the following case study.

C A S E   S T U D Y

Discovering the client's story

Stan, a nurse on a general medical unit, is caring for a 75-year-old woman, Jean, admitted for anemia of unknown origin. Preliminary investigations determined that she also had hydronephrosis of her left kidney, caused by a stricture of her ureter. The stricture was the result of chronic infection related to an ileal conduit she had in place for about 30 years. While Stan was with Jean, the urology resident came by to tell her of this finding. He advised that her only option was to have the ureter dilated under ultrasound. Jean became very upset, started to cry, and said she did not want to have the procedure. The resident told Jean that if she refused, her condition would deteriorate, and ultimately she would die. However, he explained, it was her choice; his responsibility was to inform her of her options and the risks associated with either having or refusing the procedure.

What Stan and the resident did not know was that two years earlier, Jean had experienced the same problem. The procedure was extremely painful, and following the intervention, she became septic and was seriously ill for two weeks. Just as she was recovering, a nurse accidentally removed the stent (in place to ensure the ureter remained dilated), and the procedure had to be repeated.

Issues

1. Is this resident respecting Jean's autonomy?
2. What is the ethical duty of the nurse in this case study? What actions should Frank take after observing this interaction with the resident and Jean?
3. What responsibility does Frank have to find out more about Jean's story?

Dignity

Nurses are guided by consideration for the dignity of clients. All persons deserve to be treated with respect and compassion. Disrespectful communication, disregard for client privacy, or the failure to involve patients in discussions that relate to them, violate nurses' ethical responsibility.[190] People need our care during very difficult and meaningful periods in their lives, from birth to death.

This value arises especially in relation to the dying patient. It is important that special attention be given to ensure that the process of dying is dignified, and that the emotional, psychological, and physical needs of the patient, family, and significant others are met. Nurses are obligated to ensure optimal patient comfort and pain control, to deal compassionately in situations where treatment is withdrawn, and to provide the patient and family with the opportunity for home care if and when this is possible. Based on this value, it would be the ethical obligation of the nurse to ensure, for example, that everything possible be done so that a patient does not die alone, unless he or she expresses this wish. The same priority should be given to these situations as that provided to emergencies. Assignments can be reorganized; help can be requested so that someone is with the patient.

Consider this value when reflecting on the responsibilities of the nurse in the case study that follows.

TABLE 4.3
Dignity[191]

Nurses value and advocate the dignity and self-respect of human beings.
- Nurses respect, and are sensitive to, the needs, values, and beliefs of each individual they serve.
- Nurses respect the privacy of clients.
- Nurses respect human life and the choices of persons about their quality of life, and consider these in regard to decisions about life-sustaining treatment.
- Nurses intervene when others fail to respect the dignity of human beings.

C A S E   S T U D Y

Dying—with dignity?

Ros is a community nurse who has been caring for Martha in her home for some months. They have developed a good relationship. Martha, who is 80 years old, has shared many of her life experiences with Ros. Born in Scotland, married at 16, she gave birth to three children during the Depression and the Second World War. Martha left her husband and immigrated to Canada when she was in her mid-30s. Successful in business and personally, Martha, in her own words, has "had a great life." Now in the terminal phase of lung disease, Martha is ready for—and even welcomes—death. Her one wish is to die at home surrounded by the people she loves. That is how it was in Scotland, she says.

One weekend while Ros is off duty, Martha experiences severe respiratory distress. The family panics and calls 911. Martha is subsequently admitted to the Intensive Care Unit of her local hospital, placed on a ventilator, and given aggressive treatment. When Ros returns to work on Monday she discovers this, and visits Martha in the hospital. She learns from the unit nurses that, although it is unlikely Martha will survive, the team has told the family they will keep her in the ICU and continue life support. The family agrees.

Issues

1. What responsibility does Ros have to represent Martha's interests? Do her responsibilities to Martha extend beyond the community and the home?
2. How likely is it that Martha will have a dignified death?
3. What do you think is happening with Martha's family? What help do they need?

Confidentiality

Fundamental to the nurse–client relationship is the professional obligation to respect patient confidentiality. The promise of confidentiality ensures full disclosure by the patient of information essential to achieving the goals of care.

A limitation to this rule arises if harm might result to the client or to others if confidentiality were maintained, or where statute law or legislation requires disclosure (e.g., reporting child abuse, or providing information to workers' compensation boards).[192]

Consider this value when reflecting on the responsibilities of the nurse in the following case study.

TABLE 4.4
Confidentiality[193]

Nurses safeguard the trust of clients that information learned in the context of a professional relationship is shared outside the health care team only with the client's permission or as legally required.
- Nurses observe practices that protect client/patient confidentiality and intervene when others fail to do so.
- Nurses disclose the minimum information necessary when:
  – authorized by the client,
  – there is substantial risk of harm to the client or others, or
  – there is a legal obligation.
- Nurses inform clients/patients about the limits of confidentiality and the circumstances under which confidential information would be disclosed.
- Nurses ensure that standards and policies are in place to meet this value.

Confidentiality—a sacred trust?

Anne, a public health nurse, has been visiting Barb, a young client who recently gave birth to her second child, a girl. Barb is on welfare; she and her partner have recently separated, and her relatives all live in other provinces. She plans to return to school part-time so that, in future, she can be self-reliant. Anne likes her client and has developed a sound professional relationship with her. Given Barb's isolation, Anne has extended her professional involvement.

Anne has observed Barb's strong parenting skills and her love for her children. One day during a home visit, she notices that Barb's son, Michael, has a black eye. Before Anne has the opportunity to ask about the injury, Barb starts to cry and tells Anne the injury was her fault. Michael had a temper tantrum while she was trying to settle the baby. Because the baby had slept poorly recently, Barb was very tired and "at her wit's end." She lashed out and struck Michael when he would not stop yelling.

Barb tells Anne that she has never done this before and will never do it again. Anne believes she means it. Barb asks Anne to keep this conversation confidential; if her partner were to find out, he would use the incident against her.

Issues

1. Does Anne have an ethical responsibility to keep the information Barb has shared with her confidential?
2. Are there any legal rules to guide Anne's next steps?
3. How should Anne weigh the risks of harm to others in deciding whether she should disclose the information Barb has shared in confidence?

Fairness

This value applies to both the individual patient and to society's right to health care. If the principles of the *Canada Health Act* are to be upheld, then issues related to fair distribution and equal access to health care must be constantly addressed by nurses and other health professionals. In order to gain access to the system and good health care, consumers must be knowledgeable and informed about good health practices and the health resources available to them. Ensuring fair distribution becomes a greater challenge for nurses as health care resources are diminished through budget cuts and downsizing. The structures and systems put into place in response to these changes need to ensure that fairness is maintained.

Consider this value when reflecting on the responsibilities of the nurse in the case study that follows on page 144.

TABLE 4.5
Fairness[194]

Nurses apply and promote principles of equity and fairness to assist clients in receiving unbiassed treatment and a share of health services and resources proportionate to their needs.

- Nurses provide care in response to clients' needs and are respectful of race, ethnicity, culture, spiritual beliefs, social or marital status, gender, sexual orientation, age, health status, lifestyle, or physical attributes.
- Nurses are justified in using reasonable means to protect themselves and others when violence is anticipated.
- Nurses strive to make fair decisions regarding allocation of resources.
- Nurses advocate for clients to ensure that appropriate care is available.
- Nurses promote appropriate and ethical care through involvement in development and implementation of policies and procedures designed to make the best use of resources, current knowledge, and research.

CASE STUDY

Great needs, limited resources

It is a busy night on a general medical unit in a large teaching hospital. When the shift commences there are five empty beds. Three registered nurses are responsible for the care of the remaining 21 patients. One hour after the shift commences, one of the nurses experiences a severe migraine and has to go home. The two remaining nurses develop a plan to cover the patients, until they hear that three new patients are being admitted from the Emergency Department. They call the supervisor and ask that these patients be admitted to another unit, otherwise they will need more help. There are no beds elsewhere; the only relief readily available is a registered practical nurse and a health care aide, both of whom are presently extra on another unit.

Issues

1. What other strategies should the supervisor in this situation consider?
2. If no other option is available, how should the nurses manage the resources available to them?
3. If such events occur on a regular basis, how should the hospital manage them? Who should manage these situations?

Accountability

Nurses have a professional responsibility to ensure that they are competent to practise. This requires continuing education to keep up with the many changes and improvements to nursing care, and a regular review of skills.

TABLE 4.6
Accountability[195]

Nurses act in a manner consistent with their professional responsibilities and standards of practice.
- Nurses practise in accordance with the CNA's *Code of Ethics for Registered Nurses,* professional standards, and laws pertaining to their practice.
- Nurses practise with honesty and integrity.
- Nurses safeguard the quality of nursing care and focus on expected outcomes of safe, competent, and ethical nursing practice.
- Nurses protect clients/patients from unsafe, incompetent, or unethical care, and take appropriate steps when unsafe or unethical care is observed or suspected.
- Nurses support each other in ensuring that clients are protected from incompetent, unethical, or unsafe care.
- Nurses practise within their own level of knowledge and competence and take the necessary steps (e.g., gaining additional knowledge or reassignment) when this is not possible.
- Nurses provide timely and accurate feedback to other health care providers to ensure safe and competent care, and to acknowledge excellence in practice.
- Nurses provide honest and relevant information when speaking in public forums or when testifying in court.

In non-emergencies requiring specialized skills that the nurse does not have, or where the provision of care conflicts with the nurse's moral beliefs, the nurse is required to refer that patient to another nurse. In emergencies, or where there is a lack of alternative resources, nurses may be called on to provide care.[196]

Nurses have a duty to protect clients from harm. When the facts of a situation indicate incompetence on the part of another nurse or health professional, a nurse is required to take the most appropriate action, given the circumstances, to ensure the safety of patients. When a nurse is aware of incompetence and neglects to take action, then he or she shares responsibility for the consequences of that incompetence.

When delegating responsibility to others, the nurse must be assured that this delegation is appropriate and that those delegated to (e.g., students, the family, other health care assistants) are competent to fulfil the delegated functions.[197]

Finally, the nurse must represent the profession when serving on committees dealing with health care issues. Nurses should also participate in activities that fulfil the profession's obligation to society (e.g., community groups, public organizations that shape health care policy).[198]

Consider this value when reflecting on the responsibilities of the nurse in the following case study.

The nurse's obligation

Judy is a nurse case manager with the provincial Workers' Compensation Board. She recently assumed responsibility for a worker who has been a client with the Board for about five years after sustaining a back injury on a construction site. He appears to have "fallen between the cracks" of the system: he has never returned to work, and continues to complain of pain that is being treated with large doses of Percodan and Valium. He is not receiving any other therapy, and has never attended a pain management program.

Judy phones this worker's physician to discuss strategies for future therapy. He tells her to mind her own business; he is the doctor, not she.

Issues

1. What are Judy's responsibilities to this worker?
2. Given that the physician is the primary caregiver, should Judy interfere? Should she reveal her concerns to the client?
3. What other action should Judy take?

Practice Environments

This value addresses the ethical responsibility of nursing leaders to ensure the effective management and development of nursing staff, and to ensure that adequate resources are available to secure the delivery of competent patient care.[199] As well, it deals with the ethical responsibilities related to nursing education, specifically with respect to the teacher–student relationship and to patient education.[200]

TABLE 4.7
Practice environments[201]

Nurses advocate practice environments that have the organizational and human support systems and the resource allocations necessary for safe, competent, and ethical nursing care.

- Nurses advocate health care environments that are conducive to ethical practice and to the health and well-being of clients and others.
- Nurses share their knowledge, and mentor and guide students and others.
- Nurses accurately state areas of competence and ensure that employment conditions are consistent with the values and responsibilities of the Code and the nurse's individual values and beliefs.
- When planning to participate in job action, nurses ensure the safety of clients.

This value recognizes that the work environment and the existence of appropriate resources are critical to maintaining professional standards and ethical integrity. When supportive structures and mechanisms are not in place within the work environment, it is the shared responsibility of management and staff to ensure that improvements are made.[202] For example, nurses should not accept inadequate staffing patterns that occur on an ongoing basis, when patient care is being compromised. Though circumstances may require that nurses do their best in a unique situation when resources are not available (e.g., disasters, or when several staff call in ill), inadequate staffing patterns should not be tolerated on a regular basis. It is the ethical responsibility of nurses, management, and staff to take steps to rectify this situation.

The Code recognizes that some form of job action may be necessary to achieve outcomes that will ultimately improve or guarantee a high standard of care. In these circumstances, however, it is the responsibility of nurses to ensure the safety of patients and to see that their care is not compromised. Situations where job action is initiated pose difficulties for nurses where personal and professional values may conflict.[203]

Consider this value when reflecting on the responsibilities of the nurse in the following case study.

C A S E   S T U D Y

The downsizing dilemma

Kathleen is a nursing director in a small community hospital. The president of the hospital has just informed all the directors that they will have to reduce their budget by six percent. As a leadership group, the administrators must identify strategies to find this money. Their options are clear: they must find innovative ways to reduce costs while maintaining the same level of care; or, they must close beds (i.e., reduce the volume of care) and lay off staff.

In fact, both options will require the elimination of staff. One of the administrators suggests that they could maintain the same volumes and provide good care by replacing some of the registered nurses with health care aides, who could perform basic tasks such as bathing patients and making beds.

Issues

1. How should Kathleen deal with this dilemma?
2. How can she ensure that her decisions are ethical?
3. How would Kathleen ensure that quality care is maintained? Whom should she involve in the decision making?

Summary

This chapter has reviewed the basic structures, roles, and workings of the various professional nursing bodies in Canada. We have discussed Ontario and Quebec in detail, as these bodies are the most intricate and detailed in the country; many of their principles and approaches can be applied to the regulatory bodies in other provinces. The chapter's focus has been to give the nurse some insight into the purpose and role of professional nursing organizations, and to understand their role with respect to the development of standards of practice and in the evaluation of safe, competent, ethical care.

The discussion of codes of ethics illustrates the interplay between professional standards and the ethical and legal principles that guide nursing practice. The case studies should assist in clarifying responsibilities under the *Code of Ethics for Registered Nurses*. They can provide a focus for discussion on the complicated ethical and legal dilemmas that nurses face in everyday practice.

The key points introduced in this chapter include:

- the scope of laws regulating the nursing profession across Canada
- the role, function, and responsibility of nursing governing bodies
- some of the rules and standards regulating the nursing profession
- the processes and procedures used by governing bodies relating to registration, complaints, discipline, and quality assurance
- the role of regulatory bodies in defining standards of professional practice
- clarification of the CNA's *Code of Ethics for Registered Nurses* as a guide to ethical nursing practice.

Critical Thinking

QUESTIONS FOR DISCUSSION

1. Discuss the structure and purpose of the professional nursing body in your province. How does it compare to those of other provinces?
2. What are the advantages and disadvantages of having a self-governing provincial regulatory body?
3. How does your provincial nursing governing body handle complaints against nurses? Describe the steps in its disciplinary process. Suggest ways in which the process might be improved or made more accountable to nurses and to the public.
4. What role do governing bodies play in educating nursing professionals?
5. What role should such bodies play in shaping legislation affecting nursing?
6. How do the standards of practice of the regulatory body in your province

compare with the standards within the organization where you are presently employed or receiving clinical experience? How do these standards relate to your curriculum as a student nurse?

7. How are the standards of practice in your setting measured? What mechanisms are in place to ensure these standards are maintained? Can you think of ways to improve to this process?

8. Identify the legal and ethical principles represented in the *Code of Ethics for Registered Nurses*. Are they consistent with your own ethical values? Why or why not?

References

1. *Health Disciplines Act,* RSA 1980, c. H-3.5, as amended.
2. *Health Professions Act,* RSBC 1996, c. 183.
3. Properly referred to as the "Health Professions Council" in British Columbia.
4. RSBC 1996, c. 335.
5. Supra footnote 2, section 12, and *Licensed Practical Nurses Regulation,* B.C. Reg. 71/96, section 2.
6. RSBC 1996, c. 336.
7. Supra footnote 4, section 5.
8. RSA 1980, c. N-14.5, as amended.
9. Supra footnote 1.
10. See British Columbia: *Nurses (Registered) Act,* supra footnote 4, section 2; Alberta: *Nursing Profession Act,* supra footnote 8, section 8(1); Yukon Territory: *Registered Nurses Profession Act,* SY 1992, c. 11, section 2; Northwest Territories: *Nursing Profession Act,* RSNWT 1990, c. N-4, section 2(1); Saskatchewan: *The Registered Nurses Act,* 1988, SS 1988, c. R-12.2, section 3; Manitoba: *The Registered Nurses Act,* CCSC, c. R40, section 2, SM 1989–90, c. 91, section 9; New Brunswick: *Nurses Act,* SNB 1984, c. 71, section 3; Nova Scotia: *Registered Nurses' Act,* SNS 1996, c. 30, section 3; Prince Edward Island: *Nurses Act,* RSPEI 1988, c. N-4, section 2; Newfoundland: *Registered Nurses Act,* RSN 1990, c. R-9, section 3(1).
11. See *Health Professions Act,* Bill 45.
12. See Northwest Territories: *Nursing Profession Act,* supra footnote 10, section 3; Yukon Territory: *Registered Nurses Profession Act,* supra footnote 10, section 3; British Columbia: *Nurses (Registered) Act,* supra footnote 4, section 3, section 38; Prince Edward Island: *Nurses Act,* supra footnote 10, section 9; Newfoundland: *Registered Nurses Act,* supra footnote 10, section 5.
13. See the discussion of Ontario's *Health Professions Procedural Code,* below.
14. British Columbia Act, supra footnote 4, section 44(1).
15. Alberta Act, supra footnote 8, sections 82 and 83. The appeal is heard by an Appeals Committee of the Council of the Association.
16. Yukon Act, supra footnote 10, section 52(1). The appeal is heard by an Appeals Committee of the Board.
17. Saskatchewan Act, supra footnote 10, section 34(1).
18. Manitoba Act, supra footnote 10, section 38(1).
19. New Brunswick Act, supra footnote 10, section 34(1).
20. Nova Scotia Act, supra footnote 10, section 43.
21. Prince Edward Island Act, supra footnote 10, section 27(1).
22. British Columbia Act, supra footnote 4, section 44(1)(a).
23. Ibid., sections 11 and 12; Prince Edward Island Act, supra footnote 10, sections 12 and 13; and Newfoundland Act, supra footnote 10, section 12.

24. British Columbia Act, supra footnote 4, sections 1 and 14(1); Alberta Act, supra footnote 8, sections 14 and 15 and Alta. Reg. 453/83, sections 3 and 4; Saskatchewan Act, supra footnote 10, section 19; Manitoba Act, supra footnote 10, section 7 and Man. Reg. 459/88, sections 1 and 2, amended Man. Reg. 106/95, s. 2; Nova Scotia Act, supra footnote 10, section 8(1)(a) and NS Reg. 72/97, SS 4 & 5, regulations 2 and 3; Prince Edward Island Act, supra footnote 10, sections 13 through 16 and RRPEI 1994, c. N-4, *Registration and Licensing of Nurses Regulations,* sections 2, 3, and 4; Newfoundland Act, supra footnote 10, section 8.

25. British Columbia Act, supra footnote 4, section 17; Alberta Act, supra footnote 8, sections 38 and 39; Saskatchewan Act, supra footnote 10, section 20.

26. B.C. Act, supra footnote 10, section 23(3), Saskatchewan Act, supra footnote 10, section 23(1); New Brunswick Act, supra footnote 10, sections 12(1) and 12(14); and Prince Edward Island Act, supra footnote 10, section 17.

27. British Columbia Act, supra footnote 4, sections 23 and 53; Alberta Act, supra footnote 8, sections 3(1), 5, and 107(1); Saskatchewan Act, supra footnote 10, sections 23, 24, and 42(1); Yukon Act, supra footnote 10, sections 14 and 15; Northwest Territories Act, supra footnote 10, sections 30 and 31; Manitoba Act, supra footnote 10, sections 8(1), 10(2), 50(1), and 50(2); New Brunswick Act, supra footnote 10, sections 19 and 21; Nova Scotia Act, supra footnote 10, section 25; Prince Edward Island Act, supra footnote 10, sections 15, 17, and 28; Newfoundland Act, supra footnote 10, sections 16(1), 18, 23, and 25.

28. See, e.g., Saskatchewan Act, supra footnote 10, section 26(2)(q).

29. See, e.g., Alberta Act, supra footnote 8, section 27(2).

30. Northwest Territories Act, supra footnote 10, section 29.

31. Newfoundland Act, supra footnote 10, section 22(a).

32. *Health Professions Procedural Code,* infra footnote 95, sections 85.1(1) and 85.3(4), enacted by SO 1993, c. 37, section 23.

33. Manitoba Act, supra footnote 10, section 46(2).

34. Nova Scotia Act, supra footnote 10, section 28 and NS Reg. 72/97, section 12; Manitoba Act, supra footnote 10, section 22; Yukon Act, supra footnote 10, section 24; New Brunswick Act, supra footnote 10, sections 29 and 40.1 enacted by SNB 1996, c. 82, section 7(6).

35. Newfoundland Act, supra footnote 10, sections 21(1) and (1.1), (1.2), (1.3), enacted by SN 1992, c. 28, section 1(1), and SN 1996, c. 16, section 14.

36. Yukon Act, supra footnote 10, section 24(4); Manitoba Act, supra footnote 10, sections 28, 29, and 30.

37. See, e.g., Saskatchewan Act, supra footnote 10, section 26(2); and Northwest Territories Act, supra footnote 10, section 22 (improper conduct).

38. B.C. Act, supra footnote 10, section 36.

39. *Mans v. Council of Licensed Practical Nurses (1990),* 14 CHRR D/221; aff'd. (1993), 77 BCLR (2d) 47 (CA).

40. Now renamed the *Human Rights Code,* RSBC 1996, c. 210.

41. SBC 1995, c. 37.

42. Ibid., schedule 2.

43. Ibid., section 13.

44. Ibid., section 15(1).

45. B.C. *Nurses (Registered) Act,* supra footnote 10, section 14(5).

46. British Columbia Act, supra footnote 4, sections 44 and 45.

47. This list is not exhaustive. There are many other professions regulated by this Act.

48. RSQ, c. C-26, as amended.

49. Ibid., section 12, as amended.

50. Ibid.

51. Ibid., section 16, as amended.

52. RSQ, c. I-8, section 36.

53. However, the *Professional Code,* section 87, requires the Bureau of the Corporation professionnelle des infirmières et infirmiers to make a code of ethics.

54. Supra footnote 52, section 2, as amended.

55. Ibid., section 5, as amended.
56. Ibid., sections 16 and 17, as amended.
57. Ibid., sections 18 and 19, as amended.
58. Supra footnote 52.
59. Supra footnote 48, sections 87 through 93, as amended.
60. Ibid., section 86, as amended.
61. Supra footnote 53, regulation 3.
62. Supra footnote 48, section 87, as amended.
63. Supra footnote 53, regulation 4.
64. Ibid., sections 3.03.01 through 3.06.06.
65. Supra footnote 53, sections 33 and 34, as amended.
66. Ibid., section 21.
67. RRQ 1981, c. I-8, regulation 14.
68. Supra footnote 53, section 14, as amended.
69. Ibid., section 24, as amended.
70. Ibid., sections 24, 25, and 28, as amended.
71. Ibid., section 31.
72. Ibid., sections 31.2 and 31.3, added by SQ 1989, c. 32, section 10.
73. Supra footnote 48, section 90, as amended.
74. Ibid., section 114, as amended.
75. Ibid., section 188, as amended.
76. Ibid., section 164, as amended.
77. Ibid., section 162, as amended.
78. Ibid., sections 127 and 129. A solemn affirmation is given in place of an oath (which is usu-ally sworn before God on a Bible or other holy book) in cases where a witness feels that his or her conscience would not be bound by swearing an oath to God (e.g., when a person who does not believe in God is making a complaint or giving testimony).
79. Ibid., section 128.
80. Ibid., section 116.
81. Ibid., sections 121, 122, and 123.
82. Ibid., section 130.
83. Ibid., sections 132 through 134, as amended.
84. Ibid., sections 144 and 149.
85. Ibid., sections 150, 151, 152, and 154, as amended.
86. Ibid., section 159, as amended.
87. Ibid., section 160, as amended.
88. Ibid., section 161, as amended.
89. Ibid., section 164, as amended.
90. Ibid., sections 173 and 175, as amended.
91. SO 1991, c. 18, section 18, as amended.
92. Ibid., sections 18, 19, and 20.
93. Ibid., section 24.
94. Ibid., schedule 2 (herein referred to as "HPPC").
95. SO 1991, c. 32, as amended.
96. Ibid., section 2(1).
97. Ibid.
98. Ibid., section 3.
99. Ibid., section 7.
100. Ibid., section 8.
101. *HPPC,* supra footnote 94, section 3(1).
102. Ibid., section 3(2).
103. Ibid., section 4.
104. *Nursing Act, 1991,* supra footnote 95, section 9(1)(a).
105. Ibid., section 10.
106. *HPPC,* supra footnote 94, section 10(1).

107. Ibid., section 12(1).
108. O. Reg. 653/93, section 3, amended by O. Reg. 55/94.
109. *HPPC,* supra footnote 94, section 15(1).
110. O. Reg. 275/94, amended by O.Reg. 39/98.
111. *Expanded Nursing Services for Patients Act, 1997,* SO 1997, c. 9, section 2.
112. *HPPC,* supra footnote 94, section 18(2).
113. Ibid., section 15(3).
114. Ibid., sections 21(1) and (2).
115. Ibid., section 25.
116. Ibid., sections 26, 27, and 29.
117. Ibid., section 36(1), as amended by SO 1993, c. 37, section 9, SO 1996, c. 1, Sched. G, section 27(1).
118. Ibid., section 36(2), enacted by SO 1993, c. 37, section 9.
119. *Statutory Powers and Procedure Act,* RSO 1990, c. section 22, section 10.
120. *HPPC,* supra footnote 94, section 45.
121. Ibid., section 49.
122. Ibid., section 51(1), as amended by SO 1993, c. 37, section 14(1).
123. O. Reg. 799/93, section 1, paragraph 1.
124. Ibid., paragraph 5.
125. Ibid., paragraph 7.
126. Ibid., paragraph 13. There are many more acts deemed "professional misconduct" contained in this regulation, which should be carefully consulted by the nursing professional.
127. Ibid., paragraph 9.
128. SO 1992, c. 31. This Act was repealed by SO 1996, c. 2, section 2(2).
129. *HPPC,* supra footnote 94, section 51(2), paragraphs 5 and 5.1, as repealed and re-enacted by SO 1993, c. 37, section 14(2).
130. Ibid., section 51(5), enacted by SO 1993, c. 37, section 14(3).
131. Ibid., section 57.
132. Ibid., section 59.
133. Ibid., section 68.
134. Ibid., section 72(1).
135. Ibid., section 72(2).
136. Ibid., sections 70 and 71.
137. Ibid., section 1(3), enacted by SO 1993, c. 37, section 4.
138. Ibid., sections 80 through 83.
139. Ibid., section 84. This section of the *HPPC* came into force on December 31, 1994, that is, one year after the *RHPA* came into force.
140. Ibid., section 85.1(1), enacted by SO 1993, c. 37, section 23.
141. *RHPA,* supra footnote 91, section 27.
142. See *Nursing Act, 1991,* supra footnote 95, section 4, paragraph 2.
143. Ibid., section 27(1)(a).
144. This is a controlled act under section 27(2), paragraph 5 of the *RHPA.*
145. Ibid., section 27(2).
146. O.Reg. 107/96 and supra, footnote 111.
147. *RHPA,* supra footnote 91, section 29(1)(a).
148. Ibid., section 29(1)(b).
149. Ibid., section 29(1)(d).
150. Ibid., section 29(1)(c).
151. Supra footnote 146.
152. Supra footnote 91, section 29(2).
153. Ibid., section 35(1).
154. *RHPA,* supra footnote 91, section 33, Only chiropractors, optometrists, physicians and surgeons, psychologists, and dentists or dental surgeons may use this title.
155. *Nursing Act, 1991,* supra footnote 95, section 11. The title "registered nursing assistant" and these other titles may be used only by members of the College. Despite these restric-

tions, Christian Science nurses may continue to use that title even though they may not be members of the College [section 11(2)].

156. Ibid., section 11(5).
157. *RHPA,* supra footnote 91, section 40(2); *Nursing Act, 1991,* supra footnote 95, section 13.
158. *RHPA,* supra footnote 91, section 41.
159. *HPPC,* supra footnote 94, section 92.
160. Ibid., section 93(2).
161. Ibid., section 93(1).
162. Ibid., section 93(3).
163. Ibid., section 93(4), added by SO 1993, c. 37, section 26(2).
164. *RHPA,* supra footnote 91, section 30(1).
165. See the Ontario College of Nurses web site at http://www.cno.org/nursing/
166. See the Alberta Nurses Association web site at http://www.nurses.ab.ca/setting.htm
167. College of Nurses of Ontario. (1996). *Professional standards for registered nurses and regis-
    tered practical nurses in Ontario* (p.1).
168. Ibid.
169. Ibid., p. 5.
170. College of Nurses of Ontario. (1998). *The quality assurance program: Your guide for 1998.*
171. Ibid., p. 3.
172. Ibid., p. 9.
173. College of Nurses of Ontario. (1997). *Building quality practice settings: Practice setting con-
    sultation programs. Information guide* (p. 4).
174. Ibid., p. 12.
175. Ibid., p. 7.
176. The Toronto Hospital. (1995). *Quality management reference manual* (p. 4). Toronto:
    Author.
177. Supra College of Nurses of Ontario, footnote 173, p. 14.
178. Jennings, B., Callaghan, D., & Wolfe, S. (1987, February). The professions: Public interest
    and common good. *Hastings Centre Report* (special supplement).
179. Ibid.
180. Ibid.
181. See http://www.can-nurses.ca
182. Canadian Nurses Association (CNA). (1997). *Code of ethics for registered nurses* (pp. 1–2).
    Ottawa: Author.
183. Supra CNA, footnote 182, p. 3.
184. Ibid. pp. 4–5.
185. Ibid.
186. Ibid. pp. 8–9.
187. Ibid.
188. Ibid. pp. 10–12.
189. Ibid.
190. Ibid. pp. 13–14.
191. Ibid.
192. Ibid. pp. 15–16.
193. Ibid.
194. Ibid. pp. 17–18.
195. Ibid. pp. 19–21.
196. Ibid.
197. Ibid.
198. Ibid.
199. Ibid. pp. 20–23.
200. Ibid.
201. Ibid.
202. Ibid.
203. Ibid.

Professional Competence, Misconduct, and Malpractice

LEARNING OBJECTIVES

The purpose of this chapter is to enable you to:
- appreciate the professional responsibilities and accountabilities of the nurse
- understand the ethical and legal aspects of professional competence, misconduct, and malpractice
- clarify the nurse's ethical and legal responsibilities to the patient and to other health care practitioners
- appreciate the implications of "whistle-blowing"
- apply legal rules and ethical theory to hypothetical case studies and actual situations
- explain the legal concepts of negligence, duty of care, vicarious liability, standard of care, and causation
- appreciate the significance of documentation
- clarify the criminal law with respect to standard of care and negligence
- know the role of the coroner's office and the implications of a coroner's inquest.

Introduction

As we have seen in previous chapters, society holds nurses, as regulated health professionals, to high standards of care. Nurses are accountable to the public for meeting the standards of practice for their profession, following professional codes of ethics and continuously maintaining competence. As noted in Chapter Four, the *Code of Ethics for Registered Nurses* of the Canadian Nurses Association holds nurses accountable for meeting these standards. Under the value of accountability, the Code requires that "nurses act in a manner consistent with their professional responsibilities and standards of practice." The Code makes explicit nurses' responsibility to comply with its ethical principles, and to maintain both professional and legal standards.

Society places its trust in nurses, and is clear about its expectations. The legal system measures the performance and behaviour of nurses against these professional and ethical standards. Nurses need to appreciate the significant consequences when they fail to meet these expectations. A working knowledge of the processes and legal analysis that make up a negligence action in a nursing professional setting is of immense benefit in helping nurses gain a better understanding of those consequences.

This chapter describes the legal consequences that nurses may face when failure to meet professional standards results in harm to patients or clients, and perhaps to others entrusted to their care.

Professional Competence, Misconduct, and Malpractice

The ethical and legal aspects of professional competence, **misconduct,** and **malpractice** are interrelated. Two means by which the skill and conduct of nurses are gauged are the civil law (as in the civil lawsuit) and the complaints procedures related to the disciplinary powers of the nursing regulatory bodies (as discussed in Chapter Four). By these regulatory and self-governing mechanisms, nurses are made accountable to their patients and to the public in general.

Situations may arise in which a nurse and his or her colleagues are called upon to make ethical judgements and decisions that may have unforeseen legal consequences.

Shared accountability?

Several nurses in a nursing team work and rotate together through the same schedule in a busy Intensive Care Unit (ICU) of a major hospital. Recently, one of the nurses, Kathy, has been under extreme personal stress owing to the break-up of a relationship and the death of a close family member.

Over the last four to five weeks, her colleagues have noticed occasions on which Kathy has arrived for night shift smelling of alcohol. When the other nurses raise this with her, Kathy explains that she has had a glass or two of wine over dinner with some friends. As the weeks go by, such incidents increase in frequency. At times, Kathy's speech seems slurred. The other nurses on the team hesitate to report these incidents to the nurse manager, as they do not wish to add to Kathy's stress. They hope that as she deals with her personal problems, this issue will resolve itself. To protect Kathy and to minimize the risks to her patients, she is given easy assignments and is sent on a break whenever the night supervisor visits the unit.

In this ICU, nurses are expected to perform specialized skills and are assigned certain delegated medical acts. As well, under the hospital's nursing standards policy, each nurse is subject to annual review of knowledge and skills. Kathy is three months overdue for her review. The unit teacher has scheduled this three times, but on each occasion, Kathy has cancelled, citing illness or heavy workload. It is unclear when her review can be rescheduled, since as a result of budget cuts the number of teachers available to the nurses in the ICU have been reduced.

One night, Kathy arrives smelling of alcohol. She is assigned a patient who is experiencing cardiac arrhythmias. During her shift, Kathy notes an arrhythmia on the patient's monitor, which she identifies as runs of ventricular tachycardia. In this unit, nurses have been delegated the act of administering lidocaine in response to such an arrhythmia. Kathy prepares and administers the intravenous bolus of lidocaine. A few minutes later, the patient has a respiratory and cardiac arrest. Fortunately, he is easily resuscitated.

Upon review of the patient's status, it is noted that he had in fact experienced supraventricular tachycardia, for which lidocaine is not indicated. Furthermore, one of the other nurses noticed that the empty drug ampoule contained pancuronium, not lidocaine. These drugs are contained in similar-sized ampoules, and the labelling is the same colour. Pancuronium causes paralysis and is used during general anaesthesia or with some patients who are being mechanically ventilated in an ICU. Clearly, the drug led to the patient's cardiac arrest.

Issues

1. Have the nurses in the unit an obligation to "blow the whistle" on Kathy (report her alcohol use)? To evaluate Kathy's risk to her patients?

2. What are Kathy's responsibilities for reviewing her knowledge and skills? The hospital's responsibilities?

3. What is the teacher's responsibility to ensure that Kathy's review takes place?

4. What responsibility, if any, has the second nurse to report that the incorrect drug was given?

5. What is the specific duty of the charge nurse (as distinct from Kathy's colleagues)?

6. What responsibility has the hospital to report the occurrence to the family (and the patient, if living?)

7. What is the legal, civil, and criminal liability of Kathy, the hospital, and the other nurses to the patient and his family?

8. What disciplinary action will Kathy or the other nurses face?

9. How accountable are hospitals for making resource allocation decisions that ensure the provision of safe patient care?

Discussion

This case study highlights a number of major ethical and legal challenges for nurses. What is the nurse's ethical and legal responsibility when a colleague demonstrates incompetence? What is the individual professional's responsibility to maintain competence, and what is the organization's responsibility to ensure the overall competence of staff? Further, what are nurses' responsibilities to colleagues who are in need of help?

As noted in the CNA's *Code of Ethics for Registered Nurses,* nurses have a responsibility to safeguard the quality of nursing care that clients receive, individually or with others, to take preventive and corrective action to protect clients from unsafe, incompetent, or unethical care. Nurses must also ensure that they have the skills knowledge to remain competent. When nurses suspect unethical, incompetent, or unsafe care, or doubt the safety of conditions in the care setting, they must take the appropriate steps to resolve the problem.

It is clear, then, that when we become aware of incompetence on the part of another nurse or other health professional, we are required to take action to ensure the safety of the patient. When a nurse fails to take such action, then he or she shares responsibility for any subsequent consequences of that incompetence.

Further, when health professionals delegate added responsibilities, that delegation should be appropriate and there should be assurance that those to whom the act is assigned are competent to carry out that act. In this case study, Kathy, her colleagues, and the teacher reviewing her skills had a shared professional responsibility to ensure that she was competent to care for her patients.

Individual nurses have a responsibility to maintain their professional competence, and must also maintain the minimum standards of their regulatory body. When other health facilities, such as hospitals or community agencies, impose a higher standard, then that also must be met. Here, both Kathy and the hospital bear responsibility for review of her skills. The leadership within any organization must take steps to ensure compliance with this expectation. If the employee does not respond to the requirement for reassessment or **recertification,** then reminders, counselling, and (if required) disciplinary action must take place.

With restructuring and downsizing within the health system, there is the risk that human resources perceived to be further removed from direct care can be reduced or eliminated entirely. The *Code of Ethics* clearly states that "practice environments conducive to safe, competent and ethical care" are to be maintained. As nurses we are required to collaborate with one another to ensure this environment is consistent with safe and ethical practice, and that we provide mentoring and guidance to ensure the continued competency and professional development, not only of students, but also of practising nurses. This is essential in highly technological critical care environments, where patients are vulnerable and at risk for serious harm if not cared for by a highly skilled and knowledgeable staff.

What was happening to Kathy in this case study? Did her colleagues understand the significance of her behaviour? Were they aware of the warning signs that Kathy was in crisis and needed help? Here, Kathy's colleagues, concerned about her personal situation, decided to protect her. Hoping that Kathy's crisis would resolve, they made efforts to shield her from further harm. Though one might sympathize with their concern, their strategy was counterproductive to Kathy's needs, placed the lives of patients in jeopardy, and compromised their own professional integrity.

Nurses function within a highly stressful work environment. When personal problems add to this stress, some nurses (as others in society) may become vulnerable to the misuse of substances such as alcohol or drugs to provide short-term relief of their symptoms. Some may become vulnerable to controlled substances such as narcotics, since nurses have ready access to such drugs. Nurses such as Kathy require early intervention. Rather than be concerned that she might be subject to discipline, Kathy's colleagues should be aware that support groups, counselling, and therapy are available for nurses in crisis.

Kathy's colleagues, if unsuccessful in dealing directly with her, have a responsibility both to Kathy and to her patients to take their concerns forward to the manager, a staff counsellor, or other professional or union representative. For example, a concerned and astute manager would recognize Kathy's need for help. It is better to provide counselling and therapy early on than to wait until patient care is compromised and Kathy's future career is in jeopardy.

Kathy's case highlights the responsibilities and accountabilities we share with our colleagues who are also registered nurses. But what is the nature of our relationship with other members of the team who have a narrower scope of practice, or who are not regulated or accountable to any professional body? As a framework for discussion of this question, we will focus on recent trends across Canada to alter the mix of direct caregivers in the hospital setting.

Restructuring: Implications for Registered Nurses

During much of the 1990s, the health system across Canada underwent massive restructuring, re-engineering, and downsizing. These efforts arose in response to financial pressures resulting from reductions in federal and provincial funding, and increased costs that were partly associated with introduction of innovative but expensive technology. Institutions have adopted a number of approaches to manage financial crises. Some have included reductions in length of hospital stay and a move towards home care, **utilization management** (i.e., reduced procedures, laboratory tests, etc.), case management and managed care, flatter organizational structures, **program management,** mergers, consolidations, and even hospital closures.

Many organizations focus on finding efficiencies through the redesign of work processes and workflow. Re-engineering, for example, is the "rethinking [and] redesign of [the processes by which] we conduct our business, in order to achieve improvements in quality, services, cost and speed."[1] Noted across the system, as an outcome of many re-engineering efforts, are changes in the roles of health care providers. Of concern to many nurses are the changes to the "skill mix" of staff delivering direct patient care. There has been a widespread shift from a staff consisting totally (or predominantly) of registered nurses to combinations of RNs and practical nurses, aides, and other assistants.

During the 1990s, nursing across Canada also embraced primary nursing as the ideal model of care delivery.[2] Primary nursing was believed to promote continuity of care, enhance the professional autonomy of the nurse, and ensure competent, knowledge-based practice. However, it is also perceived to be more expensive. When resources are limited as a result of staff shortages or financial pressures, there is a tendency to focus on alternatives to a staff consisting entirely of RNs. Based on the belief, or perception, that the skill and knowledge level of the RN is not always necessary, the focus is on identifying the appropriate level of provider to deliver quality care in the most cost-effective way. For example, with appropriate teaching and supervision, less qualified staff may be able to assist nurses with such tasks as bathing, bed making, and so forth. The challenge for nursing leaders is to determine the most appropriate level of staff, and to delegate appropriately in order to ensure the provision of safe, quality care. The challenge for individual registered nurses is to assign appropriately and to provide the necessary supervision.

Across the country various models have been adopted to manage economic challenges, while striving to maintain standards of care. Regardless of the model adopted, these changes have raised questions and concerns from nurses regarding their moral and legal responsibilities when working alongside caregivers with varying knowledge and skills, particularly when a professional body does not regulate them.

In response to concerns expressed by its nurses regarding changes in skill mix, the College of Nurses of Ontario produced a decision guide, *Determining the Appropriate Category of Care Provider,* for nursing leaders. Outlining a framework for registered nurses, registered practical nurses, and non-regulated care providers, the guide articulates the limits of practice for each category based on "the required level and type of knowledge, level of critical thinking, and ability to apply judgement in a given situation." This guideline is available, free of charge, from the College.[3]

Regardless of the judgement of nursing leaders in determining the appropriate level of provider, front-line nurses are still concerned about their role in assigning and supervising. Their major concerns relate to legal liability and the status of their registration with the regulatory body.

A specific area of concern is whether a registered nurse is liable for mistakes made by other professionals or non-regulated staff. If an institution follows an appropriate decision-making guideline (as discussed in Chapter Two) to determine the category of staff, then the leadership within that facility is responsible for ensuring that those staff receive the education necessary to function competently within the prescribed role, to know the limits of that role, and to know when to seek help or assistance. Thus, the leadership is accountable for the education of staff and for ensuring competence on an ongoing basis. Registered nurses then cannot be held accountable for mistakes made by others if they assign within that person's scope of practice as determined by the organization.

However, RNs would be liable, and in fact negligent, if they assigned a non-regulated staff member a task or function outside his or her scope, and if an error resulted. (Indeed, the non-regulated staff member would also be found negligent for accepting such a task.) Thus, RNs must ensure that they know the job descriptions and limits of practice of assisting personnel or non-regulated staff within their team. Nurses also have a professional responsibility to monitor the performance of these staff and to take appropriate action if they believe they are not competent to function within the scope of their role. If a registered nurse disregards concerns about the competence of others, then he or she can be liable for their actions.[4]

Negligence and the Duty of Care

General Principles

Recall the discussion of the general principles of negligence in Chapter Three. Three elements are required to prove that a person is negligent and liable to another for damages:

(1) The person who is aggrieved (the plaintiff) must demonstrate that the

person whom he or she is suing (the defendant) owed him or her a duty of care.

(2) It must be established that the defendant breached that duty of care by engaging in conduct that did not meet a reasonable standard.

(3) The plaintiff must demonstrate that he or she has suffered physical harm or damage to either person or property as a result of the defendant's breach of duty of care.

If all three of these requirements are met, the plaintiff has a case of negligence against the defendant.

Statutory Duty of Care

Most provincial nursing statutes explicitly or implicitly impose certain duties that nurses owe to patients in their care. Among these is the duty to report a fellow nurse whose conduct displays a lack of proper skill, judgement, knowledge, or training.[5] This also includes, in many provinces, a duty to report a nurse who is under the influence of alcohol or drugs.

In Ontario, for example, regulations under the *Nursing Act, 1991*,[6] define certain acts of professional misconduct: "contravening a standard of practice of the profession or failing to meet the standard of practice of the profession" is one such act;[7] failing to report an incident of unsafe practice or unethical conduct of a health care provider to that provider's employer or to the College of Nurses is another.[8]

Thus, in our case study, Kathy's colleagues clearly have engaged in professional misconduct by failing to report incidents of intoxication. In covering up a potentially harmful situation, they are ethically and legally culpable for any harm that may arise. Kathy has also breached her duty not to practise her profession while her ability to do so was impaired by alcohol.

Common Law Duty of Care

The common law also imposes a duty of care. In any negligence lawsuit involving a nurse or other health professional, the trial will essentially amount to an evaluation of the nurse's conduct and the degree to which he or she has met an accepted standard of care. The nurse, as a professional, is legally required to operate and act at a level that meets or exceeds that of a reasonably prudent caregiver or health practitioner. This, of course, implies that the nurse has a duty to maintain a level of expertise through continuing education to ensure that he or she practises in accordance with the latest standards. It would not do, for example, for a nurse trained in the 1970s to continue to operate and practise according to the standards of that decade 30 years later. These standards would be such as those laid out by the provincial regulatory body (e.g., the Registered Nurses Association of British Columbia, the College of Nurses of Ontario) and the agency or hospital in which the nurse is employed.

As the nurse in our case study is representing herself as a qualified health practitioner, she owes a duty of proper care to all her patients. This duty has been described in case law as "the duty to exercise a reasonable degree of skill, knowledge and care in the treatment of a patient."[9] Quite apart from the issue of Kathy's practising her profession while under the influence of alcohol is the issue of her having mistakenly identified the arrythmia on the patient's monitor as ventricular tachycardia, when in fact the patient was experiencing supraventricular tachycardia. Kathy has not fulfilled her duty to read and interpret the monitor signs correctly. Has she lived up to the standard of care required of her?

Case Law

An interesting illustration of the court's role in determining the standard of care and in assessing nursing conduct is found in the Nova Scotia Supreme Court decision of *Thompson Estate v. Byrne*.[10] In that case, the plaintiff, a middle-aged woman, had undergone quadruple heart by-pass surgery and was sent to the Cardiovascular Intensive Care Unit (CVICU) of the hospital following a successful operation. The patient was then placed in the care of the defendant, a nurse in the CVICU.

The defendant worked with several other nurses in this ward and, while every nurse had specific patients to care for, each would help the others as needed. While in the CVICU and while still anaesthetized, the plaintiff dislodged her endotracheal tube, which had been inserted to assist her breathing following surgery. Upon seeing this, the nurse immediately announced to her colleagues that the patient had extubated herself, and went to the plaintiff to attend to her. As in any hospital, nurses were not permitted to perform an intubation upon a patient, as only a physician could perform such a procedure. However, the patient was being "bagged" pending the re-establishment of the endotracheal tube.

The extubation occurred at approximately 16:30 h. A second nurse on duty, upon hearing the nurse's remark, called for assistance. A resident soon arrived and attempted to re-intubate the patient. With the first try, he had difficulty in locating the patient's vocal cords so that he could position the tube. He remarked that this would be a difficult intubation and requested that an anaesthetist be called to assist. The second nurse, who made the call, had difficulty locating the anaesthetist on duty. Thus, she went to the nearby Operating Room to get the anaesthetist. (This was a common means of seeking help, as the anaesthetists were usually there and the OR was near the CVICU.)

Meanwhile, the resident made a second, apparently successful attempt to re-intubate the patient. However, the tube was lodged in the patient's oesophagus, a fact that became apparent only some time later, when a respiratory technician who was "bagging" the patient noticed resistance in the flow of air and that the patient's abdomen was beginning to swell. At this point, the patient was observed to be turning cyanotic from lack of oxygen. Her heart rate had dropped, and she was given cardiac massage by the anaesthetist, who had arrived by then. It was now approximately 16:45 h, that is, 15 min since the patient had extubated herself.

The anaesthetist made a third, very difficult but ultimately successful, attempt to re-intubate the patient, and an airway was re-established by 17:00 h. The patient's colour returned to normal. Unfortunately, it was soon discovered that she had suffered severe brain damage as a result of hypoxia. She remained in a coma until she died two years later.

Her estate brought a negligence action against the resident, the anaesthetist, the hospital, and two of the nurses in the CVICU in whose care she had been placed following the heart surgery. The claim alleged that the second nurse, who had gone to get the help of the anaesthetist on the resident's instructions, had been negligent in not making sufficient efforts to obtain help promptly, and that the injury to the patient would not have occurred but for the delay in the arrival of the anaesthetist. The claims against the nurses alleged that they had failed in their duty (a) to prevent the patient from extubating herself, (b) to attend the patient properly and particularly at all times, knowing that she had attempted to remove the tube on prior occasions, and (c) to live up to standards in cardiovascular intensive care units.[11]

The claims against the doctors were dismissed for lack of evidence of negligence. However, the claims against the nurses and the hospital remained. The testimony of several doctors and one nurse educator (herself an RN) was received by the court in order to assist it in assessing the conduct of the nurses and to determine the appropriate nursing standards against which to measure that conduct.

The doctors and nursing expert were unanimous in stating that the nurses had functioned in an entirely appropriate and professional manner throughout, under very difficult circumstances. There was no duty upon the nurse, as it was judged that to find such duty would, in such circumstances, place an inordinate burden upon nurses. Of course, such a finding would depend on the size, organization, and staffing of the unit, factors that vary from institution to institution, depending upon financial and human resources. In this case, the CVICU had seven patients in seven patient beds. There was a total of five nurses on duty in the unit.

The nursing expert stated that the nursing care was comprehensive, the nursing assessments were thorough, the problems had been identified by the nurses, and the physicians were kept informed at all times. Under these circumstances, the expert felt that the nurses had not breached any standards of nursing practice in an ICU ward.[12] With respect to the nurse, the court found that she did not have a duty to do any more than she had done to obtain the help of staff physicians. Had she done more, she would have been in breach of her primary duty to stay with her patient and assist the doctor who was attempting the re-intubation.[13] The court accepted the expert's opinion, and thus found no negligence on the nurses' part.

In discussing the duty of care owed by nurses, the court stressed that health professionals are not insurers or guarantors of the success of the treatment that they undertake to provide. Thus, the standard of care to which they are held is not a standard of perfection. The court reiterated the distinction in law between carelessness in one's conduct and a genuine error in judgement. The law does not hold a professional responsible for the latter but will hold him or her responsible for the former if, in acting carelessly, harm ensues. Carelessness would be behaviour that does not accord with or conform to the approved and customary practices of similar institutions or professionals in the community (in this case, Canada).[14] In *Thompson Estate v. Byrne,* the nurses' conduct did not depart from such customary practices, as evidenced by the facts and analyzed by the expert testimony.

Application to Case Study

Similar analytical process will apply in assessing Kathy's conduct. Her actions would be re-examined with the aid of expert testimony to determine whether and how she had breached her duty of care to her patient. As the hospital is likewise under a duty to provide proper and competent medical and nursing staff to patients in its care,[15] it also would likely be named as a defendant in any subsequent lawsuit, assuming the patient had suffered harm.

Kathy and the hospital may be sued by the patient, his family, or his estate, if he subsequently died. The plaintiff might allege that the hospital had breached its duty towards him to provide proper care and to ensure competent nursing and other health care staff. Thus, the hospital could be held directly liable for any damage or injury caused by Kathy as a result of her negligence.

For example, it may be held negligent in failing to ensure adequate and safe emergency procedures and, in this case study, in failing to ensure that drugs were safely and properly stored (e.g., pancuronium may have been placed in the container labelled lidocaine). The finding of liability is also possible as the hospital, through Kathy's supervisor, failed to review Kathy's skills to ensure that she was competent and able to carry out her duties properly and effectively. She was an employee of the hospital, and her actions were under its control. This is known as the doctrine of vicarious liability.

Similarly, Kathy is under a duty to ensure that she arrives at work in a fit and proper condition. She clearly breached her duty in arriving at the hospital in an impaired state, and her condition may have placed the patient in jeopardy and contributed to the risks of harm.

Another aspect of vicarious liability as it relates to hospitals is that physicians who provide instructions to nursing staff in the care of their patients are entitled to rely on the assumption that the hospital has hired duly qualified, competent, and properly trained nursing staff. The doctors are not responsible for ensuring that the nurses carry out those instructions properly unless they have actual knowledge that the nursing staff are not competent to carry out those instructions. Thus, in cases where instructions are not properly followed, the doctor may argue as a defence that the nurse was negligent, if any claim of negligence is brought against the physician. In such a case, the instructions provided by the physician must not be negligent in and of themselves.

Professional Liability Insurance

Professionals today are held to rigorous standards of care. An increasingly litigious public will not hesitate to bring negligence lawsuits against accountants, lawyers, architects, physicians, or surgeons for any injury or damages suffered in consequence of the breach of applicable standards of professional conduct. Many health professionals who practise on their own account carry professional liability insurance to shield them from what may often be financially catastrophic negligence claims. Physicians, for instance, carry insurance from the Canadian Medical Protective Association, which is a professional group insurer set up to offer liability insurance tailored to the professional's type and scope of practice. For example, there are policies specifically designed for neurosurgeons, obstetricians, and family practitioners. Physicians and surgeons are, for the most part, self-employed and are liable for their own acts of negligence.

Most nurses in Canada are employed by publicly funded health facilities that carry negligence insurance, some with fairly large policy limits, depending on the institution's size, scope of treatments offered, claims history, and any specialization undertaken by the institution. It will be remembered from Chapter Three that health facilities, as employers, are vicariously liable for the negligent acts of their employees. This would include liability for any negligent acts committed by a nurse while in the institution's employ. The employer institution's liability is not unlimited, however. It would remain liable so long as the negligent nurse was acting wholly within the scope of his or her expressed or apparent authority. A nurse who exceeds the bounds of acceptable nursing practice and performs acts outside the normal scope of nursing would not attract liability to the employer. The nurse would remain fully liable for his or her own negligence. Nurses who are self-employed need to consider insurance coverages, therefore, to ensure adequate financial protection. The consequences of personal uninsured liability are usually devastating and can lead to bankruptcy, loss of professional status, and personal upheaval.

Moreover, insurance coverages usually include an obligation by the insurance company (usually referred to as the insurer) to defend the health professional in any ensuing litigation. This means the insurer will retain and pay for the services of a lawyer to represent and defend the professional whose negligent conduct is at issue. In some cases, the insurer will leave the choice of lawyer up to the professional involved, but this is not always the case. Other policies provide that the choice of lawyer and the source of the lawyer's instructions remain with the insurer. The professional is then required to cooperate fully with the insurer in investigating and defending the claim against him or her. This means the professional must attend any required meetings with insurance adjusters, claims representatives, and lawyers chosen to defend the claim, as well as all court appearances and examinations for discovery. (These aspects of the civil justice system are more fully discussed in Chapter Three.) Any insured professional who has knowledge of an actual or potential negligence claim against him or her is required to inform the insurer of the claim immediately and cooperate fully with the insurer if and as required.

Those policies that do not contain an obligation to defend will pay only for any negligence judgement ultimately pronounced against the professional. In the meantime, therefore, the professional must retain (hire) and pay for his or her own lawyer to defend the negligence action, though it will be recalled that these costs will be recovered from the plaintiff in the event that the suit is dismissed.

The Standard of Care and Causation

The nurse's conduct must be examined and compared to normal, competent, and reasonable standards of nursing practice to determine whether the conduct in question conformed with that expected of a reasonably competent and skilled nurse. Of course, standards of practice change over time as new knowledge and technology are introduced and become widely available. Standards also differ from one institution to another, and from one treatment setting to another. For example, the standards of practice and expectations of a nurse in a critical care setting will differ from those in a rehabilitation setting. Patients have a right to expect that a nurse employed in an ICU will have the specialized knowledge and skill required to provide the necessary care. In the case study, the fact that Kathy administered the wrong drug (and, even if it had been the drug she intended, one that was not indicated for this patient's condition) shows that she did not meet the basic standard of care with respect to the administration of medication (i.e., checking the label carefully prior to administering the drug) and thus breached her common law duty to provide reasonably competent, knowledgeable, and skilled nursing care to her patient. She is therefore negligent.

In many cases, hospitals and other health facilities that employ nurses have policies and procedures in place for the annual review of the nurses' skills. This practice would be recognized as a standard of care in any negligence suit brought against such an institution. Thus, to ensure that the hospital's duty is fulfilled, it is vital that the institution enforce nursing staff reviews. The hospital is responsible for ensuring that these reviews take place, and nurses cannot refuse to participate in them.

For example, in the case study, the nurses in the CVICU were expected to perform certain delegated medical acts, including the interpretation of arrhythmias and, when required, the administration of lidocaine. Kathy's skills should have been reviewed to ensure that she was competent and knowledgeable in the proper interpretation of arrhythmias. This inability led Kathy to conclude that lidocaine was needed when it was not.

Employers also have a common law duty to take active steps to ensure that nurses falling short of the standard come to meet the expected standard. Such steps may include counselling, additional education, and, in some cases, disciplinary measures. The duty also includes ensuring that the nurse's skills are reviewed on a regular basis (although the nurse also has such a duty). In Kathy's case, counselling would be in order, but the hospital may have to resort to disciplinary measures if Kathy persistently fails to meet the standards of practice expected of her. In cases of downsizing and budget cuts, a process would still be necessary to ensure the competence of staff. Budget cuts as an excuse would not be defensible.

In some institutions, the review of skills is completely the responsibility of the nurse. If this is the case, this stipulation should be made explicit at the outset of the nurse's employment with the institution or agency. Appropriate action must be taken if these expectations are not met.

Finally, Kathy breached her professional obligation not to work while intoxicated. Most provincial nursing statutes frown heavily upon a nurse's working while impaired. For example, in Ontario, Prince Edward Island, and Saskatchewan, practising nursing while one's ability to do so is impaired by any substance constitutes professional misconduct.[16] It would also likely constitute misconduct under the legislation of the remaining provinces and territories (even though these statutes do not expressly refer to impairment of the nurse while on duty), as it would adversely influence the nurse's ability to practise safely and properly. It may also constitute a threat to the safety of patients.

Furthermore, Kathy's fellow nurses may also be negligent. Since they know of Kathy's possible impairment when caring for the cardiac patient, they may, in permitting her to continue to provide care, be contributing to the risk of injury to that patient. It is clearly their professional and ethical duty to alert Kathy's manager of the fact that Kathy may have a drinking problem and, more importantly, that she may be under the influence of alcohol as she provides care. In some cases, failure to report improper, negligent, or unethical conduct could in and of itself constitute professional misconduct. The matter, in most cases, will then be taken up according to the disciplinary procedures and mechanisms of the provincial regulatory body (as discussed in Chapter Four).

Standards of care provide a baseline for assessment, planning, decision making, and action. They help to ensure the provision of safe and efficient nursing care within the institution or health care agency.

The case study illustrates two crucial duties that the nurse must discharge properly: (a) to assess a patient's condition correctly and (b) to ensure that the correct medication is administered when required.

Duty to Make Correct Assessment and Accurately Recorded Observations

The former of these two duties was one of several aspects of nursing conduct examined by the Ontario Court (General Division) in *Martin v. Listowel Memorial Hospital et al.*[17] This case involved negligence on the part of a nurse, two doctors, and the hospital in the birth of a child in 1981. On the day of the birth, the patient complained of discomfort; her doctor, who was subsequently included as a defendant in the lawsuit, could not be reached. The woman was sent home and told to rest and put her feet up. She later realized she was in labour and returned to the hospital, at which time the nurse on duty realized that the foetus was in distress.

When the patient's doctor was finally located by 20:00 h, he instructed the nurse to put her on her side and give her oxygen. For the next two hours, the woman was left unattended because the nurses on duty were busy with a trauma patient. The child was born spontaneously without a nurse or doctor in attendance at 20:16 h. It was a breech birth. The doctor arrived three to five minutes after the child was born. The child was found lying between the mother's legs. He was not breathing, was flaccid, had no movement, was blue in colour and cold.

The child was transferred to the neonatal intensive care unit of a larger hospital in another city, where his condition was observed to be much worse than the doctor had described. The child's circulatory system had collapsed; his entire system eventually shut down. Owing to lack of oxygen to the brain, dysfunction occurred. The court determined that the baby had suffered severe brain damage as a result of the negligence of the nurses, the doctor, and the hospital. He was left with serious physical and cognitive problems. The child was awarded damages.

It is clear that the nurses in this case were not living up to the standard of care. Given the patient was in labour and on oxygen, they should have ensured that she was attended at all times. Additional nursing staff should have been called in to deal with the overload.

Duty to Check and Ensure Proper Medication

The second duty, to ensure that the proper medication is given, was discussed in *Bugden v. Harbour View Hospital.*[18] Although the case was decided in 1947, it illustrates the duty of care required of nurses when preparing or dealing with medication. It also illustrates the fact that the physician was once entitled to rely upon a nurse's competence in the dispensing and administration of medication. This standard has changed, since physicians are now equally under a duty to ensure that the correct medication is given. The current practice is for the nurse to show the physician the medication (or, during surgery, the surgical instrument) that he or she has requested. When dispensing medication, a nurse today would normally check the bottle or ampoule up to three times to ensure accuracy. In this way, there are more opportunities to catch a mistake.

The Bugden case originated in Nova Scotia. The patient, a miner, dislocated his thumb and went to the defendant hospital to have it treated. The doctor on duty examined the thumb and decided he would reset it using a local anaesthetic. He was assisted by an experienced graduate nurse (Nurse A.), whom he asked to give the patient morphine and atropine. This she did. He then decided to have x-rays taken of the thumb prior to beginning the resetting, and asked the nurse to get Novocain (a local anaesthetic).

Nurse A. immediately went to another part of the hospital and asked a second nurse (Nurse B.) for Novocain. Nurse B. gave Nurse A. a labelled bottle, but neither she nor Nurse A. examined the label. Nurse A. took the bottle back to the doctor who, without checking it, filled his syringe with the solution it contained and injected it into the patient's thumb. Upon seeing that the thumb was not yet properly anaesthetized, he injected more of the solution. A total of 4 mL of this solution was injected into the patient. The doctor then proceeded to set the thumb.

A short while later, Nurse A. noticed that the patient looked ill and called the doctor, who attempted an unspecified treatment that failed. Thirty minutes later, the patient died. It was subsequently discovered that the bottle from which the doctor had filled his syringe and which was thought to contain Novocain in fact had contained epinephrine hydrochloride, a heart stimulant (also known as adrenaline). A 4-mL dose of this drug was fatal: the patient had died of heart failure as a result of the error.

The patient's wife sued in negligence for damages, naming the doctor, the hospital, and the two nurses as defendants. The Supreme Court of Nova Scotia stated that where it was the duty of several persons to guard against danger, any one of them who failed to take precautions could not escape by saying that another person should have caught his error.[19] The court elucidated upon the duty of care of each nurse involved in this case and stated:

> Persons who are in charge of dangerous things under which category, I think, drugs are included are under a duty to handle them with such care that harm will not arise to those who depend upon their skill. At the least they must exercise reasonable care to avoid such harm.... The liability in any particular case arises from the foreseeability of damage, and the duty to take care.[20]

In this case, the court noted that it was impossible for a competent nurse not to realize that if adrenaline were used instead of Novocain, the danger of death would be great. There was, therefore, a duty upon each nurse to avoid what in fact happened. The failure of Nurse B. to verify that she was giving the correct drug did not absolve Nurse A. from a similar duty. Although Nurse B. was not directly involved in treating the patient, she was the nurse in charge of drugs at the hospital and owed a duty to all potential patients to ensure that they were given the proper medication. Since drugs are articles dangerous in and of themselves, there is a duty upon anyone handling them to take precautions so that others coming into proximity with them are not hurt.[21]

Both nurses, as well as the hospital, were found negligent. The doctor escaped liability in that expert evidence from other doctors indicated it was reasonable for him to rely on Nurse A. to give him the proper medication. It would have been unreasonable to impose upon the doctor a duty to supervise nurses who were hospital employees (not his own) while treating patients. As we have said, the standard of care today in such a situation has been increased to require the nurse to show the bottle or container of medication to the physician or other person administering it. Further, there would probably be an obligation today on the physician to check the medication as well.

In another Ontario case, *Fiege v. Cornwall General Hospital et al.*,[22] a nurse was found negligent when she improperly administered an injection of Talwin into the left buttock of a patient. The nurse, contrary to standard procedure, administered the injection directly into the site of the patient's sciatic nerve, causing the patient an injury. The trial judge concluded that it was improper for an injection to be made over the sciatic nerve and that if the plaintiff's injury could be attributed to this injection, the nurse was negligent in administering it.[23]

Criminal Law Sources of Liability

The criminal law also holds significant consequences for nurses and other health practitioners who act carelessly or with recklessness. In Chapter Three, we mentioned the *Criminal Code* provisions concerning the omission to do that which a health practitioner has undertaken to do. Section 216 of the *Criminal Code* states:

> 216. Every one who undertakes to administer surgical or medical treatment to another person or to do any other lawful act that may endanger the life of another person is, except in cases of necessity, under a legal duty to have and to use reasonable knowledge, skill and care in so doing.

In specific relation to the practice of nursing, this places an obligation upon people who represent themselves as qualified and competent nurses to ensure that their skills and education are adequate to perform properly the treatment that they are called upon to administer. The section excludes cases of necessity, which imply emergency or life-threatening situations. Here, however, a nurse would not normally act to administer such treatment if there were a more qualified practitioner, such as a physician, available to administer (for example) emergency surgery. Otherwise a nurse, acting in good faith, could proceed if he or she performed to the best of his or her ability. The legal policy here is to encourage people to render emergency treatment to those in urgent need of it. In some extreme cases, such treatment could include surgery under circumstances where the aid of a qualified surgeon was unavailable.

Criminal Law Standard of Care

A person who represents herself or himself as a duly qualified health practitioner will, if serious injury or bodily harm ensues, be held to the standard of the reasonably qualified practitioner. The decision of the British Columbia County Court in the case of *R v. Sullivan and Lemay*[24] illustrates this point. Although that case involved two midwives, the principle discussed is equally applicable to nurses. In that case, the midwives were assisting in a home birth. The child died as a result of their negligent delivery, and they were each charged with criminal negligence causing death (with respect to the infant) and with criminal negligence causing bodily harm (to the mother, as a result of their negligent delivery procedures).

In addressing the standard of expertise to which the defendants would be held, the court said that the midwives' conduct constituted a lawful act that might endanger the life of another person within the meaning of this section. Therefore, they were under a legal duty to have and use reasonable skill, care, and knowledge in performing the delivery, and their conduct would be held to the standard of a competent childbirth attendant, even though they had no formal training as midwives.

Criminal Negligence

Section 219 of the *Criminal Code* defines criminal negligence thus:

> 219(1). Every one is criminally negligent who (a) in doing anything, or (b) in omitting to do anything that it is his duty to do, shows wanton or reckless disregard for the lives or safety of other persons.

The "duty" of which this section speaks is a duty imposed by law, either statute law or common law.[25] This section must be read in conjunction with section 217 of the Code, which states:

> 217. Every one who undertakes to do an act is under a legal duty to do it if an omission to do the act is or may be dangerous to life.

Thus, if a nurse fails to perform some act that is part of his or her nursing procedures and duties, and as a result someone dies or suffers serious bodily harm, the nurse's omission may be characterized as criminally negligent and would constitute a criminal offence of either criminal negligence causing death, or criminal negligence causing bodily harm, depending on the impact on the patient. Before the conduct could be characterized as negligent, however, it would have to demonstrate a marked or substantial departure from conduct that one would expect from a reasonable and competent nurse. There would have to be extreme carelessness, or recklessness (i.e., a complete disregard for consequences of one's actions), or such grave and serious omission as to show that the nurse failed to recognize obvious risks or, if aware of those risks, that he or she chose to take them anyway, "reckless" and oblivious to the consequences. Such a formulation in the law shows how extreme and outrageous the carelessness must be in order to be judged criminally negligent. (In the case study, Kathy's intoxication and failure to see she was administering the wrong drug might be classified as reckless behaviour.)

Necessity for Causation

By definition, criminal negligence must cause death[26] or bodily harm[27] to another. In many cases, impairment has been a factor in finding drunk drivers criminally negligent when they have operated motor vehicles while under the influence of alcohol and have either hurt or killed others in accidents. In such cases, the fact that the accused was intoxicated of his or her own volition is evidence that may lead a court to decide that the driver acted with wanton or reckless disregard for the lives or safety of others.[28] Intoxication is therefore a relevant factor in determining whether a person acted wantonly or recklessly.

Application to Case Study

In Kathy's case, the fact that she was impaired would be relevant in a charge of criminal negligence causing death. The fact that her intoxication rendered her incapable of appreciating the probable consequences of her actions would not be a defence. Whether a conviction could be successfully obtained, however, would depend on whether the mistake in administering the wrong drug demonstrated a wanton or reckless disregard for the life or safety of the patient. Even if Kathy's conduct was negligent according to civil law, if it was not negligent according to this criminal law standard, she would not be convicted of criminal negligence. Even if Kathy's conduct was found to be grossly negligent in a civil law context, that conduct may not be sufficient to show the degree of wanton or reckless disregard required to convict her of criminal negligence. The patient would have to suffer some harm, or die.

There is a substantial difference between being negligent in a civil lawsuit and being criminally negligent. The latter type of negligence requires conduct that exceeds what one would normally expect of a reasonable person (in this case, a reasonable nurse). The intent of the accused is irrelevant. It is sufficient that the accused acted in such a manner as to demonstrate that he or she either recognized the obvious risk of danger to another and took that risk anyway, or that he or she ought reasonably to have foreseen such a risk and failed to do so.[29] In other words, the accused was completely indifferent to the risks that his or her actions posed to the life or safety of others who might reasonably be expected to be so affected.

The Provincial Coroner's and Medical Examiner's Systems

In every province, the consequences of an unexplained death must be investigated with a view to determining its causes and identifying ways to prevent similar occurrences in the future. The coroner's and medical examiner's systems of the various provinces merit discussion, as these are concurrently integral components of both the criminal justice system and provincial constitutional responsibility for administering justice within the province. Thus, if there is any evidence of serious negligence on the part of nursing or medical staff that is attributed to the death of a person, an inquest may be ordered by a coroner, or a court, to determine all possible causes and circumstances of the death. It is therefore important for nurses to have a basic understanding of both the coroner's and medical examiner's systems in use across Canada, since nurses may be called upon to testify at such inquests.

The **coroner's inquest** is primarily a fact-finding and investigatory endeavour. In earlier times, a coroner's court could also find criminal or civil responsibility; however, the modern coroner's inquest is not a criminal trial. There is no accused person. In some provinces, the coroner has the authority, upon conclusion of an inquest, to order the arrest of anyone who has been found by the coroner to be responsible for the death of any person whose death forms the subject of the inquest.

Ontario, Quebec, New Brunswick, Prince Edward Island, Saskatchewan, British Columbia, the Yukon Territory, and the Northwest Territories use the traditional coroner's system adopted from English common law. The remaining provinces have moved away from this system to a more modernized medical examiner's system. Both systems, however, are broadly similar in their workings as a means to investigate suspicious deaths. In the medical examiner's system, the function of holding an inquiry is usually left to a judge, or, in the case of Alberta, the Fatality Review Board.[30]

A detailed review of each province's system is beyond the scope of this book. However, Ontario's system will serve as an example. Under Ontario's *Coroner's Act*,[31] a Chief Coroner for Ontario is appointed to supervise a number of coroners throughout the province. Each such coroner will be appointed for a particular region, and each is a legally qualified medical practitioner. A coroner appointed for a specific region is required to live in that region.

Under the Act, everyone who has reason to believe that a person has died:

(1) as a result of violence, misadventure (e.g., an accident), negligence, misconduct or malpractice;
(2) by unfair means;
(3) during pregnancy or following pregnancy in such circumstances to which the death could be attributed;
(4) suddenly and unexpectedly;

(5) from disease or sickness for which the person was not treated by a legally qualified medical practitioner;

(6) from any cause other than disease; or

(7) under circumstances that require investigation

must report the death either to a coroner or to the police.[32] Similarly, if a person dies while in a home for the aged, a children's residence, a home for
retarded persons, a mental institution, a nursing home, or a public or private
hospital to which the person was transferred from one of those previously
mentioned institutions, the person in charge of such institution must notify
the coroner in writing of the death.[33] Pending an order from the coroner, no
person may in any way alter the condition, or interfere with the body, of the
deceased.

Once notified, the local coroner will issue a warrant to take possession of
the body as part of his or her investigation. The investigation and fact finding into the circumstances of the death begin at this point. The coroner has
the power to enter into any place where the death occurred, inspect and
extract information from any records or writings relating to the deceased, and
seize anything that he or she believes is material to the purposes of the investigation.

In cases where someone has died under care of a health facility or agency,
it is likely that the coroner would seize the deceased's medical records immediately upon being notified of the death. This is a precaution to preserve the
character of the evidence and to avoid the possibility of additions being made
to such records that might obscure the medical circumstances and condition
of the deceased at the moment of death.

It is important, therefore, to ensure that records are made as contemporaneously as possible with the act being recorded. The nurse involved in the
care of the deceased is at the very least a potential witness to the circumstances surrounding the treatment, care, and condition of that person
immediately prior to the death. At most, such a nurse may be called upon to
testify at the coroner's inquest and will have to rely upon the records to
refresh his or her memory as to the events leading up to the death. Questions
asked of witnesses in such cases may be quite detailed and require precise
interpretation of the nursing notes and other records. Therefore (as we will
discuss further in Chapter Nine), the necessity of making clear and accurate
records as close as possible to the time when the nursing act was performed
cannot be overstressed.

If the coroner deems it advisable, he or she can order an inquest to be
held into the circumstances of the deceased's death. Otherwise, the matter
will proceed no further.

If an inquest is held, the coroner will convene a hearing, in some
provinces, with the aid of a jury (usually smaller than a criminal trial jury of
twelve). The jury's function is to aid in making recommendations as to any
improvements to procedures, policies, and standards that may help to prevent similar occurrences.

The inquest will usually proceed along the same lines as a trial. However, the inquest is not a criminal trial; there is no prosecution and no accused. The Crown attorney may be a participant, and any other parties who are material witnesses or participants in the events leading up to the person's death may be called to testify at the inquest.

A person cannot be compelled to testify at an inquest once he or she has been charged with a criminal offence. If a person is called to testify, he or she will have the right to the aid of a lawyer. However, the lawyer's involvement may be limited to advising on answers to questions and the rights of the witness. In most provinces, the witness has the right not to have any evidence that he or she gives at an inquest used against him or her in any ensuing criminal proceedings. This is to ensure that the witness's rights (under the Canadian *Charter of Rights and Freedoms*) against self-incrimination are maintained. This does not mean, however, that the witness has the right to refuse any proper questions put to him or her. A refusal to answer may place that witness in danger of being found in contempt of court, a judgement that carries with it fines and a possible jail term.

The inquest is more relaxed in terms of following the strict rules of evidence normally applied in a court. However, coroners tend to follow such rules, especially in recent years.

In provinces with a medical examiner's system, the medical examiner takes the place of the coroner. Such a person is appointed by the provincial government and is usually a trained physician, given the medical complexities and technicalities that tend to be the focus of such inquests. Historically, however, coroners were laymen, untrained in medical matters. In the past few decades there has been a trend away from lay coroners, and now most are physicians. The procedures across the country are fairly similar, except that in some provinces (such as Nova Scotia and Manitoba) the inquest may be held by a provincial court judge. The investigative and inquiry functions are thus kept separate.

Once the inquest is concluded, the coroner, or judicial officer conducting the hearing, may give a decision (taking into consideration any recommendations made by the jury) on the causes of the deceased's death, and anything that could have been done to prevent it. For example, if the inquest is into the death of a patient at a hospital, the coroner's jury might recommend changes to certain policies or procedures that it feels may have contributed to the death. Further, if as a result of the coroner's decision, anyone is suspected of criminal responsibility, it is possible that criminal charges may be laid in the wake of the coroner's decision. The criminal justice process would then take over to determine the guilt or innocence of any accused person.

Summary

This chapter has demonstrated the complexity of the interrelationship between nursing practice, ethics, and the legal system. The significance of the expectations society has for nurses is documented in the serious consequences nurses may face when these expectations are not met. It is critical for nurses to appreciate the seriousness of these responsibilities and the extent to which their performance is measured based on these professional, ethical, and legal standards. The professional responsibilities and accountabilities of nurses are made explicit by society in order to safeguard and protect the interests and well-being of vulnerable persons entrusted to their care. Society, through the legal systems, does not view these responsibilities lightly and evaluates nurses' actions and behaviours relative to the high standards imposed by the public and the profession.

The key points introduced in this chapter include:

- the professional responsibilities and accountabilities of the nurse
- the ethical and legal aspects of professional competence, misconduct, and malpractice
- the nurse's ethical and legal responsibilities to the patient and to other health practitioners
- the implications of "whistle-blowing"
- legal rules and ethical theory as they apply to hypothetical case studies and actual situations
- the legal concepts of negligence, duty of care, vicarious liability, standard of care, and causation
- the significance of documentation
- the criminal law with respect to standard of care and negligence
- the role of the coroner's office and the implications of a coroner's inquest.

Critical Thinking

These case studies are for further reflection, discussion, and analysis. As you review each case, consider the following questions as well as those specific to the case.

1. Have the nurses in these cases violated any ethical or legal standards?
2. If so, what are these standards?
3. Is there risk of any civil or criminal liability?
4. How could these situations have been prevented?

CASE STUDY: NO HARM DONE?

Susan is the only RN on the night shift at a small home for the aged. She is working with Marie, a health care aide. Susan has worked with Marie on many occasions; she respects her judgement and her caring approach to the patients. One night Susan asks Marie to clean Mrs. White, an 80-year-old patient with Alzheimer's, who had just been incontinent. After helping Mrs. White, Marie leaves the room to dispose of the soiled linen. Unfortunately, Marie forgets to put up the bed rail and, during her absence, Mrs. White slips to the floor.

Marie and Susan check Mrs. White, who does not appear to have sustained any injury, and return her to bed. Marie is very concerned about the incident and pleads with Susan not to report it to their manager, Mr. Glove. Mr. Glove recently chastised her over a similar incident, which she did not believe was her fault, in which another patient fell after climbing over the bed rails. Also, Mrs. White's daughter worries a great deal about her mother's care. Marie is afraid she will be in serious trouble.

Susan is unsure what to do. She knows how punitive Mr. Glove can be; she also does not want to get Marie into trouble or worry Mrs. White's daughter unnecessarily.

QUESTIONS

1. What should Susan do?
2. Would Susan also be accountable for this accident, since she is the registered nurse and Marie is not a regulated health care provider?

CASE STUDY: WHO IS RESPONSIBLE?

Mikhaila is a public health nurse (PHN) who has been asked to follow a high-risk mother who was just discharged from hospital only 24 h after delivery. Terry is single, on welfare, and also has a two-year-old son. The hospital nurse has suggested that Terry remain in the hospital another day or two since she wants to be assured that Terry is able to provide appropriate care for the baby. Though Terry had experience with her previous child, the nurse has observed that she is somewhat uncomfortable while bathing and feeding the baby. In hospital, Terry could get some rest; her two-year old would stay with neighbours until she came home.

The unit manager thinks the nurse is overreacting. The unit is also tight for beds. The nurse therefore requests an early visit from the PHN. Although Mikhaila is very busy, she manages a quick visit. Everything seems fine, though Terry is tired and says she is having difficulty feeding the baby.

Mikhaila promises to return the next day; however, the next morning she phones in ill. The unit is unable to send another nurse until the following day. When this nurse arrives she finds everything in chaos. The two-year-old is screaming and seems to have a cold. Terry is very stressed. The new baby has been vomiting and is obviously dehydrated. The nurse calls an ambulance; the baby is taken to the closest Emergency Department, where she is stabilized.

QUESTIONS

1. Who is ethically, and legally, accountable for the potential harm to the baby: the hospital, the hospital nurse, Mikhaila, the public health unit, the system, or Terry?
2. How could this situation have been prevented?

CASE STUDY: SHOULD SHE HAVE STOPPED?

Gail is driving home after a very busy 12-h shift in the Cardiovascular Intensive Care Unit. She is five minutes from home and is looking forward to spending the evening with friends. As she rounds a corner, she sees a multi-vehicle accident. She slows her car and observes a number of people rushing to help. Reassured that appropriate assistance will be provided, Gail continues home.

The next day she arrives at work to discover that she is assigned to care for one of the accident victims, a 20-year-old man who sustained serious chest trauma resulting in a tear to his aorta. Delays in the arrival of paramedics resulted in problems with early management of his airway. Now, though surgery has corrected the tear, it is unclear whether inadequate oxygenation to his brain will result in permanent brain damage. Gail feels responsible and wishes she had stopped to help.

QUESTIONS

1. Did Gail have an ethical (or legal) responsibility to provide assistance to the victims of this accident? Is there a difference between her legal and moral responsibilities?
2. What choice would you have made?

QUESTIONS FOR DISCUSSION

1. What systems are in place in your facility to guard against negligence?
2. What standards would the courts use in deciding whether a registered nurse had been negligent?
3. What actions would you take if you realized you made a mistake? How would your organization respond?

References

1. Hammer, M., & Champy, J. (1994). *Reengineering the corporation.* New York: Harper Business.
2. Glandon, G.L., Colbert, K.W., & Thomasma, M. (1989). Nursing delivery models and RN mix: Cost implications. *Nursing Management, 20,* 30–33.
3. College of Nurses of Ontario. (1997). *Determining the appropriate category of care provider.* Toronto: Author. Available (in English and French) from: Publications, College of Nurses of Ontario, 101 Davenport Rd., Toronto, ON M5R 3P1; or from www.cno.org
4. See O. Reg. 799/93, section 1, paragraph 25.
5. See, e.g., Alberta: *Nursing Profession Act,* RSA 1980, c. N-14.5, section 103(1); Ontario: supra footnote 4; Saskatchewan: *Registered Nurses Act, 1988,* SS 1988, c. R-12.2, section 26(2)(k); Manitoba: *Registered Nurses Act,* RSM 1987, c. R40, CCSM, c. R40, section 46(1).
6. Supra footnote 4.
7. Ibid., section 1, paragraph 6.
8. Ibid., paragraph 25.
9. *Thompson Estate v. Byrne et al. (1993),* 114 NSR (2d) 395, at p. 423 (SCTD).
10. Ibid.
11. Ibid., p. 397.
12. Ibid., p. 421.
13. Ibid., p. 424.
14. Ibid., citing *McCormick v. Marcotte,* [1972] SCR 18, at p. 21, per Abbott J.
15. *Kolesar v. Jeffries* (1974), 59 DLR (3d) 367, at p. 376.
16. Ontario: supra footnote 1, section 1, paragraph 6; Saskatchewan: supra footnote 1, section 26(2)(n); Prince Edward Island: Reg. No. EC504/89, section 2(a)(ii).
17. (Unreported; May 29, 1998.) Doc. No. Kitchener 5499/82 (Ont. Gen. Div.); additional reasons at (unreported; December 3, 1998) Doc. No. Kitchener 5499/82 (Ont. Gen. Div.).
18. [1947] 2 DLR 338 (NSSC).
19. Ibid., per Doull J., at p. 30.
20. Ibid., pp. 340–341.
21. Ibid., citing *Dominion Natural Gas Co. v. Collins,* [1909] AC 640 (JCPC), at pp. 646–647.
22. (1980) 30 OR (2d) 691 (HCJ).
23. Ibid., per Carruthers J., at p. 692.
24. (1986), 31 CCC (3d) 62; 55 CR (3d) 48 (B.C. Co. Ct.), appeal dismissed on other grounds (1988), 43 CCC (3d) 65; 65 CR (3d) 256; 31 BCLR (2d) 145 (CA).
25. *R v. Coyne (1958),* 124 CCC 176; 31 CR 335 (NBCA).
26. *Criminal Code of Canada,* RSC 1985, c. C-46, as amended, section 220.
27. Ibid., section 221.
28. See *R v. Anderson (1985),* 35 MVR 128, at p. 133 (Man. CA).
29. *R v. Sharpe (1984),* 12 CCC (3d) 428; 39 CR (3d) 367; 26 MVR 279 (Ont. CA).
30. Alberta: *Fatality Inquiries Act,* RSA 1989, c. F-6, as amended.
31. RSO 1990, c. C.37.
32. Ibid., section 10(1).
33. Ibid., section 10(2).

Six

Consent to Treatment

LEARNING OBJECTIVES

The purpose of this chapter is to enable you to:
- understand the foundation of consent in law and ethics
- explain the principle of autonomy and its role in consent
- appreciate the concept of competence or capacity
- understand the tort of battery
- explain the concept of informed consent
- clarify the various types of, and approaches to, consent
- understand the rights of patients to refuse consent to medical or health care
- describe the nurse's role in ensuring that informed consent takes place
- apply the legal rules and ethical theory to hypothetical case studies and real case law
- understand the consent challenges with respect to the incompetent adult and to children
- clarify professional responsibilities in emergency situations
- understand the concept of proxy or substitute consent
- review consent legislation in the various provinces.

Introduction

Much of what we do as nurses involves direct interaction with the mind, body, and spirit of another. Many nursing actions require physical touch. Though intended to promote recovery, or to relieve pain and suffering, such actions are not without risk, and could result in pain or harm.

Legally, to touch another person without permission constitutes battery. As discussed in previous chapters, individuals in Canadian society have the right to determine the course of their lives (so long as they cause no harm to themselves or others), as well as the right to privacy.

The intimacy and integrity of the nurse–client relationship demand that nurses ensure protection of the rights of their patients and clients. This is achieved through standards, policies, guidelines, legislation, and rules regarding consent—the last of which is the subject of this chapter.

Consent in Law and Ethics

As discussed in Chapter Four, the *Code of Ethics for Registered Nurses* requires that nurses respect and promote the autonomy of clients. Nurses ensure that autonomy is respected by assisting clients in expressing their values and health needs, and by ensuring that they have the right information and support in order to make informed decisions and choices. The Code is clear that it is the nurse's responsibility:

- to involve the client in health planning and decision making;
- to provide truthful and accurate information to assist clients in making decisions on their own behalf;
- to ensure that timing and context are right, and that clients are receptive to this information;
- to discuss with clients their condition and health care options;
- to practise within relevant legislation;
- to be sensitive to the nurse's position of power and potential to influence clients;
- to respect the decisions of clients even when the nurse does not believe a decision is based on the client's best interests;
- to involve competent clients in decision making as much as possible;
- to respect advance directives and the legitimacy of substitute decision makers.

Based on the principle of autonomy, these responsibilities stress the significance of informed choice. Recognizing that consent may be given in writing or verbally, or simply implied (for example, holding out an arm to have blood drawn), a valid consent must be based on the relevant information required to make that choice. Consent must be free from coercion, and it must be made by someone capable of that level of decision.

The following case study highlights the legal and ethical challenges associated with consent.

CASE STUDY

Whose decision?

Doris, a widow 75 years of age, lives alone in a suburban bungalow that she and her late husband owned for 30 years. Her few close friends have died in the past few years. She has two grown children, a son and a daughter, who both live in another city. Over the past six or seven months, Doris's general health has declined. She has lost weight, has grown weak, and finds it difficult to leave home to go about her daily activities.

One week, Sam, her postman, notices that Doris's mail has not been taken in for two days. Sam is concerned; he knows Doris's daily routine, and she always informs him when she plans to go out of town. He knocks on the door but receives no answer. Alarmed, Sam calls the police, who, upon arrival at Doris's home, discover her lying semi-conscious on the kitchen floor.

Doris is rushed to hospital. The attending physician makes a preliminary diagnosis of gastrointestinal bleeding and, since it is an emergency, orders a blood transfusion to stabilize her. A few days later, when Doris is awake and alert, the physician in charge of her case advises her that he wants to do further investigations. Though she is apparently alert and competent, the nurses caring for Doris have noted some occasions when she seems confused as to her surroundings and does not know what day it is.

When the physician tells Doris that her condition urgently warrants further tests, she becomes agitated and upset. She fears that the doctors will discover cancer and that she will soon die. Consequently, she refuses to authorize any further tests. The members of the team know that any number of easily treated factors could be causing the bleeding, and they are concerned that Doris's refusal of further investigation and treatment is not in her best interests. Some nurses question whether Doris, in her present state of mind, is capable of making such a decision.

The team wishes to involve her children, but Doris refuses to give any information that would enable contact. She does not want her family involved; she feels she has always been able to take care of herself and does not wish to worry her children.

Over the next few days, the team finds evidence that Doris's bleeding is recurring. Something must be done soon or she may die.

Issues

1. Does Doris have the mental (and hence legal) capacity to make the decision to accept or refuse treatment?
2. Has Doris been given adequate opportunity to make an informed decision with respect to consent to treatment?
3. May the nurses or other team members legally and ethically disclose information pertaining to Doris's condition to her children, assuming they are able to contact them through their own efforts?
4. What are the competing ethical interests in this situation, and how can they be resolved?
5. May the team proceed with the investigation of Doris's condition on the assumption that she is not capable of giving or withholding consent?
6. What legal procedures must be followed to obtain permission to proceed with further investigation of Doris's condition, assuming she is not mentally competent?

Discussion

In this case study, it is clear that the health care team cannot proceed legally without Doris's consent. If they do so, they may be liable for battery, as there is absolutely no consent here, let alone an informed one. Although the nurses and physicians are genuinely motivated by good faith and have Doris's best interests at heart, they are not free to substitute their own judgement and proceed on their own authority. Even if Doris is not mentally competent to consent (which is unclear, based on the details given), this would still not authorize the team to proceed of its own accord.

The law and practice in this area require that, as a first step, a nurse or physician must explain the procedures and their importance, as well as the risks of forgoing them, to Doris. Also, Doris needs to be given enough time to make her decision. The team needs to respond to her questions and clarify any misconceptions. Nurses can play a role in exploring with patients the factors that might motivate their decisions (e.g., fear, past experiences, misconceptions). If Doris does consent, any subsequent withdrawal of that consent must be respected by the team members.

Rights

As we saw in Chapters Three and Four, in Canada the rights of patients extend to personal autonomy, and the right to be informed of all risks material to a particular medical procedure, including the risks, both real and probable, in forgoing such treatment. (A material risk is one that a reasonable person would wish to know in deciding whether to consent to or forgo a given medical procedure.) These rights include the right of a patient not to be subjected to any treatment to which he or she has not given a free and informed consent if mentally capable, and the moral right to be treated with respect, dignity, and courtesy by all health professionals. Legal rights are enforceable by the courts via the lawsuit. Moral rights are guaranteed by professionals who deem these part of their ethical and professional duty.

Autonomy

As described in Chapter Four, the principle of autonomy supports the capable and competent patient's right to determine and act on a self-chosen plan. Informed consent represents autonomy and ensures the individual's right to the information required to make personal decisions about health care. Nurses are obliged to respect the choices of their patients. However, there are situations when nurses may face a conflict between respect for the individual's wishes and their obligation to help their patients and protect them from harm.

Patients have the right to refuse consent to treatment, regardless of whether that treatment is in their best interests. It is the duty of the nurse to support the patient through such decisions. It is also the nurse's duty to ensure that the patient has the information required to make such choices, as well as sufficient time to reflect on the alternatives available. Whether or not the nurse is part of an informed consent process, he or she is obligated to advocate for the patient where the patient has not been duly informed, or where the patient's wishes have not been respected.

Patient autonomy is the hallmark of free and informed consent to treatment. It is recognized in both civil law and common law throughout Canada. In Quebec, for example, the *Civil Code* proclaims this principle. Article 3 declares that every person possesses personality rights, which include the right to life, the right to personal integrity and inviolability, and respect of name, reputation, and privacy. This last-mentioned right of privacy is interesting in that it implies that individuals have the right to make decisions about their life and affairs free of governmental scrutiny and interference (except as permitted by law). This right to privacy is likewise implied in the United States Constitution, and has been used to strike down laws restricting abortion rights in that country.

If a patient is mentally competent, the law requires health practitioners, including nurses, to respect any decision he or she makes, no matter how potentially harmful that decision may be to the patient. Yet, autonomy can be meaningful only when patients are given full and complete information as to their medical condition, the risks which that condition poses, and the benefits and drawbacks of any proposed treatment that health professionals may offer. The risks, material facts, and alternatives, including the consequences of non-treatment, must be explained to the patient.

For example, if a patient refuses to ambulate, or to practise deep breathing and coughing exercises prior to surgery, the nurse must explain the benefits and risks of such procedures and the consequences of not doing them. The explanation must be respectful and courteous, and the nurse must give the patient an opportunity to change his or her mind. Such interventions as injections, medications, and so forth cannot be forced on a competent patient.

Suppose a patient is in the final phases of metastatic cancer: the cancer has spread to her bones, and she is in severe pain. The care plan is to turn her every two hours to prevent pressure sores and to minimize the likelihood of pneumonia. Turning causes her great pain such that she requires additional sedation, which causes extended drowsiness. Should the nurses give this patient the choice of being turned or not? Are there alternatives? As long as the patient understands, and is willing to accept, the consequences of not being turned, her decision is valid. She may choose to refuse turning in order to avoid the pain and the need for increased sedation.

If the patient is ill informed, or is misled by the information provided, any consent given is, in law, no consent at all. He or she may have decided differently if informed fully and properly. Hence, that patient's right to autonomy will have been infringed, as he or she has not been able to make a free and informed decision as to whether to undergo or forgo treatment.

Respect for the patient's autonomy is likewise compromised when, in the absence of consent, the health professional presumes to decide whether treatment should proceed. This includes decisions as to what is and is not a material risk, all of which should be disclosed to the patient. (There are exceptions to the need for such consent in emergencies, as we will see later in this chapter.)

Features of Consent

Lack of Consent (Battery)

As discussed in Chapter Three, battery is a category of intentional tort, and is legally defined as the touching of another, however slight, without that person's consent. Thus, it is an unwanted intrusion on the physical person of another. In a health care context, the administration of any medical treatment, surgical procedure, nursing action, diagnostic test, or other such intervention, no matter how necessary or beneficial to the patient's health and well-being in the health practitioner's opinion, is forbidden unless the professional who is administering the treatment has obtained the patient's prior consent; or, unless the patient has suffered a serious injury that renders him or her unable to give consent, and a lack of prompt medical attention would result in serious bodily harm or death.

It is a fundamental principle of ethics and the law that people who are mentally competent have the right to their bodily integrity and personal autonomy respecting health care treatment. This right applies even to mentally incompetent persons to the extent that their wishes, when they were competent, are known. If the patient is not competent, his or her prior wishes, as expressed to others or in an **advance directive** (discussed in Chapter Seven), must be respected to the greatest extent possible. The final decision as to whether any nursing care, medical treatment, or plan of care should or should not proceed rests with the patient. The nurse or other health practitioner who proceeds without the patient's consent runs the risk of being found liable in a civil lawsuit for battery or, if he or she has carelessly informed the patient and harm results, for negligence.

Table 6.1 on page 186 sets out the required conditions of a truly informed consent.

Types of Consent

There are two basic types of consent: expressed and implied. Expressed consent is a clear statement of consent from the patient. No specific wording is

---

TABLE 6.1
Conditions for informed consent

- The consent must be given voluntarily. There must be no coercion or undue pressure from another person to obtain that consent.
- The patient must be told of all material and possible risks inherent in a proposed procedure, together with its benefits and drawbacks, as well as the risks of forgoing the treatment.
- The consent given must be specific to the proposed treatment or procedure. For example, a consent to an appendectomy does not authorize the removal of other infected or diseased tissues unrelated to that condition.
- The consent must specify who will perform the procedure or treatment. If a patient has consented to its performance by a particular specialist, this would not authorize the substitution of another, less qualified, or different type of health practitioner.
- The patient must be legally capable. A minor under a certain age may not be legally qualified to consent, depending on the province.
- Similarly, in most provinces, mental incompetence renders persons legally incapable of consenting unless they are capable of understanding the nature and consequences of the procedure, notwithstanding their mental condition.

---

required; an expression such as, "Okay, nurse, go ahead" is sufficient. Many provinces require that a written consent also be obtained as evidence that the patient has consented to a medical procedure or treatment. It is important to remember that the patient has the right to withdraw consent or revoke (cancel) a previously given consent at any time, even orally, provided he or she is mentally competent to do so.

Implied consent is inferred from a patient's conduct. For example, a nurse advises a patient whose hand has just been punctured by a rusty nail that she will be administering a tetanus vaccine as a precaution to prevent "lockjaw." The patient then holds out his arm to receive the injection. Clearly, through this action, he has consented to the treatment without written or verbal means.

Record and Timing of Consent

Many nurses may be concerned when no expressed written consent is found in the patient's chart and the patient is ready for surgery and perhaps already sedated. Must a written consent be obtained in this instance? The written consent form itself does not stand alone; it is merely documentary evidence. What matters is the fact that an informed consent has been given. If the physician has documented somewhere in the patient's chart the fact of the patient's consent and the disclosure relating to the risks, consequences, and benefits of the procedure, this will usually be sufficient. Moreover, the written consent can be revoked at any time by the patient provided he or she is mentally competent to do so.

Written Consent Forms

The blanket consent form used in some health care institutions should not be solely relied upon, since it may not be specific to the particular procedure or treatment. The health professional should document the fact that the procedure was explained to the patient along with its risks and consequences, and that the patient verbally consented. In many cases, the gravity of the situation or the risks in delaying treatment may preclude the obtaining of a signed consent; thus, documenting the fact of an informed consent is very important. Any such note should be signed and dated by the physician. It can also be signed by the health professional who is present at the time when such disclosure is made to the patient.

Case Law on Consent

Informed Consent

The most celebrated case dealing with the requirement of informed consent to medical treatment is *Reibl v. Hughes*.[1] In the Reibl decision, the plaintiff suffered from a blocked left carotid artery. Accordingly, he was booked for an elective internal carotid endarterectomy, which was performed by the defendant, a neurosurgeon. During the surgery, or immediately thereafter, the plaintiff suffered a stroke which resulted in unilateral paralysis, impotence, and permanent disability. The plaintiff sued the neurosurgeon for negligently performing the operation and for the surgeon's failure to inform him adequately of the risks of the surgery.

The case ultimately reached the Supreme Court of Canada, where the court held that the surgeon was liable in that he had indeed failed to inform the plaintiff of all material risks attending the surgery. In this case, although there was a real risk of stroke, paralysis, and possible death, the surgeon had told the patient only that it would be better for him to have the surgery. Furthermore, as the plaintiff had difficulty with the English language, it was incumbent upon the surgeon to ensure that the information conveyed was fully understood.

If such disclosure is not made, the health practitioner risks being found liable for negligence. The complete failure to obtain any consent at all, or the obtaining of consent through fraud, would leave the practitioner open to a civil suit for battery.

Refusal of Consent for Religious or Other Reasons

Along with the issue of informed consent is that of an instruction or limitation by which the patient refuses consent to certain procedures or treatment on moral or religious grounds. The Ontario Court of Appeal dealt with such a case in its decision in *Malette v. Shulman*.[2] In that case, the plaintiff had been seriously injured in a motor vehicle accident and rushed to a nearby hospital. She had sustained serious injuries to her head and face and was bleeding profusely. The physician on duty in the Emergency Department, who attended her upon her arrival, determined that she would need blood transfusions to maintain her blood volume and pressure lest she succumb to irreversible shock. The surgeon who examined her prior to x-rays being taken also determined that she would require a blood transfusion. She was barely conscious at the time.

Meanwhile, shortly after the patient's arrival at the hospital, a nurse discovered a card in the patient's purse printed in French, signed by the patient, identifying her as a Jehovah's Witness. The card read:[3]

NO BLOOD TRANSFUSION!

As one of Jehovah's Witnesses with firm religious convictions, I request that no blood or blood products be administered to me under any circumstances. I fully realize the implications of this position, but I have resolutely decided to obey the Bible command: "Keep abstaining ... from blood." (Acts 15:28, 29)

However, I have no religious objections to use the non-blood alternatives, such as Dextran, Haemaccel [sic], PVP, Ringer's Lactate, or saline solution.

The card was brought by the nurse to the attention of the physician who had first seen the patient.

Before x-rays could be completed, the patient's blood pressure dropped markedly, her respiration became increasingly distressed, and her level of consciousness dropped. She continued to bleed profusely. At that moment, the physician determined that a blood transfusion was necessary to preserve her life. He decided to administer the transfusion to her personally and on his own responsibility, notwithstanding the card that had been brought to his attention.

Usually, nurses would administer a blood transfusion pursuant to an order drawn up by a physician. The question then becomes: What is the legal obligation of a nurse to follow a physician's order when he or she knows that order to be contrary to the patient's wishes and that the patient has not consented to such treatment? In such a case, the law would apply equally to the nurse as well as to the physician. Both must respect the patient's wishes, and may not proceed to administer treatment to which consent has been withheld, no matter how necessary that treatment, or how irrational the patient's decision may seem.

Returning to the Malette case, shortly after the physician administered the transfusion, the patient's daughter arrived at the hospital and became furious when told that blood transfusions had been administered to her mother. She affirmed her mother's instructions that no blood be given to her, and signed a document specifically prohibiting the giving of further blood to the patient, saying that her mother's faith forbade blood transfusions and that she would not wish them.

Despite these objections, the physician refused to follow the daughter's instructions. In his professional opinion, transfusions were absolutely necessary to save the patient's life, and it was his professional duty to ensure that she receive them. He did not believe that the card signed by the patient expressed her current wishes. He could not be sure that she had not changed her religious beliefs, or that she had been fully informed of all the risks of forgoing a blood transfusion. (Again, if a nurse were carrying out an order for a blood transfusion under similar circumstances, despite the fact that he or she may have similar misgivings about the instructions, that nurse would be bound by the patient's limitations on consent to treatment.)

The plaintiff recovered fully from her injuries. Despite this, she brought a lawsuit for battery, negligence, and religious discrimination against the physician and the hospital. Her action was allowed, and she was awarded damages on the grounds that blood transfusions had been administered against her specific wishes and that this constituted a battery upon her. The physician appealed this judgement in the Ontario Court of Appeal.

The Court of Appeal reviewed the law dealing with informed consent. It found that the common law recognized the right of a patient to refuse consent to medical treatment, and that this right was paramount to the health practitioner's professional opinion about what might be best for that patient. The Court stated that, while it is true that informed consent is not required in emergencies where the patient is unable to give consent (and the physician has no reason to believe that the patient would refuse consent if conscious or able to do so), in the presence of clear instructions such as those contained in the Jehovah's Witness card in this case, the physician was not free to disregard the patient's instructions. There is no corresponding doctrine of "informed refusal" requiring or authorizing a health practitioner to proceed with emergency treatment where the practitioner has not been able to inform the patient of all the consequences and risks of refusing treatment.[4]

The Court upheld the trial judge's finding that there was no rational basis or evidence upon which the physician could found a belief that the card was not valid or that the patient's religious views had changed. Hence, there was no justification for the doctor's refusal to adhere to the patient's advance instructions. The treatment having thus been administered without the patient's consent, the Court of Appeal upheld the finding of liability for battery against the physician.[5]

Of course, the Court made clear the fact that, in this case, it was not deciding the enforceability of advance directives regarding euthanasia or withdrawal of treatment. The patient here asked only that her spiritual beliefs be respected, and she was willing to risk death for them. She did not wish to die, as she consented to the use of non-blood alternatives. This case illustrates a limit on the doctrine of emergency treatment wherein the requirement for consent is waived. It further reinforces the principle that a patient's wishes are the final say on whether treatment shall be administered, no matter how necessary to life that treatment may be.

Withdrawal of Consent

The Supreme Court of Canada reviewed the law of informed consent in a situation where the patient withdrew consent during a medical procedure to which she had previously consented. Although this case involved an action for battery and negligence against the attending physicians, the principles contained in this decision and developed by the Supreme Court are equally applicable to nursing professionals.

In *Ciarlariello v. Schacter,*[6] the court was asked to consider whether a doctor still owed a duty of disclosure to a patient of all material risks inherent in a medical procedure where the patient withdraws a previously given informed consent during that procedure.[7] The plaintiff was asked to attend at a hospital for the purpose of undergoing the first of two angiograms meant to determine the exact location of a suspected aneurysm. On the patient's arrival at the hospital, the physician who was to administer the test explained the risks inherent in the procedure, including possible blindness, paralysis, and death. Although the plaintiff's first language was Italian and her English was poor, she claimed at that time to have understood the doctor's explanation. The plaintiff's daughter acted as interpreter during these explanations. The patient thereupon signed a consent to the tests. Despite this, the doctor had misgivings as to the free and informed nature of the consent.

The doctor therefore destroyed the patient's consent and asked her to go back to her family to consult with them. This she did, and later returned with a consent signed by her daughter. The patient took the test; it failed to reveal the aneurysm conclusively but indicated a possible site. The doctors in charge of her case decided that a second angiogram would likely pinpoint the site of the aneurysm.

In the meantime, the plaintiff suffered a second severe headache indicating a "re-bleed" of the aneurysm, and it was decided that a second angiogram was needed. The patient consented to this second test. Beforehand, a second radiologist (who had worked with the radiologist who administered the first test) carefully explained the test to her, including all possible material risks (skin rash, and on rare occasions, blindness, stroke and/or paralysis, death). He stated that the patient appeared to understand, and proceeded with the angiogram.

During the procedure, the plaintiff began moaning and yelling. She began to hyperventilate and flex her legs. She calmed down sufficiently to tell the doctor, "Enough, no more, stop the test." The test was stopped, and both radiologists proceeded to examine her complaint that her right hand was numb. She was unable to move it or grasp with it. Her left hand was also slightly weak. Gradually, the strength returned to her left hand and both arms, though her left hand remained weak. Her sensory perception was normal. Both radiologists concluded that the residual weakness in her left hand was due to her hyperventilating. Both expected the weakness to be temporary. The rest of her motor function appeared to return to normal.

At this point, the plaintiff became quiet and cooperative. The first radiologist took over the test and explained to her that one more area needed investigation and that this procedure would take five more minutes. She asked the plaintiff if she wished to continue the test, to which the plaintiff replied: "Please go ahead." The final injection of dye was administered, during which the plaintiff suffered an immediate reaction, rendering her a quadriplegic. She sued all the doctors involved in treating her for damages for negligence and battery. She died soon after her lawsuit came to trial, and her family and estate continued the suit.

This case is of some relevance to nursing in that it illustrates that a patient has the right at any time to withdraw consent to treatment. Such withdrawal may occur in difficult circumstances, as in the Ciarlariello case, and it is important for the health practitioner to ascertain whether the consent has been withdrawn. This may not always be clear. A professional who continues to administer treatment, regardless of a patient's instructions to stop, risks being found liable to the patient for battery. In the Ciarlariello case, the patient clearly withdrew her consent. She had given an informed consent within the requirements laid down in *Reibl v. Hughes*.[8] Thus, the doctors had not been negligent in explaining the risks of the procedure to her.

A further issue with respect to resumption of treatment after consent to it has been withdrawn is also crucial. The criteria laid down by the court governing the health professional's actions in such a case include a consideration of whether the risks have changed materially during the procedure, and whether a reasonable patient would wish to know of such changes.[9] In the Ciarlariello case, there was no evidence that the patient's condition had deteriorated such that she could not properly consent to the resumption of the treatment. Thus, her consent to resume the tests was valid.

As discussed in Chapter Three, one of the elements that must be proven in a negligence action is that the plaintiff's injury must have resulted from the defendant's breach of duty towards the plaintiff. In an action for negligence such as that in *Reibl v. Hughes* or *Ciarlariello v. Schacter,* the question becomes whether a reasonable person in the plaintiff's position would still have consented to the procedure if he or she had known the information and risks that the health practitioner failed to disclose.

In *Ciarlariello v. Schacter,* the court found that the plaintiff's consent was an informed one and that there was no negligence on the doctors' part. It also found that, as the risk of quadriplegia resulting from an angiogram was far less than the risks of not locating the aneurysm, a reasonable patient in the plaintiff's position would still have consented to the procedure.

Competency, Consent, and Substitute Decision Makers

Incompetent Adults

To return to our case study, before her children can be consulted, Doris's attending physicians must determine whether she is mentally competent to make an informed decision respecting the diagnostic tests. If Doris is competent, her wishes that her children not be contacted must be respected.

In cases involving elderly patients, the initial and seemingly irrational refusal to consent may not necessarily be evidence of mental incompetence. The nurse or other practitioner must remain patient (if the situation is not urgent or life-threatening). Elderly clients are often fearful of impending illness. Many may have friends or relatives, even a spouse, who have recently succumbed to a serious illness. For example, a patient whose brother has died of cancer may fear that he himself will be stricken with the disease. This fear may paralyze some people's thinking. They may be in a state of denial and may rationalize their refusal to consent on the basis that "if cancer is not detected, then that means I don't have it." This may be what is going on in a patient's mind when he or she says: "No! I don't want to go through those tests; leave me alone, I'm all right!"

The law allows any mentally competent adult to refuse consent to medical treatment. How, then, can the mental capacity of a patient be determined? Some have suggested the following test: "... can the patient appreciate the nature and consequences of the proposed treatment so as to be capable of rendering an informed judgement?"[10] A method of testing for this appreciation is to explain to the patient, carefully and in detail, the risks and nature of the proposed procedure and then to ask the patient to repeat his or her understanding of the risks and treatment, while carefully noting the responses and words used.[11] On this basis, the health practitioner is then able to form an opinion of the patient's ability to appreciate the nature, risks, and consequences of the proposed procedure.

Of course, patients may be capable of making decisions concerning some matters yet not others, and their mental capacity may fluctuate over time. Even when the patient has stated an intention that the procedure should commence but has displayed an irrational or confused understanding of that procedure, the health practitioner should be reluctant to proceed. If the patient's responses demonstrate a mental incapacity to comprehend the nature of the risks of the procedure, however beneficial it may be to the patient, the practitioner should not proceed without the consent of an authorized substitute decision maker.

In some provinces, any health professional faced with a question of administering treatment to a mentally incompetent patient must obtain the consent of the patient's spouse, parent, a person in lawful custody of that patient, or the patient's next of kin.[12] If no such persons are available, and the situation is not an emergency, a physician may have to obtain the consent of the patient's guardian, appointed under statute (e.g., Ontario's *Health Care Consent Act, 1996* or a substitute decision maker designated by the patient pursuant to the *Substitute Decisions Act, 1992*.[13] Under such a law, a court may be asked by any interested party, usually a spouse or relative, to appoint a person to act in the patient's best interests, including the giving or withholding of consent to medical treatment. This committee then has the authority to consent to any medical treatment on behalf of the patient, who will legally have been found incompetent by the court. In such a case, the physician may obtain the necessary consent from the committee.

For example, the Quebec *Civil Code* provides that where a person is incapable of giving consent, such consent may be given by a curator (or tutor, in the case of a child). A curator in Quebec is similar to a committee of the person in some common law provinces. He or she (or they) are appointed by the court to act in the incapable person's best interests and to ensure proper care for that person. In the absence of a curator, the person's spouse or, if there is no spouse or the spouse cannot consent, a close relative or adult showing a special interest in the patient may give consent.[14] If such a person (including the patient) either cannot consent or refuses consent, a health professional in Quebec cannot proceed with such treatment until and unless he or she obtains an order from the court authorizing such procedure.[15]

For example, suppose a patient in the later stages of Alzheimer's disease is rushed to the Emergency Department suffering from sharp abdominal pain. The patient's son is with him and has been appointed committee over the person of his father. The father exhibits classic symptoms of Alzheimer's: he is confused and incoherent, and at times does not recognize his son. The emergency team will have to obtain the son's consent to tests and treatment for the father. In such consultation, the son should be encouraged to make any decisions as his father would have made them when he was competent.

Children

There are likewise competency issues with respect to children. In some provinces, a child who is old enough and mature enough to understand the nature and risks inherent in a medical procedure is given the right to consent to such treatment of his or her own accord.

Ontario's *Health Care Consent Act, 1996* provides that the wishes of any mentally capable person 16 years of age or older with respect to medical treatment must be adhered to.[16] In Quebec, any child over the age of 14 may give consent freely without need for recourse to his or her parents or guardians.[17] However, if such a child refuses consent, a court order is necessary before treatment may proceed, even if the health professional has obtained the consent of that child's parent or guardian.[18]

A Children's Aid Society (CAS) may apply to a court to have a child in need of protection made its ward so that it can make treatment decisions on that child's behalf. This has been done in cases involving parents who had refused medical treatment for their children on religious grounds. If the refusal places the child's life at risk by denying life-saving treatment, the court can deem such a child a "child in need of protection" and can authorize the CAS or other such body (in some provinces, the director of child welfare) to give the required consent where it is in the child's best interests.

Emergency Treatment

In all cases, the law in all the common law provinces and Quebec allows physicians and other health professionals to administer treatment in an emergency where the patient's consent cannot be obtained. Such a situation might arise because of the nature of the injuries or illness, or because no time can be spared in administering such emergency treatment. Health professionals acting in extreme emergencies will be absolved of any liability for administering treatment, provided there is no gross negligence on their part.

Proxy Consent

The common law traditionally did not allow proxy consent to treatment—that is, a consent granted by a third party designated by the incapable person (when capable) to make decisions on his or her behalf. The only situations in which third-party consent was recognized was in the case of parents consenting on behalf of minors and committees appointed over mentally incompetent persons. However, situations may arise where the patient is unable to consent, not because of some current or progressive mental infirmity, but owing to a physical condition, for example, coma.

A proxy decision maker is clearly desirable in such situations. In our case study, the medical team would have to resort to a proxy if Doris were not competent to give or withhold consent.

The following discussion of recent legislative reform of the common law in this area focusses on Ontario's legislation, as it is presently the most detailed such legislation in Canada.

Legislative Reform of the Common Law Respecting Consent to Treatment

The main components of the Ontario legislation affecting consent to treatment are contained in the *Health Care Consent Act, 1996*[19] and the *Substitute Decisions Act, 1992.*[20]

The *Health Care Consent Act, 1996* enshrines into statute law the existing common law requirements for an informed consent to treatment, as discussed above. It preserves the right and duty of health care providers to restrain or confine persons when necessary to prevent serious bodily harm either to themselves or to others.[21] The Act requires all health practitioners (including nurses) to ensure, firstly, that the patient to be treated is capable of consenting, and secondly, that the patient in fact consents. If the patient is not capable, the health practitioner must obtain the consent from another person authorized to give consent under the Act.[22] The Act also provides for other consents by patients to admission to a care facility, such as a nursing home, or to personal assistance services, such as assistance with dressing, hygiene, eating, grooming, and so forth.[23]

Ontario's statute defines informed consent in much the same way as discussed earlier in this chapter: that is, it allows the consent to be expressed or implied, provided that (a) an informed consent has been given, (b) it relates to the treatment proposed, (c) it is voluntary, and (d) it has not been obtained through fraud or misrepresentation.[24] Consent is informed if, before giving it, a patient received information about the nature of the treatment, its expected benefits, material risks, material side effects, alternative courses of action, and the consequences of not having the treatment.[25] A health practitioner (which under this Act includes a nurse) is entitled to presume that consent to a treatment includes consent to variations or adjustments in the treatment or the continuation of the treatment in a different setting, provided the benefits, risks, and material side effects of such alteration do not differ significantly from those of the original treatment.

This provision has a practical purpose. It would be quite impractical to require the health practitioner to obtain renewed consent, along with having to restate all the information required, every time a course of treatment was altered in even the slightest way. This legislative provision also addresses the issue that arose in *Ciarlariello v. Schacter* (discussed on page 190), where there were few or no significant changes to the risks and side effects from one angiogram to the next.

The legislation also defines when a person is capable of giving consent. A person is capable if he or she understands the information given that is relevant to making a decision concerning the treatment, and can appreciate the reasonably foreseeable consequences of a decision or lack thereof. A person is always presumed to be capable unless a health practitioner has reasonable grounds to believe that he or she is not.[26] For example, a health practitioner could not assume that a patient was capable if he or she were to observe erratic or confused behaviour in the patient, or a lack of lucidity or rationality, even before the patient had actually been judged incapable by a health practitioner. Although such an observation would not necessarily mean the patient was incapable to give consent, a health practitioner could not legally proceed on such basis. The statute provides that persons can be capable with respect to certain treatments and incapable for others, and capable and incapable at different times.[27] This provision addresses concerns that arise when a capable person has not yet given consent and then later may no longer be capable, for example, while under heavy sedation. It also addresses such situations as Alzheimer's patients who have periods of lucidity, only to relapse into a confused state moments later.

The health practitioner in charge of the patient's care is responsible for determining whether the patient is capable or incapable of consenting to a proposed treatment. If the patient's capacity to consent returns after another person has made a decision with respect to the patient's treatment, the patient's own decision to give or refuse consent will govern.[28]

If the physician examining the patient determines that he or she is not capable of consenting to treatment, the patient must be informed of that fact and of the consequences of such a finding in accordance with the guidelines laid out by the governing body of the practitioner's profession. For nurses, this would be the guidelines set out by the College of Nurses of Ontario.[29] Once the health practitioner has determined that the patient is incapable (or, if before the treatment is begun, the practitioner is informed that the person intends to apply to the Consent and Capacity Board for review of the finding of incapacity, or has applied for appointment of a representative to give consent to treatment), the practitioner must not begin treatment or must take steps to prevent such treatment being given. The practitioner must then wait (a) until 48 h have passed after first being informed of the application to the Board, (b) until the application is withdrawn, (c) until the Board has rendered a decision in the matter and the practitioner knows of no appeal from such decision, or (d) until the period for appealing the decision of the Board has passed.[30]

The Consent and Capacity Board is an administrative tribunal (as discussed in Chapter Three). Its role is to hear appeals from findings of incapacity by health practitioners. It also hears applications brought on behalf of incapable persons for the appointment of representatives who can give consent to treatment in specific situations. In the event that the health practitioner has found a patient incapable of giving consent, the patient has recourse to this tribunal if he or she does not agree and still believes himself or herself capable of giving consent. This mechanism protects patients' autonomy and prevents abuses of patients' rights, for example, in a case where a non-consenting patient might be subjected to treatment that is not in his or her best interests or is unnecessary. Without such review, a person might be incorrectly deemed incapable of giving consent and may then be subjected to treatment to which he or she would not consent, simply because a health practitioner was of the opinion that the patient lacked capacity.

Any decision of the Board can be further appealed to a court. The court has the power to order the treatment to begin, even before hearing the appeal, if it is satisfied that the treatment is necessary and will likely substantially improve the patient's condition, and that any delay in administering the treatment poses a serious risk of rapid deterioration to the person's health.[31] Of course, nothing prevents the health practitioner from giving emergency treatment when it is not possible for the patient to give consent, and the patient is at risk if treatment is not given promptly.[32]

Ontario law formerly provided for the appointment of "rights advisers" to meet with incapable persons in order to provide them with as much information as to their rights in such situations, but this law was repealed in 1996 with the passage of the *Health Care Consent Act, 1996*.[33]

Where an incapable person has appointed an attorney who is acting under a validated power of attorney for personal care or a court-appointed guardian of the person (see next two sections), such an agent can give the required consent, but only in accordance with the instructions, limitations, and authority contained in the power of attorney or court order.[34]

Where a substitute decision maker has been chosen, the known wishes of the patient must be taken into account and must govern the substitute's decision to give or refuse consent to treatment. The wishes may be contained in the power of attorney itself or any other document, or may be known orally. Such documents are commonly known as **living wills** because they provide directions on behalf of the maker after that person has lost the ability to make those decisions on his or her own behalf. If there are no known wishes requiring the giving or refusal of consent to a given treatment, the substitute decision maker must make the decision in the patient's best interests and in accordance with the incapable person's values and beliefs. In particular, the substitute must consider whether:

- the proposed treatment will likely improve the patient's condition or well-being;
- the proposed treatment would prevent the patient's condition or well-being from deteriorating, or
- reduce the extent to which (or the rate at which) the patient's condition or well-being is likely to deteriorate;
- the patient's well-being or condition would likely improve, remain the same, or deteriorate without the treatment;
- the benefits of treatment outweigh the risks; and
- a less intrusive or restrictive treatment would be as beneficial as the one proposed.[35]

The Act establishes a hierarchy of alternative substitute decision makers.[36] The persons set out in this list may give or refuse consent only if no person described in the next higher ranking (in descending order of priority, from one to eight) is available and meets the requirements of the Act:

(1) a guardian appointed by the court under the *Substitute Decisions Act, 1992*;
(2) an attorney for personal care acting under a validated power of attorney for personal care that confers that authority;
(3) the incapable person's representative, appointed by the Board, if the representative has authority to give or refuse consent;
(4) the incapable person's spouse or partner;[37]
(5) the incapable person's child, or parent, or a Children's Aid Society or other person lawfully entitled to give or refuse consent in place of the parent (this does not include parents having only a right of access over the

child, and does not include the child's parents if a Children's Aid Society is lawfully entitled to give or refuse treatment in the parents' place);

(6) the person's parent with only a right of access;

(7) the person's brother or sister;

(8) any other relative of the incapable person.

For example, in our case study, let us assume that Doris has not signed a power of attorney appointing an attorney for personal care, nor has any guardian or representative been designated for her; however, she has a younger brother living across town. Let us further assume that a hospital staff psychiatrist has been asked to examine Doris, and that he has determined that she appears to be suffering from some form of senile dementia, possibly Alzheimer's disease. A determination is made that Doris is not capable of giving or refusing informed consent. In such a situation, Doris's children would clearly be entitled to make the decision provided they can be located and are willing, capable, and available to give such consent, and that no higher-ranking person is available. Doris's brother could give consent, but only if her children could not be found or were incapable or unwilling to assume responsibility for making such a decision.

Other requirements are that the substitute decision maker be: at least 16 years of age; capable with respect to the treatment; not prohibited by court order or separation agreement from having access to the incapable person or giving or refusing consent; available, and willing to assume the responsibility of giving or refusing consent.[38] In the event of a conflict between two or more persons mentioned in any of the categories listed above, each of whom claimed to have authority to give consent, the person who ranks highest prevails. If two persons of equal ranking disagree about whether to give or refuse consent, the Public Guardian and Trustee may give or refuse it.[39]

With respect to minors, parental wishes will not necessarily govern situations where a minor 16 or older refuses treatment, even if the treatment is necessary. The Act provides that the wishes of a minor over the age of 16 to give or refuse consent to treatment must be respected. Unlike the former *Consent to Treatment Act, 1992,* the *Health Care Consent Act, 1996* does not explicitly set out a minimum age for consent. Rather, the guidelines that would likely govern would be the person's capacity to understand the proposed treatment, its risks, benefits, and consequences. A child under 16 might be capable of giving an informed consent if he or she were of sufficient intelligence and maturity to appreciate the consequences of his or her decision and all the relevant information surrounding the proposed treatment.

Emergency treatment poses a special challenge for the health practitioner, and the Act provides special rules for such situations. If a patient is found incapable, in the health practitioner's opinion, with respect to proposed treatment necessary to alleviate severe suffering, or the patient is at risk of serious bodily harm if the treatment is not administered promptly, and it is not possible to find a substitute decision maker without delaying such treatment, then the practitioner may administer the treatment. He or she may do so even when an application has been made to the Consent and Capacity Review

Board for the appointment of a representative to give such consent on the patient's behalf.

The authority to proceed extends to any examination of the patient or diagnostic procedures (if these are reasonably necessary) to determine whether the patient is at risk of serious bodily harm or is experiencing severe suffering. The emergency treatment can continue for as long as is reasonably required to find someone who can give the necessary consent from among the list of persons authorized to do so. The Act obliges the health practitioner to ensure that a continuing search is made for any substitute decision makers willing to assume responsibility to give or refuse consent. In the event that the patient becomes capable once again, his or her wishes govern.

The health practitioner is also required to note in the patient's chart the opinions required by the Act to permit treatment without consent in an emergency.[40] If the health practitioner has reasonable grounds to believe that the incapable patient, while capable and after the person reached the age of 16, expressed a wish to refuse treatment with respect to the circumstances, the practitioner may not administer treatment. Thus, for example, if the patient is unconscious, and an attorney for personal care advises the practitioner that this patient once expressed the desire that no blood transfusions be administered in an emergency, the practitioner may not administer such treatment.[41] Notwithstanding a refusal of consent by someone in the above list, the practitioner may proceed if he or she continues to believe that the treatment is necessary to alleviate suffering or avoid serious bodily harm, and that the person refusing the consent has done so against the patient's previous wishes, or has not acted in the patient's best interests in accordance with the guidelines and considerations enumerated in the Act. The authority to proceed as discussed above extends to having the person admitted to a hospital or psychiatric facility for treatment. The only exception is a person's objection to admission primarily for treatment of a mental disorder. This provision was included to cover situations in which a person might be forced to undergo psychiatric treatment against his or her will. There are separate procedures for admission of mental patients to psychiatric facilities set out in the *Mental Health Act*.[42] These include legal safeguards to ensure that otherwise mentally healthy persons are not detained against their will in psychiatric institutions.

Attorneys for Personal Care

With respect to substitute decision makers or attorneys for personal care, Ontario's *Substitute Decisions Act, 1992* provides that a person over the age of 16 may exercise power of decision on behalf of an incapacitated person who is also at least 16 years old.[43] In most cases, the parents of an incapacitated adolescent would presumably continue to make treatment decisions and give the necessary consents, as is currently the case. The determining factor under this statute for incapacity (thus the need for a substitute decision maker) is similar to that under the *Health Care Consent Act, 1996;* but in this case, the patient must be unable to understand information regarding his or her health care, nutrition, shelter, clothing, hygiene, or safety, or be unable to appreciate the reasonably foreseeable consequences of a decision (or lack of decision) respecting these matters.[44]

Under this statute, there are two methods of providing a substitute decision maker for an incapable person. The first is an appointment of a person or persons in a written document (called a **power of attorney for personal care**) in advance of the person (usually referred to as the **grantor**) becoming incapable. Those named in the power of attorney are authorized by the grantor to make decisions concerning personal care on his or her behalf.[45] The person named in the power of attorney (the attorney[46]) for personal care may be the grantor's spouse, partner,[47] a relative, or another. It cannot be anyone who provides health care to the grantor for compensation or who provides residential, social, training, or support services to the grantor for compensation.[48] This provision is important, since in some situations the grantor may be tempted to name his or her physician, or a respected and trusted nurse, as an attorney. The legislation prevents any such conflict of interest from arising. However, critics point out that a nurse may be one of the more knowledgeable persons relative to care and treatment issues concerning the incapable patient, and thus a practical and beneficial choice of attorneys. This provision may therefore be viewed as a questionable limitation on the incapable patient's rights to choose and appoint an attorney.

The attorney may act only in accordance with this statute and the limitations stipulated by the grantor in the power of attorney. In the case of a person who has neither a trusted friend, partner, spouse, nor relatives to name as attorney, he or she can name the Public Guardian and Trustee of Ontario (with that person's permission, obtained prior to signing the power of attorney).[49] This is a government official charged with ensuring that mentally incompetent persons, orphaned children having no legal guardians, and their property are cared for, and their legal rights protected, when there is no one else available to act in their interest.

Powers of attorney for personal care in Ontario no longer need to be validated, as was the case before amendments to the *Substitute Decisions Act,* which came into force in 1996. A power of attorney for personal care is a fully and legally valid document from the moment the grantor becomes incapable to make treatment decisions and give consent to treatment within the requirements of the *Health Care Consent Act, 1996* and the *Substitute Decisions Act.*

Of course, the grantor making the power of attorney must be mentally capable of giving it. The test for determining this capacity is: Does the grantor understand whether the proposed attorney has a genuine concern for his or her welfare, and does the grantor appreciate that he or she may need to rely on the attorney to make decisions?[50] The power of attorney for personal care can be revoked at any time, provided the grantor is mentally capable when he or she does so. The grantor must also have had the capacity to make decisions with respect to any instructions contained in the power of attorney for personal care.

The formalities for making a legally valid power of attorney for personal care in Ontario are not complicated, but should be carefully observed. Otherwise, there is a risk that the power of attorney might be declared invalid by a court. The power of attorney for personal care must be signed by the grantor in the presence of two witnesses, who cannot be any of the following: the proposed attorney or that person's spouse or partner; the grantor's spouse or partner; a child of the grantor, or a person that the grantor has treated as if that person were his or her child; someone whose own property is under a guardianship (this prevents a potentially incompetent person from being a witness); or a person under 18 years of age.[51]

Prior to March 1996, witnesses to the signing of a power of attorney for personal care could sign the document only if they had no reason to believe that the grantor was incapable of making the power of attorney or was incapable of giving the instructions provided in that document. They would then have been required to certify that they had no such belief. This certification is no longer required; it proved too stringent a requirement, and thus made finding willing, able witnesses difficult. In many health facilities, patients often make such powers of attorney on short notice and usually, members of the health care staff are called upon to witness the grantor's signature. Many had been reluctant to do so because in most cases, they were not qualified to form an opinion as to the grantor's capacity, or did not have sufficient opportunity to observe the grantor's behaviour and demeanour in order to form such an opinion. This hardship was drawn to the attention of the Ontario Legislature's Standing Committee on the Administration of Justice which, in hearings held in February 1996,[52] considered amendments to the *Consent to Treatment Act, 1992* and the *Substitute Decisions Act, 1992.* Consequently, the need for witnesses to certify that they had no reason to believe the grantor was incapable was eliminated. Likewise, the validation of the power of attorney for personal care is no longer required since the March 1996 amendments.

The power of attorney for personal care now takes effect to provide the attorney with full authority to make a decision respecting the grantor's personal care if the *Health Care Consent Act* authorizes the attorney to make the decision, or if the attorney has reasonable grounds to believe that the grantor is incapable of making the decision. This is subject to any contrary provisions in the document.[53] For such provisions to be legally effective, however, an assessor must certify, within 30 days of the signing of the document, that the grantor was capable when he or she signed it. In addition, the grantor must also sign a statement certifying that he or she understood the effect of these provisions, and that the power of attorney can be revoked (cancelled) only if, in the 30 days before the revocation, an assessor has made a statement that the grantor was capable when the revocation was signed and which sets out the facts on which the assessor has based that opinion.

The legislation allows maximum protection for the grantor. For example, the grantor has the right to request the attorney's assistance in arranging an assessment by an assessor who may be a physician, a psychologist, or a psychiatrist, as designated by government regulation to make such an assessment. The assessor is responsible for determining whether the grantor is in fact incapable with respect to some, if not all, treatment decisions. The attorney is not required to make such arrangements, however, if the person was assessed within six months prior to the request for an assessment.[54]

The *Substitute Decisions Act, 1992* also allows grantors to specify the method by which the person's capacity is to be determined. In addition, it may provide the attorney with the authority to use such reasonable force as is necessary to determine the grantor's capacity, to confirm whether the grantor is incapable of personal care, to take the grantor to any place of treatment, or admit the grantor to such place and detain and restrain him or her there for the duration of the treatment.[55]

Court-appointed Guardians of the Person

The second method of providing a substitute decision maker under the *Substitute Decisions Act* in Ontario is through an application to the court for the appointment of a guardian of the person.[56] This route is more difficult. In such an application, the court must consider whether there is an alternative course of action for making decisions that does not require the court to declare the applicant incapable of his or her own personal care. Such an alternative may be less restrictive of the patient's decision-making rights than appointing a guardian.[57] Thus, the legislation is aimed at encouraging alternatives to court proceedings in these matters.

Any person may bring the application for the appointment of a guardian, which conceivably might include the applicant's physician, a close friend, relative, spouse, partner, or any person who has an interest in the applicant's care. In any event, the appointed guardian cannot be someone who provides health care for compensation,[58] but may include the applicant's attorney for personal care. The exception to this is in a situation where there is no other suitable person who can act as guardian.[59] Such an appointment could expand the attorney's decision-making power over and above the authorization contained in the power of attorney for personal care. If it is made in a court order for full guardianship, it might include the power to determine the person's living arrangements, shelter, and safety; take charge of any lawsuits by or against the applicant; gain access to personal information about the applicant; make decisions about the applicant's health care, nutrition, and hygiene; give or refuse consent to medical treatment on the person's behalf pursuant to the *Health Care Consent Act, 1996;* make decisions about the applicant's employment, education, training, clothing, and recreation, and any other duties and powers specified in the order. In short, a full guardianship may (depending on the exact provisions of the court order) grant power to the guardian over all facets of the incapable person's life.

Before appointing a guardian, the court must find that the patient is in fact incapable according to the definition outlined above. The appointment of the guardian may be for a limited time, or may have such conditions attached to it as the court considers appropriate. In deciding the application, the court must consider (a) whether the proposed guardian is the attorney under a power of attorney, (b) the incapable person's wishes, to the extent that these can be ascertained, and (c) the closeness of the relationship between the person applying for the guardianship and the incapable person.

A partial guardianship order may be made when the court considers the patient incapable with respect to some, but not all, aspects of personal care and health. In such a case, the guardianship order will specify those matters in which the guardian has the power to make decisions, leaving other matters to the patient's own discretion. In this way, any court order can be tailored to be as unobtrusive as possible to the incapable patient's life, while still affording the protection of a competent guardian to make crucial decisions on his or her behalf.

Duties of Guardians and Attorneys for Personal Care[60]

The philosophy behind the law is to involve the incapable person in the process of consent to the greatest extent possible in the circumstances. This accords with the basic principle of autonomy, discussed in Chapter Two. Thus, both guardians and attorneys are required to exercise their powers diligently and in good faith, and to explain their powers and duties to the incapable person. His or her wishes, made while capable, must guide the guardian or attorney when faced with decisions relevant to these wishes. The guardian or attorney must make diligent efforts to ascertain the existence and substance of prior wishes. The most recent wish made while the person was capable must prevail over an earlier such wish. To determine these prior wishes, the guardian or attorney must take the incapable person's values and beliefs into account. In addition, the guardian must consider whether his or her decision is likely to improve the quality of the incapable person's life, prevent that quality of life from deteriorating, and reduce the extent to which (or rate at which) the person's quality of life is likely to deteriorate. Further, he or she must weigh the relative risks and benefits the person is expected to obtain from the decision against those that may arise from an alternative decision.

If it is not possible to make a decision in accordance with an incapable person's wish, or if such wishes or instructions cannot be determined, the guardian or attorney must make the decision in the person's best interests. The least restrictive and least intrusive course of action under the circumstances must be chosen and, in making any decision, the guardian should foster the incapable person's independence as far as possible. The guardian should involve the person to the greatest extent possible, and should likewise consult with the person's family, friends, and health care providers. Here, nurses caring for such patients have an opportunity to make their perspectives and views known and to contribute to the quality of care. Unlike attorneys for personal care, however, court-appointed guardians of the person must have written guardianship plans to which they must adhere. Guardians and attorneys are also required to maintain records of all decisions affecting the incapable person.

Manitoba and British Columbia

Manitoba's substitute decision-maker legislation, the *Health Care Directives Act*[61] (in force as of July 23, 1993), is fairly similar to that of Ontario. In Manitoba, the document signed by the grantor is called a **directive**, and the grantor is referred to as the maker of the directive. The person who is appointed to be the substitute decision maker is the **proxy**.

The Manitoba Act is silent on court-appointed guardians; however, this area is covered through other legislation. The directive need not be witnessed so long as the maker has signed it. However, the Manitoba Act does permit another person to sign for the maker in the maker's presence and in the presence of a witness. Neither the person who signs for the maker nor the witness may be nominated as proxies in the directive. This is intended to cover directives made by blind persons or others who, though mentally competent, are physically unable to sign the document.

British Columbia recently passed an *Adult Guardianship Act*[62] and a *Representation Agreement Act,*[63] which establish procedures respecting substitute decision making, similar to those of the Ontario and Manitoba statutes. The *Adult Guardianship Act* provides for the appointment of a guardian or substitute decision maker on behalf of the incapable person. Under the *Representation Agreement Act,* a competent adult also has the right to appoint a substitute decision maker (called a representative) to make treatment and care decisions on his or her behalf. The document making the appointment is called a representation agreement, which must be signed by the patient's representative (unlike Ontario's or Manitoba's legislation). The signatures of each party to the agreement must be witnessed by two persons. The representative of the incapable person is also supervised by a monitor whose duty it is to ensure that the representative carries out all his or her obligations under the agreement and in accordance with the wishes of the incapable person (as expressed when he or she was capable). British Columbia's legislation is similar to Ontario's, but was not yet in force at the time of writing.

British Columbia has also recently passed the *Health Care (Consent) and Care Facility (Admission) Act,*[64] which codifies much of the law on informed consent and is broadly similar to Ontario's *Consent to Treatment Act, 1992.* As was formerly the case in Ontario, the British Columbia legislation provides for the participation of an "advocacy organization" on behalf of an incapable person, but at a later stage. In British Columbia, an advocate becomes involved only if major treatment (e.g., surgery, major diagnostic testing or investigation) is contemplated, and then only if other substitute decision makers (such as the person's spouse, including same-sex spouses, or a child, parent, or other relative) dispute among themselves what treatment should be administered.

British Columbia's legislation also provides for consent to admission to a health care facility only upon acceptance of a proposal from the institution outlining the activities and programs that are offered and its treatment policies. A substitute decision maker may accept such a proposal on behalf of an incapable person. No person may be admitted to a facility in British Columbia without acceptance of such a proposal.

Other Provinces and Territories

Several other Canadian jurisdictions, notably Newfoundland, Prince Edward Island, Saskatchewan, and the Yukon Territory, have also recently passed legislation respecting advance directives.[65] Of these, only PEI's legislation actually codifies the law respecting consent to treatment as does Ontario's *Health Care Consent Act, 1996*. The statutes of the other three jurisdictions only purport to deal with substitute decision makers and advance directives provided by subsequently incapable persons. The PEI statue, interestingly, makes legal any advance directive made before the law was passed.[66] This acknowledges that the practice of making so-called living wills arose before the law had a chance to catch up with societal change. The directive in PEI can set out the maker's wishes with respect to treatment, or may be limited simply to appointing a proxy, or it may do both.

The PEI statute, like Ontario's, sets out what does and does not constitute treatment under that Act. Included in this list are: an examination or assessment conducted under PEI's *Adult Protection Act, Mental Health Act, Public Health Act, Public Trustee Act,* or any other statute respecting capacity or guardianship of the person; the assessment or examination of a person to determine his or her general health and condition; the taking of a person's health history; the communication of an assessment or diagnosis; the admission of a person to a hospital or other facility; a personal assistance service; a treatment posing little or no risk of harm; counselling that is primarily in the nature of advice, education, or motivation; and any other act prescribed by regulation. The provisions in this statute are subject to any contrary provisions in the *Mental Health Act* and the *Public Health Act* of PEI.

PEI's statute sets out specific "consent rights," including the right to give or refuse treatment on any grounds, including moral and religious grounds, even if the person's death results as a consequence.[67] A person is also permitted to have a trusted adviser, referred to as an "associate," to assist him or her, and has the right to select the practitioner and form of treatment on any grounds. The provisions respecting the giving of consent and prohibitions on administering treatment without consent are similar to Ontario's. The requirements for determining capacity and whether consent is informed are also similar; however, a person may waive the right in writing to receive information as to the nature of the proposed treatment.[68] In determining capacity, a health practitioner must inform the patient of his or her right to the assistance of an associate, and must take into account the associate's assistance.

PEI also provides for specific persons to act as substitute decision makers in decreasing order of priority, as is the case in Ontario.[69] The order is quite similar to Ontario's legislation, save for the lack of any provision for a "partner," although farther down the list, mention is made of "a person whom the health practitioner considers to be the patient's trusted friend with close knowledge of the person's wishes."[70] A substitute decision maker is not authorized by the Act to give consent to electric shock therapy, the removal of non-regenerative tissue from the patient, an abortion except in cases where there is likely immediate danger to the life or health of the patient, sterilization not medically necessary for the protection of the patient's health, or a procedure whose primary purpose is research except where the research is for the patient's own benefit. This is somewhat different from Ontario's legislation, which does allow consent to electric shock therapy where consent is required under the *Health Care Consent Act, 1996.*

In most other respects, PEI's legislation is quite similar to Ontario's, but it does not provide for a Consent Capacity Board. In Both Ontario and PEI, health practitioners acting on the basis of an apparently valid consent are shielded from legal liability for their actions. Neither is a substitute decision maker or associate (in PEI) liable for a decision made while acting in good faith and in accordance with the law. "Good faith" means that the person must have an honestly held belief that the patient is either capable of giving an informed consent, or incapable of doing so, and acts appropriately.

While in Ontario two persons must witness the making of a power of attorney for personal care, only one witness is required in PEI. A complaint with respect to the proxy in PEI may be filed with a public official designated by the Minister of Health and Social Services by any interested person.[71] A proxy cannot delegate the authority to make decisions to anyone else. Further, a decision by a proxy under an advance directive takes precedence over a decision made by a court or any other person, including a guardian, unless the directive provides otherwise. A directive made outside PEI is still valid in that province if it meets the requirements of the PEI legislation, or accords with the laws of the province (or other country) where it was made (and the maker was habitually resident in that other province or country).

Saskatchewan's *Health Care Directives and Substitute Health Care Decision Makers Act* is fairly similar to the other Acts described above, but does not purport to codify completely the common law relating to informed consent.[72] It provides for the making of health care directives in a similar manner. It is notable in its provision that it does not authorize a decision, in a directive, by a proxy or guardian (which is prohibited by criminal law), or the use of a directive to consent to active euthanasia or assisted suicide. Given the recent decision involving Robert Latimer in Saskatchewan,[73] this provision sends a strong message respecting that province's view of this matter.

In Saskatchewan, the proxy must be an adult, that is, a person over the age of 18 years. However, the maker of a health care directive may be anyone who is capable and over 16 years of age. As in PEI, only one witness is required to the making of a health care directive.

The legislation in the Yukon Territory is also fairly similar to that of other provinces.[74] It provides that a regular power of attorney becomes an "enduring power of attorney" if it is in writing, signed by its donor, dated, and contains a provision that it is to continue in force after the donor's incapacity or is to take effect at such time.[75] The Yukon statute also provides that certain notes on the enduring power of attorney be included in it. These notes relate to the donor's appreciation of the nature of the document, the powers it grants to the attorney, when it takes effect, and when (and under what circumstances) it can be cancelled. A lawyer must attest in writing that the donor understands the document, was competent when he or she signed it, and was an adult, and that the power was given freely and voluntarily. The legislation does not explicitly set out what powers or restrictions may be contained in the enduring power of attorney. The attorney is prohibited from renouncing his or her appointment once it has taken effect without the permission of the court. Consent to treatment in the Yukon Territory is dealt with under that territory's *Health Act,* insofar as the attorney as substitute decision maker is concerned. Newfoundland's statute is similar to that of the remaining jurisdictions.

Summary

This chapter has focussed on the ethical and legal foundations of consent and has given examples to clarify their application in practice. Many challenges exist for nurses seeking to protect their clients' autonomy: advances in technology, the complexities within the health care system, constantly changing legislation, increasing emphasis on individual choice, and concerns regarding potential litigation, to name but a few. Further, legislation pertaining to consent is constantly being revised to achieve a balance between respecting client choice and protecting people from harm.

Consent policies, rules, and legislation are very much based on the principle of autonomy, which recognizes that a capable and competent individual is free to determine and act in accordance with a self-chosen plan. Other equally important ethical principles, such as beneficence and non-maleficence, that nurses must consider, at times may compete with this principle (as suggested in the case study in Chapter Four).

Each clinical environment or institution in which nurses work needs to establish nursing guidelines relative to consent. Processes should be in place, such as ethics committees, to assist nurses and other members of the team to deal with problematic cases. Ongoing education, peer review, and continuous quality improvement are necessary to ensure that our standards are constantly high.

There are many complex dynamics involved in dealing with ill, vulnerable patients. Nurses must take seriously their role in caring for and supporting these clients, and protecting them from harm.

The key points introduced in this chapter include:

- the foundation of consent in law and ethics
- the principle of autonomy and its role in consent
- the concept of competence or capacity
- the tort of battery
- the concept of informed consent
- the various types of, and approaches to, consent
- the rights of patients to refuse consent to medical or health care
- the nurse's role in ensuring that informed consent takes place
- how the legal rules and ethical theory apply to hypothetical case studies and real case law
- consent challenges with respect to the incompetent adult and to children
- professional responsibilities in emergency situations
- the concept of proxy or substitute consent
- existing new and impending consent legislation in the various provinces.

Critical Thinking

These case studies are for further reflection, discussion, and analysis. As you review each case, consider the following questions as well as those specific to the case.

1. Have the nurses in these cases violated any ethical or legal standards?
2. If so what are these standards?
3. Is there risk of any civil or criminal liability?
4. How could these situations have been prevented?

CASE STUDY: OLD ENOUGH TO CHOOSE?

Ronnie is a 13-year-old girl with acute lymphocytic leukemia, presently in the paediatric unit of a large tertiary cancer centre. Her leukemia was diagnosed when she was eight, at which time she had several rounds of chemotherapy. She was successful in achieving a remission, but as her form of leukemia was severe the team asked her parents to consider a bone marrow transplant. Her brother, Robert, two years older than she, was a perfect match. The bone marrow retrieval was scary for Robert, as it required a general anaesthetic and he experienced much pain afterwards. However, his pain and suffering was nothing like Ronnie's. In preparation for the transplant she received additional high doses of chemotherapy and underwent total body radiation. A short time after the transplant, the new marrow started to reject her body (graft versus host disease).

Ronnie recovered, and the last five years have been great for her. Now, however, she has relapsed. The team is proposing more chemo, and possibly another transplant.

Francine is Ronnie's primary nurse; they have known each other since the beginning of Ronnie's illness. Ronnie tells Francine that, although she knows her parents favour more treatment, she herself is tired and has "had enough." Further, two friends whom she met in hospital underwent similar treatment, and ultimately died anyway. Although Ronnie wants only to go home and spend time with her family and friends, she plans to go ahead with the treatment because she does not wish to upset her parents.

QUESTIONS

1. What are Francine's responsibilities to Ronnie?
2. Is Ronnie old enough and competent to make this choice? Would her parents be able to overrule her decision?

CASE STUDY: AN INFORMED DECISION?

Elizabeth is an 86-year-old Hungarian woman who is followed regularly by a nurse practitioner, Nori, who works within a family practice unit. Elizabeth came to Canada with her husband in 1956. They had had an unsettling time during the Second World War and the subsequent revolution in Hungary. They looked forward to a new life in Canada and ultimately became very successful. Elizabeth's husband died about 10 years ago; she now lives alone in a condominium, but is visited regularly by her children and grandchildren.

Elizabeth has just shared with Nori reports from recent studies undertaken on her gall bladder. Elizabeth has some narrowing of her bile duct, and the surgeons are recommending dilatation under laparoscopy. Elizabeth has declined. She has survived for 86 years without surgery and doesn't want to break her "record." She would prefer to "take her chances."

Nori is concerned. She knows the procedure is straightforward, and that without it, Elizabeth will experience pain, and may possibly become septic. Elizabeth is otherwise healthy, and this decision could affect the quality of her life.

QUESTIONS

1. Should Nori try to convince Elizabeth to go ahead with the procedure? What should she do?
2. Do you think Elizabeth is making a competent decision? What are her legal rights?

QUESTIONS FOR DISCUSSION

1. Identify 10 nursing interventions where the patient/client's consent is implied.
2. In what circumstances should nursing interventions require a more explicit consent?
3. Provide some examples where the principle of beneficence is in conflict with the person's right to chose. How might this dilemma be resolved?
4. Your patient is about to go for surgery for an exploratory laparotomy. He has received his pre-operative teaching and was seen by the surgeon the evening before. The family has come a long distance to be with him the morning of his surgery. It is only after you give him the pre-operative sedation that you notice the actual consent form has not been signed. What would you do? What would be the practice in your facility if this were to occur?
5. Should parents be permitted to give or refuse consent for their children regardless of the circumstances? Why or why not? Should the child's best interests govern? Are there any legal avenues open to ensuring that the child's best interests are considered?
6. It is a busy evening, and one of your elderly, confused patients is restless and keeps trying to climb over the bed rails. You believe your only option to pro-tect this patient is to restrain her. As you prepare to do this, the patient—appearing lucid for the moment—states she wishes simply to sit up in the chair. She says she doesn't want to be tied down. What do you do?
7. You are a nurse in the obstetrical wing of a busy teaching hospital. A woman comes in for a pelvic examination under general anaesthetic a few days prior to her due date. A young nursing student comes to ask whether he can observe the examination. What do you tell the patient? Can you assume the patient knows that such students will observe procedures as part of their training? What are the risks of proceeding without properly informing the patient and obtaining her consent?

References

1. [1980] 2 SCR 880; (1980) 14 CCLT 1; 114 DLR (3d) 1; 33 NR 361.
2. (1990), 72 OR (2d) 417 (CA), aff'g. 63 OR (3d) 243; 47 DLR (4th) 18; 43 CCLT 62 (HCJ).
3. Ibid., p. 419.
4. Ibid., p. 432.
5. Ibid., p. 434.
6. [1993] 2 SCR 119, aff'g. (1991), 44 OAC 385; 76 DLR (4th) 449; 5 CCLT (2d) 221 (CA), aff'g. (1987), 7 ACWS (3d) 51 (Ont. HCJ).
7. Ibid., per Cory J., p. 123 (SCR).
8. Supra footnote 1.
9. Supra footnote 6, p. 139.

10. This is a formulation suggested by G. Sharpe (1986), *The law and medicine in Canada* (2nd ed., p. 77). Toronto: Butterworths.
11. Ibid.
12. Infra footnote 13.
13. *Substitute Decisions Act, 1992*, SO 1992, c. 30, as amended by SO 1994, c. 27, sections 43(2), 62; SO 1996, c. 2, sections 3–60; *Health Care Consent Act, 1996*, SO 1996, c. 2, Sched. A. *The Consent to Treatment Act, 1992* was repealed and replaced by the *Health Care Consent Act, 1996*.
14. *Quebec Civil Code*, article 15.
15. Ibid., article 16, paragraph 1.
16. *Health Care Consent Act, 1996*, supra footnote 13, section 1(c)(iii).
17. Quebec *Civil Code*, article 14, paragraph 2.
18. Ibid., article 16, paragraph 2.
19. Supra footnote 13.
20. Ibid.
21. Ibid., *Health Care Consent Act, 1996*, section 7.
22. Ibid., section 10(1).
23. Ibid., sections 2(1) "personal assistance service," 4(1).
24. Ibid., section 11.
25. Ibid., section 11(3).
26. Ibid., section 4.
27. Ibid., section 15.
28. Ibid., section 16.
29. Ibid., section 17.
30. Ibid., section 18.
31. Ibid., section 19.
32. Ibid., sections 18(4), 25(1).
33. The *Advocacy Act, 1992*, SO 1992, c. 26, which provided for rights advisers as patient advocates, was repealed when the *Health Care Consent Act, 1996* came into force.
34. *Health Care Consent Act, 1996*, supra footnote 13, section 20.
35. Ibid., section 21(2).
36. Ibid., section 20(1), (3).
37. A "partner" is defined in section 20(9) of the *Health Care Consent Act, 1996* as one with whom the incapable person has lived for at least one year and with whom he or she has a close personal relationship of primary importance to both their lives. This would apply to homosexual couples.
38. *Health Care Consent Act, 1996*, supra footnote 13, section 20(2).
39. Ibid., section 20(6).
40. Ibid., section 25(5).
41. Ibid., section 26.
42. *Mental Health Act*, RSO 1990, c. M.7.
43. *Substitute Decisions Act*, supra footnote 13, sections 43 and 44.
44. Ibid., section 45.
45. Ibid., section 46(1).
46. The term "attorney" is not used in this legislation in the sense commonly understood to mean "a lawyer." The person appointed as attorney need not be a lawyer, and his or her office, as such, should not be confused with that of a lawyer who is a practising member of the provincial bar.
47. Supra footnote 37.
48. *Substitute Decisions Act, 1992*, as amended, Supra footnote 13, section 46(3).
49. Ibid., section 46(2).
50. Ibid., section 47(1).
51. Ibid., sections 10(1), (2), and 48(2).
52. Ontario Standing Committee on the Administration of Justice, hearings, *Hansard*, February 1996.

53. *Substitute Decisions Act,* supra footnote 13, section 49, as amended.
54. Ibid., section 55(1), as amended.
55. Ibid., section 59(3).
56. Ibid., section 55(1).
57. Ibid., section 55(2).
58. Ibid., section 57(1), as amended.
59. Ibid., section 57(2.1).
60. Ibid., sections 66 to 68, as amended.
61. *Health Care Directives Act,* SM 1992, c. 33, CCSM, c. H27.
62. RSBC 1996, c. 6, not yet in force.
63. RSBC 1996, c. 405, not yet in force.
64. RSBC 1996, c. 181.
65. *Newfoundland: Advanced Health Care Directives and Substitute Health Care Decision Makers Act,* SN 1995, c. A-4.1; Prince Edward Island: *Consent to Treatment and Health Care Directives Act,* SPEI 1996, c. 10; Saskatchewan: *The Health Care Directives and Substitute Health Care Decision Makers Act,* SS 1997, c. H-0.001; and Yukon Territory: *Enduring Power of Attorney Act,* SYT 1995, c. 8.
66. Ibid., PEI statute, section 1(e) "directive."
67. Ibid., section 4.
68. Ibid., section 6.
69. Ibid., section 11(1).
70. Ibid., section 11(1)(f).
71. Ibid., section 27.
72. Saskatchewan Act, supra footnote 64.
73. *R v. Latimer (1997),* 121 CCC (3d) 226 (Sask. QB).
74. Yukon Act, supra footnote 64.
75. Ibid., section 3(1).

Ethical and Legal Issues at the Extremes of the Life Continuum

LEARNING OBJECTIVES

The purpose of this chapter is to enable you to:
- understand recent advances in reproductive science and technology
- appreciate the legal, social, and ethical dimensions that arise out of these advances
- appreciate some of the legal and ethical issues surrounding death and the process of dying
- distinguish among the legal definitions of death, euthanasia, and assisted suicide
- articulate the legal and ethical issues surrounding tissue donation and organ transplantation
- understand the legal and ethical implications of withdrawal of treatment
- appreciate the use and legality of advance directives (living wills)
- consider some possible redefinitions of death.

Introduction

Some of the most challenging ethical, legal, and emotional issues in health care today are associated with the beginning and the end of the life process. Recent, extraordinary advances in medical technology have made it possible to manipulate the reproductive process at one end of the life continuum and, at the other, to extend life in cases where death would once have been certain. Traditionally, we have been awed by birth and fearful of death. These remain life's greatest mysteries.

Is it better to be born than never to exist? Is it the right of every human being to have a child? If so, does that right extend to control over the characteristics and attributes of our children? Reproductive and genetic technologies now exist that can overcome infertility, eliminate genetic anomalies, and manipulate and control the characteristics of the children produced. This power to manipulate the creation of life has the potential to reshape our society and to redefine future generations.

Nurses who work in settings where these technologies are used face profound social, psychological, and emotional issues, and are challenged to question their own values and beliefs about life and the creative process. Nurses in other areas, such as neonatal intensive care, may struggle with the consequences of these technologies when caring for increasing numbers of premature infants and multiple-offspring births. As there are many divergent perspectives on reproductive technologies, it is important for nurses to understand a broad spectrum of views.

Our fear of death has led to a heavy emphasis on finding ways to extend life at all costs. Yet, there is also a cost when extending life diminishes the quality and dignity that give life meaning. When a person dies in hospital—for example, in an Intensive Care Unit—the very technology that extends life may distance caregivers from the person. Indeed, he or she may ultimately die in isolation. In such a setting, nurses are challenged to find new ways to preserve people's autonomy and dignity. In assisting the dying patient, we must afford that person as much comfort, respect, and freedom from anxiety and pain as possible. Special consideration must be given to the needs of the family or significant others in coping with their impending and subsequent loss.[1]

In a multicultural society such as Canada's, patients come from many religious and cultural backgrounds, and will view the process of dying and death from these varying perspectives. Nurses must be sensitive to these differences and respectful of individuals' values and beliefs.

This chapter will examine the complex ethical and legal issues that relate to both extremes of the life continuum: reproductive technologies, and death and dying.

Reproductive Technologies

Over the past decade, significant scientific and technological advances have been made in the area of reproductive technologies. In fact, many of these have been available for some time, such as techniques in fertility control, management of labour and childbirth, and screening procedures to monitor foetal development.[2]

Fertility control includes methods to prevent conception or implantation of embryos, as well as to terminate pregnancy—for example, the diaphragm, the intra-uterine device, the condom, sterilization, abortion, and contraceptive drugs such as "the pill."[3]

In recent decades, the management of labour and childbirth has moved from the home to the hospital setting. Giving birth was once a family-oriented process in which the mother was assisted by female relatives, friends, or midwives; today, the medical model places childbirth in the control of physicians and other health professionals. Technologies that have been developed to control the process of labour and delivery include forceps deliveries, caesarian sections, induced labour, and monitoring of the foetal heart rate.[4]

Indeed, foetal development can now be monitored from the very early stages of pregnancy. A majority of women now undergo ultrasound at some point during their pregnancy; high-risk and older pregnant women often experience amniocentesis. The purpose of these procedures is to identify defects in the foetus early in development, either to facilitate a decision regarding the termination of a pregnancy or to take action to correct problems or to prevent complications.[5]

Newer Technologies

Among the most controversial new reproductive technologies are those aimed at promoting pregnancy by overcoming or bypassing infertility. While many hitherto infertile couples have embraced these techniques, the options available raise profound social, legal, ethical, and emotional questions. These technologies have thrust us into previously uncharted territory, related to the creation of life itself.

The need for these technologies stems from the basic human desire—or powerful cultural pressures—to procreate.[6] Infertile couples or individuals seem prepared to accept the physical, psychological, and emotional risks associated with these interventions for the sake of having a child, even though the chances of success are still quite low.[7] With an increase in the incidence of sexually transmitted disease,[8] and with today's tendency for couples to marry late (after their careers are established), infertility problems have increased. Pelvic inflammatory disease (PID; a consequence of sexually transmitted diseases) often results in blocked fallopian tubes, a major cause of infertility in women. Even in healthy females, fertility diminishes after the age of 30.[9] The incidence of infertility in Canada (8.5%) affects approximately 500 000 people between the ages of 18 and 44.[10]

The birth of the first "test-tube" baby, Louise Brown, in 1978 heralded the beginning of the proliferation of reproductive innovations, including **donor insemination (DI), assisted insemination (AI), in vitro fertilization (IVF), cryopreservation, ovum and embryo donation,** and **surrogacy.** Advanced genetic technologies have also developed that include sex selection, embryo research, prenatal diagnosis, and human embryo cloning.

There are varying views on whether infertility is a disease (and therefore a medical condition), or whether its influences are primarily social in nature.

Infertility as a Medical Condition

This view associates infertility with a medical problem, related to a dysfunction of the body, specifically, the reproductive system. From this perspective, infertility is an important health issue requiring medical solutions, especially infertility treatments,[11] to "fix" the problem.

Infertility as a Social Condition

Infertile couples seeking assisted reproduction have a strong desire to have a child as closely related to them, genetically, as possible.[12] This view holds that the desire or need to have children is socially constructed or influenced. The stigma and emotional pain experienced by infertile couples results from the strong pressure placed on married couples, and most especially women, to bear children.[13]

Descriptions of some of the newer developments in reproductive technologies follow.

Therapeutic Donor Insemination

Therapeutic donor insemination (TDI) is the oldest form of assisted reproduction available. Sperm from healthy donors (often students, who are paid a fee) are introduced into the fertile woman's uterus. This approach is used when the male partner is infertile, or when a single woman, or a lesbian couple, wants a child without association with the biological father. Sperm donors are required to undergo extensive screening for infection and genetic disease. The program is totally anonymous: donors and recipients know nothing about one another.[14]

A similar procedure may also be used when the male partner has a low sperm count; thus, a process to concentrate sperm is necessary for conception to occur. When the male partner's sperm is used, the technique is called assisted insemination (AI). AI may also be an option for couples if the male partner has to undergo treatment/therapy that may cause infertility, an unfortunate side effect of some chemotherapy and radiation treatments. Here the sperm may be frozen (cryopreserved) for later use.[15]

Donor insemination (DI) technologies raise ethical questions associated with confidentiality, disclosure, screening, and the nature of relationships. Presently, the donor insemination process is confidential. Advocates for this approach suggest that the numbers of donors would decrease if donors' identities were to be revealed to the recipients and their children. Other concerns arise associated with disclosure to the child regarding the nature of the conception, and questions about the identity of the biological father, especially if subsequent medical problems of a hereditary nature arise. In the case of freezing sperm for later use, what happens if the male partner dies? Who owns the sperm? Should they be destroyed, or does the female partner have the right to use them for the purpose of conception? There is great debate about these questions, but little consensus on their resolution.

In Vitro Fertilization

In vitro fertilization (IVF) was developed to overcome various physical problems associated with infertility that do not respond to traditional forms of artificial insemination. These conditions include mechanical obstructions resulting from damaged or absent fallopian tubes, endometriosis, intractable ovulatory problems, unexplained infertility, and some forms of male infertility resulting in low sperm count.[16]

IVF is a process whereby fertilization occurs outside the body and without intimate contact. The procedure involves a series of interventions that include the use of drugs to hyperstimulate the ovaries to produce excess eggs, followed by the laparoscopic aspiration of these eggs with the guidance of ultrasound. The retrieved eggs are then mixed with the partner's (or donor's) sperm in a petrie dish in the laboratory. After approximately 48 h, about three of the successfully fertilized eggs (embryos) are transferred into the woman's uterus. The remaining embryos may be cryopreserved and, if necessary, used at a later date, although this practice raises questions about what to do with any remaining frozen embryos.[17]

Cryopreservation

The number of embryos transplanted into the uterus is usually limited to three, in order to maximize the rate of success and to limit the risk of multiple births. Any additional embryos are usually maintained in liquid nitrogen for future use, if necessary. This minimizes the need for further invasive procedures that are involved in the retrieval of eggs, and reduces costs. Most programs limit the duration of storage, either based on a certain number of years, the onset of a client's menopause, or the break-up of a relationship. However, only about 50% of embryos survive the thawing process.[18] Sperm can also be frozen for future use.

Egg Donation

This is a variation of IVF used to enable pregnancies in women with normal uteruses but non-functioning ovaries. The eggs are donated from healthy, usually younger, donors, who undergo ovarian stimulation, or from women with normal functioning ovaries who are participating in the IVF program. The recipient undergoes the transfer component of the process once the partner's (or donor's) sperm fertilizes the egg.[19] The donor may be known to the recipient or may be part of an anonymous donor program.

Embryo Donation

Since cryopreservation techniques now enable the freezing of embryos for use in the future, dilemmas arise out of what to do with these when they are no longer needed or wanted by the couple. There is apparently a growing inventory of surplus embryos. The options are to destroy them, to use them for research purposes, or to donate them to other couples.[20]

When is there a need for embryo donation? This option may be desirable when neither partner is fertile but the woman has sufficient uterine capacity for pregnancy and childbirth. It may also be an option for older, single women who are no longer producing eggs, for lesbian couples for whom sperm donation has not worked, and for couples who cannot afford IVF or egg donation.[21]

A number of ethical issues arise out of the question of whether embryo donation or "adoption" should be considered for couples where both partners are infertile. Unique ethical issues relate to whether the process should be treated similarly to adoption, with similar legal processes, screening, and rules. For example, should recipients undergo the same social and psychological testing to ensure they are fit parents?[22] Further questions relate to whether the donor couple should be informed about the outcome (positive or negative) of the donation, and whether their anonymity should be maintained.[23]

Gestational Surrogacy

Surrogate or gestational mothers bear a child for another couple or individual. The gestational mother may be the biological mother (through sperm donation of either the male partner or a donor), or may carry the embryo of the couple, an embryo donated by another couple, or one created from a donor egg and donor sperm. This approach may be considered when infertile couples have experienced multiple failures with IVF, or when the woman has a medical condition that limits pregnancy, an anatomical condition that causes repeated spontaneous abortions, or has undergone a hysterectomy.[24]

Though surrogacy is not a technology itself, the many possible approaches to it raise complex ethical and emotional issues. These arise from the sheer number of parties involved (the infant, the surrogate mother, the infertile couple, society as a whole). Other issues related to surrogacy involve concerns regarding the surrogates' own reproductive future, producing offspring with whom they will not be involved; the appropriateness of the recipients to raise the child; the process of informed consent; and the possibility of coercion, especially when financial remuneration is a factor.[25]

The following case study highlights only a few of the complex ethical issues associated with reproductive technologies.

Parenthood—a right or a privilege?

Marion is a 30-year-old woman with cystic fibrosis who is involved in a lesbian relationship with Sandra, 15 years her senior. They would like to have a child. Sandra has been tested and determined to be infertile. Though Marion is fertile, her medical condition places her at high risk during pregnancy and delivery.

Sandra is a successful lawyer, and Marion inherited some money from her parents. Since the couple can afford the technology, they present themselves at an infertility clinic, where they are interviewed by a nurse and an infertility specialist.

Marion and Sandra ask for IVF. They would like eggs from Marion's ovaries to be retrieved and fertilized by donor semen. Once there is successful fertilization, they would like the embryos transplanted into Sandra's healthy uterus. Since Marion is concerned about passing on the genes for cystic fibrosis, they also request genetic testing on the embryos, and the destruction of any having those characteristics.

Issues

1. What kind of counselling and advice would you give this couple?
2. What ethical and social questions does this case raise for you?
3. What are the rights of the various parties: the couple, the nurse and physician, the potential donor, and the offspring?

Discussion

This case highlights the extent of ethical challenges associated with this new science. On the surface it would appear that only good can result from this couple's request. They would have the privilege of parenthood, and the resulting child or children would have the opportunity of life. Yet, a number of questions have raised debate in this area.

What are the rights of the two women in this case study? Is procreation a right or a privilege? What are the rights of the potential child? Should criteria be established to screen potential parents? Should this couple's status as lesbians be a factor? What about the fact that one parent, Sandra, is older, and that Marion is likely to have a short life expectancy because of her disease? Should the donor have any say relative to potential recipients of his sperm? What should Sandra and Marion tell their child, or children, when asked about the biological father? Should the donor process remain private and anonymous? Is it fair that this technology is available only to affluent people? Should health professionals be using genetic technology to screen out abnormalities such as cystic fibrosis, or further, to manipulate physical characteristics such as sex, or hair and eye colour? (People with even minor disabilities are concerned about the negative social attitudes that may emerge as we attempt to create "perfect" humans.) Is it right to destroy defective embryos? Who would be the

legal mother of this child? Who would have custody if the two women separated? What should be done with the surplus embryos? If the couple chose to
donate them, should the recipients be told about the potential for genetic
abnormalities? If the embryos produced an abnormal child, would Marion and
the medical team bear any legal liability? Would that child have the right to
know about his or her origins and other siblings?

   The issues that arise from these technologies are endless. The answers are
not clear. The potential impact on future generations is daunting.

New Reproductive and Genetic Technologies: Setting Boundaries, Enhancing Health

A Royal Commission on New Reproductive Technologies was initiated in 1989
to examine the social, medical, legal, ethical, economic, and research implications of these new technologies.[26] The mandate of the Royal Commission,
which issued its final report in November 1993, was to recommend policies
and safeguards, and to direct special attention to the implications for
women's reproductive health and well-being and the prevention of infertility.[27] The Royal Commission made 293 recommendations that focussed on the
prevention of infertility, the management of assisted reproduction, sex selection for non-medical reasons, prenatal diagnosis techniques and gene
therapy, judicial interventions in pregnancy and birth, and the use of foetal
tissue.[28]

   In response to the report, the federal government established a moratorium on the use of specific practices, established an advisory committee, and
proposed a legislative framework intended to "protect the health and safety
of Canadians, ensure the appropriate treatment of human reproductive materials and ... protect the dignity and security of all persons, especially women
and children."[29] The strategy was to manage reproductive and genetic technologies through a plan that would prohibit unacceptable technologies and
develop a legislated regulatory process to manage technologies deemed
acceptable.[30]

   The moratorium announced in July 1995 focussed on nine problematic
areas.[31] The following practices were proposed to be prohibited:

- sex selection for non-medical purposes;
- buying and selling of eggs, sperm, and embryos;
- germ-line genetic alterations;
- ectogenesis (maintaining an embryo in an artificial womb);
- cloning of human embryos;
- creation of animal–human hybrids;
- retrieval of sperm or eggs from cadavers or foetuses for fertilization and
  implantation, or research involving the maturation of sperm or eggs
  outside the body;
- commercial preconception or surrogacy arrangements.

In the proposed legislative framework, additional practices were added:[32]

- transfer of embryos between human and other species;
- use of human sperm, eggs, or embryos for assisted reproduction or research without the informed consent of the donors;
- research on human embryos 14 days or more after conception;
- creation of embryos for research;
- offering to provide or to pay for prohibited services.

In June 1996, bill C-47 was introduced in the House of Commons.[33] While it did not progress farther than the first-reading stage, it included the foregoing prohibitions. The government once again reintroduced these in the form of amendments to the *Criminal Code of Canada*. At the time of writing, they had been introduced at first reading and were not yet law.

Given this legislative vacuum, it would not, strictly speaking, be illegal to perform any of these acts, since there is currently no criminal sanction against these practices. It is hoped that these prohibitions will soon become law; otherwise, serious ethical and legal dilemmas will ensue. These practices will be difficult to change once they are established.

Ethical Perspectives

Feminist Views

Reproductive technologies are primarily practised on women's bodies and have implications for women's reproductive autonomy; thus, they are of strong interest to feminist thinkers. Feminists argue that the focus of the related ethical discussions has been too narrow, avoiding the broader social implications of these technologies' introduction.[34] According to Sherwin, a Canadian feminist, these practices must be evaluated "within the broader scheme of oppressive social structures."[35] She argues the need to explore the possibility that new approaches to reproduction will bring about "profound cultural change" and that their social, political, and economic effects also need to be evaluated.[36] The lower social and economic status of many women may make them susceptible to the risks associated with reproductive technologies (especially the high risk of failure, and the unknown future effects of the drugs used to hyperstimulate the ovaries). We need also to evaluate those social influences that contribute to the expectations placed on people, especially women, to procreate. Although the intention of these technologies is to give couples or individuals the right to reproductive choice, some feminists are concerned that, in practice, the actual control will belong to others, specifically the male-dominated medical profession.[37]

Additional concerns arise from the potential to commercialize and, therefore, commodify women's reproduction. This possibility was underlined by the placement of an advertisement in a University of Toronto newspaper a few years ago, seeking a white female, between the ages of 23 and 32, who was willing to donate her eggs for money. This ad was published in spite of the moratorium established by the Royal Commission. In fact, the going rate for egg donors in the United States in 1995 was about US$2400.[38]

Implications for Children

A number of known and unknown risks exist for the children who are produced through reproductive technologies. Thirty percent of IVF deliveries are multiple births; thus, these babies are at high risk for low birth weight or problems during delivery.[39] Further, little is known regarding the long-term effects on the children of the drugs used throughout the procedure.

The future holds legal uncertainties regarding family relationships, since there may be situations where the legal parenthood of the child is unclear, or is challenged. Inheritance, custody, access, and support issues may be raised in future years.[40]

Most parents choose to keep their use of DI secret from family members, friends, and the child, who is usually presented as the biological offspring of both social parents. This practice has been encouraged in the past by many infertility programs.[41] This conspiracy of silence means that many children born as a result of assisted reproduction do not even know the circumstances of their birth.[42]

With regard to sperm donors, the present practice is to maintain the anonymity of the donor with regard to the recipient parents and the child. Thus, if children conceived in this manner were made aware of the circumstances of their birth, they would not (as is the case with adoption) be able to find or contact their biological fathers. Anonymity is usually a factor in a male's decision to donate semen. There might be many legal and emotional difficulties for future donors if this practice were to change.[43]

Consent

As we saw in Chapter Six, informed consent requires that the client be totally informed of all material risks and benefits and that the process be free from coercion. Factors influencing consent in the area of reproductive technologies include the emotional nature of the process, and the psychological effects on both recipients and donors. This is especially important when surrogates or donors are friends or relatives. They may be subjected to personal pressures to participate. Full disclosure of all risks and uncertainties related to the procedures must be provided to recipients and to donors.

Financial Incentives

A major concern, for feminist thinkers in particular, is the potential exploitation of poor and middle-class women as breeders for the upper class.[44] Feminists note that, while women now can make their own reproductive choices, they are still forced to make these decisions under social conditions that remain controlled by men, and that stress the importance of female fertility.

Presently there is no payment to female egg donors, although typically they are not required to bear the costs of the procedures. Ironically, men have long been paid for semen donation—a far less invasive procedure. Defenders of this practice claim that payment only covers expenses, and that without such payment, the rate of donation would decrease.

Many current reproductive technologies are expensive and are not covered by the Canadian health care system. Thus, they are limited to those who are able to pay, creating inequity of access.[45] Further, concerns may arise in the area of embryo donation when the decision to donate may be influenced by the prohibitive costs associated with cryopreservation.[46]

Psychological Impact

What must be remembered is that reproductive technologies are new, evolving, and imperfect. Success rates are low, leaving potential parents at risk for feelings of extreme loss and grief. Nurses must help their clients deal with the pain associated with grief and mourning, as well as the psychological effects arising from the technological processes.

These processes place a great burden on the relationships of the people involved. The drugs used to stimulate ovum production can cause emotional lability. The regimentation of the process, and the coldness of the environment for procreation, is at the opposite extreme of the normal private and intimate experience. Fear of failure adds further strain. All these factors must be considered in the care that nurses provide. Nurses need to understand the issues and be prepared to support and guide their clients through a difficult, emotionally charged process.

With the introduction of each new technology in this field, more possibilities, and more ethical questions, emerge. As we reflect on the explosion of reproductive and genetic technologies it is worth reflecting on the following statement by Dr. Bernard Dickens, a legal ethicist from the University of Toronto:

> One may recall ... the words perceptively written in 1966 about artificial insemination, which were proven true ... and have significance in other reproductive means ... : "Any change in custom or practice in this emotionally charged area has always elicited a response from established custom and law of horrified negation at first; then negation without horror; then slow and gradual curiosity, study, evaluation, and finally a very slow but steady acceptance."[47]

Death and Dying

Today, even the process of dying has become more complex. In many hospitals, patients are no longer said to "die"; instead, they have "cardiac arrests." They may be denied the privilege of dying surrounded by family and friends, or of dying in their own home. Today's advanced technology even allows parts of human bodies to continue after death through organ donation and transplantation. This is possible because the body can be kept alive well beyond the point at which our capacity to interact with the world is gone. Recently, various special-interest groups have begun to demand that patients be given back their right to die, or at least, the right to decide how that dying process will unfold. Consequently, health professionals have been obliged to explore and redefine the distinction between life and death.

The issue of withdrawal of treatment first gained prominence in the mid-1970s with the case of Karen Ann Quinlan in the United States.[48] More recently, the cases of Sue Rodriguez[49] in British Columbia, Robert Latimer[50] in Saskatchewan, and Nancy B.[51] in Quebec have renewed and re-energized controversy over the ethical and legal justifications for and against euthanasia, withdrawal of treatment, and physician-assisted suicide. In the United States, pathologist Dr. Jack Kevorkian publicly admitted assisting the deaths of a number of patients using the "suicide machine" that he designed and built; at the time of writing, he had been convicted of first-degree murder in Michigan following broadcast of a videotaped assisted suicide on a well-known U.S. current affairs program. Here in Canada, the federal government has promised a full legislative debate and public hearings on the issue, but these have yet to take place.

A special committee of the Senate of Canada was established in February 1994 "to examine and report on the legal, social and ethical issues relating to euthanasia and assisted suicide."[52] The intention of this study was to assist members of Parliament in preparing for the legislative debate on these issues, and to seek opinions regarding them. The committee presented to the Senate a number of recommendations related to palliative care, pain control and sedation practices, withholding and withdrawal of life-sustaining treatment, advance directives, assisted suicide, and euthanasia.

Today's heightened awareness of euthanasia arises partly from advances in health care technology, and partly from the growing number of patients with terminal conditions (such as cancer and AIDS), in which the quality and dignity of the dying process are a concern.

Euthanasia and Assisted Suicide

There is an important distinction between euthanasia (or assisted suicide) and withdrawal of treatment. In euthanasia, active steps are taken to help end the life of a patient who requests this. Such a request might arise in the case of irreversible injury or terminal illness, when the patient has deemed his or her quality of life unacceptable. This may be due to complete loss of mobility and the ability to perform even the most basic tasks of everyday life (as in the case of patients with amyotrophic lateral sclerosis [ALS], or the extreme confusion and incapacity to communicate typical of Alzheimer's disease), or severe and unendurable pain that requires heavy medication, rendering the patient too sedated and disoriented to take an active part in life.

In assisted suicide, the patient is mentally competent to decide to end his or her life because of its deteriorating quality, yet is too debilitated by illness to act on this decision without the assistance of a third party (e.g., a physician, nurse, relative, or friend).

In withdrawal of treatment, nothing active is done to end the patient's life; rather, all treatment necessary to sustain life is withdrawn, and nature is permitted to take its course. Indeed, it is this approach, previously labelled "passive euthanasia," which the Quebec Superior Court adopted in the Nancy B. decision, discussed in Chapter Three.

The following case highlights some of the legal and ethical challenges associated these issues.

CASE STUDY

A cry for help?

Joan, a 40-year-old mother of two teenage children, was diagnosed two years ago with ovarian cancer. She has always been independent and active, a devoted mother who ran a corporate law practice and participated in civic organizations.

Early in her illness, Joan was treated with chemotherapy, radiotherapy, and surgery. For a time, the cancer seemed to be in remission. However, after a year, the cancer metastasized to her liver and lower intestines. Since then, Joan has been in and out of hospital receiving various treatments. Over the last two months, her health has deteriorated such that she is in constant and intense pain, especially in her bones. During her last admission to hospital, the team decided that nothing they could do would slow the growth of the tumour. After discussions with the team and her family, Joan decided to enter a home palliative care program that provides her with home care services, a pain control protocol, and a home care nurse. As well, Joan's husband Bob has taken leave of absence from work to remain at home with his wife.

For the past few weeks Joan's condition has remained unchanged, although the pain is becoming difficult to control and she suffers frequent bouts of nausea and constipation (side effects of the medication). She has become despondent and distressed with respect to her loss of dignity and the effect her illness is having on her family.

One day Joan exclaims to the home care nurse: "I've had enough! I can't stand the pain; I've become a burden on my husband and children. Please help me end it!"

Issues

1. What can the home care nurse do in this situation (a) legally and (b) ethically?
2. What alternatives are available to the nurse?

Discussion

Sometimes, patients, families, and caregivers are asked to choose between extending a painful, undignified life, or death. Even when the best palliative care is available, not all pain and suffering can always be relieved. When death is preferred, the means towards achieving that choice may place caregivers and family under great moral stress—for example, in the case of withholding food and fluids at a patient's own request. These decisions become even more difficult when the patient is no longer competent and has left no advance directive. Hence, it is not surprising that questions regarding advance directives, withdrawal of treatment, euthanasia, and assisted suicide have surfaced in recent years.

Many ethical principles ground decisions about these issues. Often, these principles conflict. On the one hand, we have the principle of autonomy, or respect for the rights of individuals to make decisions that affect their lives. But the law places limits on that autonomy and draws the line when it comes to individuals' determining how and when their lives will end. In such cases, the principle of autonomy conflicts with the principle of the sanctity of life, which for many is an absolute principle—that is, it cannot be overridden in any circumstances.

Nurses placed in such situations undergo extreme emotional and moral distress. Whether in the institutional or the home setting, they are often in closer contact with the patient and family than any other health professional. Consequently, they empathize with the physical, emotional, and spiritual experience of the patient and family. Conflict occurs when the patient's wishes, the nurse's loyalty to the patient, and the principle of beneficence (e.g., concern over providing a good, and avoiding harm when pain control and symptom relief fail) clash with the principle of sanctity of life and the law. These situations, more than any others, represent true dilemmas that nurses face in their practice, and provide a poignant reminder that what is legal may not, for some, be what is right.

This case study is a moving example of a situation that challenges the ethical and professional integrity of the nurse and the nature of the nurse–patient relationship. We are encouraged to empathize, that is, to enter into the patient's way of seeing and being, so that the nurse can feel what the patient feels and can understand the situation from the patient's perspective. A nurse working closely with a patient such as this might understand the patient's pain and be sensitive to her request. Regardless of their ethical values and beliefs, most nurses would feel frustrated by their limited ability to reduce the patient's physical and emotional pain, and to respect and support her wishes.

Nurses have a duty to care for the physical, emotional, and psychological needs of the patients and families entrusted to them. The CNA's *Code of Ethics for Registered Nurses* expresses the following responsibilities:

> Nurses treat human life as precious and worthy of respect. Respect
> includes seeking out and honouring clients' wishes regarding quality of

life. Decision-making about life-sustaining treatment carefully balances these considerations.[53]

Nurses advocate health and social conditions that allow persons to live with dignity throughout their lives and in the process of dying. They do so in ways that are consistent with their professional role and responsibilities.[54]

The nurse in this case study cannot assume that Joan has thought through all the issues and choices available to her and has made a reasoned decision to end her life. The nurse caring for Joan has a responsibility to explore with her the reasons behind this request. Has it arisen out of fear and uncertainty about the future and how her death will occur? Has her pain become unbearable? Does she believe she is a burden to her husband and family? Is she angry about her illness and its inevitable outcome? Is she frustrated with the growing lack of control she has over her life? Finally, does she believe she has little or no dignity left?

Based on the reasons behind Joan's request, the nurse may be able to intervene to assist in making her remaining life, and her dying, more tolerable. Although Joan is already receiving palliative care, perhaps her symptoms can be managed more effectively; for example, she may require better pain control.

Patients dying of cancer can tolerate extremely high levels of pain medication. Nurses should ensure that such patients receive the level of analgesia they require while attempting to minimize the related complications of drowsiness, confusion, constipation, and diarrhoea. Patients should be given choices regarding the level of pain control they receive. Some may elect to experience some pain in order to remain lucid and to continue communicating with others. For other patients, the pain may be so severe that they want it controlled even if that means falling into a semi- or unconscious state. Nurses may be concerned that high levels of pain medication may bring about or hasten the patient's death. From an ethical perspective, the nurse's primary obligation is to respect the patient's wishes and to provide a good by minimizing the pain, which may or may not hasten death. The obligation to provide palliative care and adequate pain control is also supported in law.[55]

Joan's nurse should assist her in taking control over the time she has left. There are ways that her family and caregivers can give her back some control. Perhaps she needs more opportunity to talk about her feelings and the meaning this experience has for her. Joan's husband and family may have similar needs; the nurse could help them talk about these matters with Joan.

There may be many other nursing interventions that might help Joan. Occasionally, there is nothing else nurses can do to relieve a patient's physical and emotional suffering. It is in these situations that we face one of the most challenging ethical and legal dilemmas in health care today.

Legal Perspectives

Euthanasia

Euthanasia, or "painless death," is defined as an act that brings about the immediate death of a terminally ill patient. Commonly referred to as "mercy killing," it is seen as a means to end the suffering and pain of patients who otherwise would experience a difficult, undignified death. It is viewed as an act of compassion, as the intention is to do a good by relieving pain and suffering.

Today's heightened awareness of euthanasia arises partly from advances in health care technology, and partly from the growing number of patients with terminal conditions (such as cancer and AIDS), in which the quality and dignity of the dying process are a concern. The recent court case involving Saskatchewan farmer Robert Latimer's conviction for the second-degree murder of his severely disabled daughter is a case in point.[56] After his conviction, following a second trial ordered by the Supreme Court of Canada, he was sentenced to time served plus two years in jail, notwithstanding the fact that the minimum sentence for second-degree murder is imprisonment for life without possibility of parole for at least 10 years. The sentencing judge held that to sentence Mr. Latimer to the minimum term specified in the *Criminal Code* would have constituted cruel and unusual punishment under the circumstances and violated his constitutional right to be free from such punishment. The Court granted Mr. Latimer an extremely rare (and equally controversial) constitutional dispensation from the legally mandated sentence for this offence. In so doing, the judge recognized the agonizing choices and decisions that Mr. Latimer made in the face of his daughter's suffering. Some argue that the Latimer decision signalled a turning point in the law's attitude towards euthanasia. Mr. Latimer's sentence was subsequently overturned on appeal by the Crown to the Saskatchewan Court of Appeal, which substituted the minimum 10-year sentence mandated by the *Criminal Code*. At the time of writing, the case is on further appeal to the Supreme Court of Canada.

Similarly, the situation involving Dr. Nancy Morrison in Nova Scotia has focussed attention on the divergent views between the legal system and the public at large on this issue. Dr. Morrison enjoyed a groundswell of public support for her cause after she was charged with the murder of a terminally ill cancer patient. Charges against Dr. Morrison were dropped at a preliminary hearing owing to insufficient evidence that she had done anything to hasten the patient's death. The Crown has since stated it would not appeal a recent ruling dismissing its application to reinstate the charges. Subsequently, Dr. Morrison accepted a reprimand from her provincial College of Physicians and Surgeons.

The attention given to patients' rights and respect for patient autonomy has provoked questions regarding the right to die and the right of patients to choose the time and means of their death.

Some who argue against euthanasia base their reasoning on the principle of sanctity of life and the traditional rules and laws prohibiting the taking of life except in situations of self-defence or war. (Strong advocates of this principle would argue that even in these circumstances, it is unacceptable to kill.) Others are concerned about the potential for abuse if euthanasia were permitted. It would be difficult to limit the act to situations where patients were terminally ill and actively dying; conceivably, it might extend to the chronically ill, the infirm, the elderly, and the demented. This is the "slippery slope" argument.

Those who support euthanasia believe that not all life is worth living. They believe that when someone is dying and it is no longer possible to eliminate their physical, emotional, and psychological pain, then euthanasia should be permitted at the request, and with the consent, of the competent patient. Supporters believe that sanctity of life is not an absolute principle and can be overridden out of respect both for patient autonomy and for the dignity of human life. They believe that, since death will occur anyway, euthanasia only makes that process more compassionate and dignified. If rules were in place to control euthanasia, as they are in the Netherlands, they argue, then the potential for abuse would be lessened.

Assisted Suicide

Suicide is defined as the act of taking one's own life. In assisted suicide, the person lacks the means of completing the act and requires the assistance of someone else. For example, an accomplice might provide the patient with a lethal dose of medication, or help the patient to ingest it. This issue has arisen in cases where patients with a chronic disease have desired the means to control the time of their death prior to falling into a state where such action is no longer possible. An example is the patient with amyotrophic lateral sclerosis (ALS) who wishes to live as long as possible, yet not end up in a state of total paralysis, dependent on artificial ventilation. Such persons would require assistance to commit suicide, since generalized weakness would limit their ability to do this on their own.

The arguments for and against assisted suicide are similar to those of euthanasia. However, those who support assisted suicide also argue that by not providing assistance, we set limits on disabled people's autonomy by denying them the opportunity to perform an act that able-bodied persons are capable of doing.

Public Opinion on Euthanasia and Assisted Suicide

A number of polls have been conducted to determine the public's attitudes with respect to euthanasia and assisted suicide. These polls indicate that the level of support for physician assistance in relation to euthanasia or assisted suicide for terminally ill patients ranges from 54% to 75%.[57] A poll published in the *Canadian Medical Association Journal* (March 1994) found that 65% of respondents supported active euthanasia for patients experiencing severe pain and terminal illness. However, these same respondents (63%) expressed concern that the legalization of euthanasia might lead to its use in other situations. Only 34% were against euthanasia in all situations.[58]

Since nurses are representative of society at large, it is unlikely that their views differ statistically from the opinions expressed in this survey. Some nurses hold strong views on one side of the debate; others are confused by the shades of grey and the arguments on both sides. Regardless of their perspective, all nurses experience moral distress in these situations, which are likely to increase in future years.

The Current Law in Canada

The case of *Rodriguez v. British Columbia (Attorney General)*[59] received much public attention. Sue Rodriguez was diagnosed with amyotrophic lateral sclerosis (ALS), a progressive disease of the nervous system that eventually results in complete paralysis and loss of the ability to speak, swallow, or breathe without a respirator. The patient afflicted with ALS gradually loses control of all bodily functions. Finally, even the heart succumbs to paralysis, and the person dies. Throughout the course of the disease, the patient's mind remains clear. The ability to reason is unaffected by the deterioration of the nervous system, although the disease can take a heavy emotional toll on patient, family, and friends. The disease is accompanied by painful muscular spasms, though these can be controlled to some degree with medication.

Mrs. Rodriguez was married and the mother of a young son. At the time of her Supreme Court hearing, she had been given a life expectancy of between two to 14 months (without the assistance of a respirator).[60] Her concern throughout was that, while she wished to live as long as possible, she did not wish to live through the last and most debilitating stages of ALS and die as a result of asphyxiation. Fearing complete loss of control over her bodily functions, and hence the ability to end her own life when she wished to do so, she brought an application before the Supreme Court of British Columbia for an order declaring section 241(b) of the *Criminal Code* unconstitutional.

Section 241(b) makes it an offence, punishable by up to 14 years' imprisonment on conviction, for anyone to counsel, aid, or abet another to commit suicide, whether or not the suicide is successful. Mrs. Rodriguez sought a declaration on the grounds that the effect of that section was to deprive her of several of her rights under the Canadian *Charter of Rights and Freedoms*, namely, life, liberty, security of person,[61] equality before the law,[62] and freedom from cruel or unusual treatment.[63] She argued that the effect of the law was to deprive her of control over her body and her life. Further, she argued that section 241(b) prevented her from obtaining the assistance of another person in ending her life when she could no longer do so on her own, and that this subjected her to cruel and unusual treatment at the hands of the state. Finally, she argued that since suicide was no longer a criminal offence in Canada,[64] she was being discriminated against and treated unequally by the law solely by reason of her physical disability, because she was effectively being prevented from doing that which able-bodied people could do legally.

Mrs. Rodriguez's application was dismissed by the Supreme Court of British Columbia and again by the B.C. Court of Appeal. A final appeal to the Supreme Court of Canada was heard on May 20, 1993, and the Court rendered its decision in September of that year.

The Court delivered a five-to-four decision against Mrs. Rodriguez's application. The closeness of the vote illustrates the difficulty of the issues and the lack of consensus in the courts. The majority of the judges felt that while the effect of section 241(b) was to impinge on Mrs. Rodriguez's right to life, liberty, and security of person, such intrusion was not contrary to the principles of fundamental justice. The majority also felt that her right to equal treatment was violated, but that this was permitted as being a "reasonable limit which [was] demonstrably justified in a free and democratic society."[65] The minority judges opined that both her right to life, liberty, and security of person, as well as her right to equality before the law, had been infringed, and that the infringement by the state through section 241(b) could not be justified in any way under the Charter. Thus, they felt that the section could not stand as valid under the Constitution and that therefore, Mrs. Rodriguez should be free to seek assistance in committing suicide when she wished it.

Mr. Justice Sopinka, writing the decision for the majority, undertook a historical review of the ethical and legal principles behind the legislative prohibitions against both suicide and assisted suicide. The chief ethical principle that he identified was the state's and society's concern for the sanctity and value of human life and human dignity,[66] as well as society's role in protecting those who are vulnerable and who could be coerced or encouraged, in a moment of weakness, to commit suicide. The purpose of section 241(b) was to protect such members of society. In recent times, the concept of protecting human life at all costs has become tempered with limitations premised on personal independence and dignity and with quality-of-life considerations.[67] Further, the common law has recognized the right of an individual to withdraw or withhold consent to medical treatment, even where such lack of treatment would likely result in death. Mr. Justice Sopinka's decision relied on the decision of the Supreme Court of Canada in *Ciarlariello v. Schacter*,[68] the decision of the Quebec Superior Court in the case of *Nancy B. v. Hôtel-Dieu de Québec*,[69] and the decision of the Ontario Court of Appeal in *Malette v. Shulman*.[70]

The majority judgement suggests that the law recognizes a form of passive euthanasia, for example, inadvertently hastening a terminally ill patient's death by administering larger and larger doses of pain medication where the intent was to control pain. Another example might be withdrawing (with the patient's consent) all treatment and artificial means to prolong life where such treatment has become therapeutically useless. The distinction between passive and active euthanasia is thus seen as a basis for upholding the law's continued prohibition against assisted suicide.

In response, the majority judgement of the Supreme Court notes that the law has always had great aversion to the participation of one person in the death of another, but passive euthanasia is considered acceptable because artificial means to prolong life are withdrawn on the patient's request and death ensues as a natural consequence. While some have criticized the distinction between passive and active euthanasia as artificial (since both take place with the full knowledge that death will ensue),[71] in the case of passive euthanasia the exact time of death cannot be known, and death does not result directly from the actions of another. Critics of the active/passive distinction and proponents of euthanasia also note that the outcome in either situation is ethically the same, but that in a case where treatment is merely withdrawn, death can come more slowly and may be more painful.

Another legal concern that justifies maintaining the blanket prohibition on assisted suicide, in the majority's opinion, is that of preventing abuse, together with the difficulties in formulating guidelines and conditions under which assisted suicide would be legally permissible. Mr. Justice Sopinka cited a working paper of the Law Reform Commission of Canada[72] that points out examples of mass suicides, or of one person taking advantage of the depressed state of another to encourage him to commit suicide for the other's financial gain, as reasons justifying the continued prohibition. Further, he reviewed the record in the Netherlands, which has the most liberal guidelines on euthanasia and physician-assisted suicide, and noted evidence (without stating his source) of a disturbing rise in cases of involuntary active euthanasia (which is not permitted by those guidelines).[73] Thus, the "slippery slope" argument, in the opinion of the majority, justifies a complete prohibition on physician-assisted suicide. To Mr. Justice Sopinka, to hold otherwise would "send a signal that there are circumstances in which the state approves of suicide."[74]

The minority justices wrote equally compelling dissenting opinions. The Chief Justice, Mr. Justice Lamer, opined that section 241(b) of the *Criminal Code* infringed on the rights of disabled persons such as Sue Rodriguez because it effectively deprives them of choosing suicide, an option available to able-bodied persons.[75] Thus, they were not being treated equally before the law as guaranteed under the Charter. Lamer also relied on the fact that it is a fundamental aspect of personal autonomy in the common law that citizens have the right to make free and informed decisions about their bodies and to consent (or withhold consent) to specific medical treatment, even when to do so would likely result in death.

The next consideration was whether such violation was "a reasonable limit, demonstrably justified in a free and democratic society" within the meaning of section 1 of the Charter. Here Mr. Justice Lamer undertook an interesting review of the values and objectives of the prohibition against

assisted suicide. He pointed out that the repeal of the attempted-suicide prohibition by Parliament in 1972[76] reflected its belief that self-determination
was now a paramount factor in the regulation of suicide. Thus, if no outside
interference with an individual's decision could be shown, then that person's
attempting suicide would no longer be a criminal offence.[77]

With respect to the "slippery slope" argument, His Lordship felt that
despite the concern that decriminalizing assisted suicide would leave the
physically disabled vulnerable and open to manipulation by others, this still
would not justify depriving a disadvantaged group (i.e., the disabled) of
equality before the law, specifically, the right to determine the circumstances
in which they end their life. In Mrs. Rodriguez's case, there was no evidence
of such vulnerability and plenty of evidence of her free consent.[78] He thus
concluded that the limit placed by section 241(b) of the *Criminal Code* upon
Sue Rodriguez's right to equality was not reasonable and could not be justified under the Charter.

Hence, the section was constitutionally invalid. However, he was inclined
to suspend the declaration of unconstitutionality for one year, until such time
as Parliament could address the issue and either enact legislation that would
deal with assisted suicide in cases such as Sue Rodriguez's, or simply enact no
constitutional legislation to replace section 241(b). This effectively meant
that, while the law was unconstitutional, it would nevertheless remain in
effect for one year so that the "floodgates" would not be opened, thus negat-
ing the objective of protecting the vulnerable from the influence and coercion
of others in consenting to assisted suicide.

In the meantime, he would have granted Mrs. Rodriguez an exemption to
compliance with section 241(b), provided that:

(1) she had applied to a superior court for authorization;
(2) she had been certified by her attending physician and a psychiatrist to be
competent and had made her decision freely and voluntarily, and that at
least one physician be with her when she commits assisted suicide;
(3) the physicians also certify that (a) she is or will become physically incapable of committing suicide unaided and (b) they have informed her of
her continuing right to change her mind about terminating her life;
(4) notice and access be given to the Regional Coroner at the time;
(5) she be examined daily by the physicians;
(6) the exemption would expire 31 days after the date of the physicians' certificate in (1) above; and
(7) the act actually causing her death must be her act alone, unaided by
anyone else.[79] The conditions were described as having been designed
with Mrs. Rodriguez's circumstances in mind. However, Mr. Justice
Lamer advanced them as guidelines to future applicants in similar circumstances.

The approach taken by two of the dissenting justices (Madam Justice
McLachlin, who wrote the dissent, and Madam Justice L'Heureux-Dubé, who
concurred in that dissent) is also interesting. Madam Justice McLachlin felt

that security of person entails personal autonomy, which protects the dignity and privacy of individuals with respect to decisions surrounding their own bodies.[80] Part of that autonomy involves the right of the person to decide what is best for him or her. There was thus no rational basis upon which to deny Mrs. Rodriguez a right that was freely available to others who were more able-bodied than she.

Application to Case Study

The nurse in Joan's situation clearly is not entitled to assist her to commit suicide, given the Supreme Court's pronouncement on this issue. Section 241(b) is constitutional and prevents the nurse from actively assisting Joan to end her life. It is legal, however, for the nurse to assist in pain control and to make Joan as comfortable as possible. Even if the nurse wished to proceed and help Joan, she runs the risk of being found out and criminally charged. The sentence recently handed out to Robert Latimer by a sympathetic Saskatchewan judge, and currently under appeal, cannot realistically afford comfort and encouragement to the nurse.

Withdrawal of Treatment

The following case study focusses on a more common dilemma faced by health care professionals.

CASE STUDY

Who speaks on my behalf?

A patient in the Critical Care Unit, Mr. C., is 70 years old and has end-stage cardiac disease. He is intubated and dependent on medication to sustain adequate blood pressure. Though his case is seemingly futile, the medical team plans to continue aggressive therapy. One of the patient's sons would like treatment to be withdrawn. The patient's wife and daughter disagree. Mr. C. is unable to speak for himself and made no decisions respecting care in advance, while competent. The treatment plan and the rules of the unit mean visiting is kept to a minimum of 10 min/h.

Issues

1. In the absence of direction from the patient, how should the health care team make their decision?
2. Who has the right to make the decision in this situation?
3. Would an advance directive have helped? How?
4. What are the responsibilities of Mr. C.'s nurse?

Discussion

Situations like the one described in this case study often give rise to conflict among family members, and this is stressful for all involved. The health care team may feel torn between their primary focus—the best interests of the patient—and the competing interests of the family. Decisions regarding withdrawal of treatment are more difficult when the patient is incompetent and unable to participate. Unfortunately, this is often the case in Intensive Care Units. The nurse may experience moral distress when the wishes of the most appropriate next-of-kin or substitute decision maker conflict with what the nurse believes is in the patient's best interest. This distress is alleviated if the nurse is confident that decisions regarding care are based on the previously expressed wishes or values of the patient.

Legal Perspectives

In this case study, the facts that the treatment being administered is futile and that the patient seems near death raise an interesting legal point with respect to withdrawal of treatment. The Quebec Superior Court's decision in *Nancy B. v. Hôtel-Dieu de Québec* dealt with the legality of a lucid patient's request not to be subjected to further medical treatment when that person deems such treatment no longer appropriate. (The details of this case are reviewed in Chapter Three.) This ruling was made in the context of Quebec's *Civil Code,* which places ultimate responsibility for treatment decisions with the patient. Thus, consent-to-treatment issues (as discussed in Chapter Six) may be inseparable from the issue of withdrawal of treatment.

In point of fact, withdrawal of treatment in these circumstances is supported by the common law. For example, in the United States, the Superior Court of New Jersey ultimately supported the concept of withdrawal of treatment in the case of Karen Ann Quinlan. The problem is that the common law has historically been hesitant to recognize the right of a spouse or next-of-kin to make treatment decisions on behalf of an incapable person. In Manitoba, this situation has been remedied in the *Health Care Directives Act;*[81] in Nova Scotia (to an extent), in the *Medical Consent Act;*[82] in British Columbia, in the recently enacted *Adult Guardianship Act*[83] (not yet in force at the time of writing); and in Ontario, in the *Substitute Decisions Act, 1992,*[84] which enables another person to make decisions on behalf of those who cannot make them for themselves. Alberta has similarly passed the *Personal Directives Act.*[85]

At present, in provinces without specific legislation on this subject, the practice is to accept treatment decisions made by an incapable person's spouse or, if there is no spouse, that person's closest living relative. For example, the patient's closest living relative may make the decision on the basis of what the patient would have wished. This means that the proxy (the person making the decision for the incapable patient) must make every effort to determine what the patient's wishes would have been.[86]

In the case study, the conflict between the son on the one hand, and the wife and daughter on the other, suggests that the matter may have to be resolved in court through guardianship proceedings (as discussed in Chapter Six). The guardian(s) would be authorized to make treatment decisions respecting the patient. This is a sad, costly, and needless development. Otherwise, it is fairly certain that the law would not interfere with the decision to withdraw treatment in such a case, especially where such treatment is demonstrably futile. However, as we have said above, it draws the line at positive acts in the nature of assisted suicide.

In the majority of cases, the resolution should not end up in court. It is the health care team's responsibility to meet with the family to weigh the alternatives and to explore their feelings and views. It is important that the family be fully informed of all the medical facts relevant to the patient's situation. It is also helpful to share with them a framework that might assist them to reach consensus on the best course of action.

Through discussion, the family might remember occasions when Mr. C. expressed thoughts on what he would want in such a situation as this—for example, a comment made about a similar case on television or in the newspapers. Or, they might talk about Mr. C.'s lifelong values in order to get some sense of his likely decision, were he capable. With the support of the health care team, clear communication, and time, most situations like this can be resolved.

Advance directives are always helpful in cases of incompetence. In future, it is likely that these will play a greater role in treatment decisions, especially when legislative reform in such provinces as Ontario, PEI, Newfoundland, Saskatchewan, and the Yukon Territory encourages them.

Advance Directives (Living Wills)

An **advance directive** is a person's instruction regarding decisions about care if he or she is ever rendered incompetent. Advance directives can take the form of verbal discussion with someone whom the person has identified as a substitute decision maker.

This practice does not have legal sanction in all provinces. However, it is legally recognized in Ontario in the *Substitute Decisions Act, 1992*.[87] It is also recognized in Manitoba under the *Health Care Directives Act*,[88] in Nova Scotia under the *Medical Consent Act*,[89] and in Alberta pursuant to the *Personal Directives Act*.[90] Substitute-decision legislation has been passed in British Columbia (the *Adult Guardianship Act*[91] and the *Representation Agreements Act*), but is not yet in force. The former statute contemplates an application to a court for the appointment of a guardian or substitute decision maker. Despite differences in the law from province to province, a living will is still a useful document.

A written advance directive may be obtained in the form of a living will, a document that enables a patient to specify his or her informed choices well in advance of requiring such care. The living will takes effect only when the patient is incapable of making decisions. People with living wills usually update and revise them on a regular basis. Regardless of whether they are sanctioned by law, living wills are a useful resource for health professionals.

The University of Toronto Joint Centre for Bioethics has published and distributed a comprehensive living will (excerpted in Appendix B). This tool defines the salient points of a living will and frames a process whereby an individual can make informed choices with respect to possible health care situations in the future.

There are two components to this living will. An *instruction directive* allows the person to specify which life-sustaining treatments he or she would not wish in various situations. The *proxy directive* allows individuals to identify a substitute decision maker, should they ever be rendered incompetent.

Individuals who complete the living will are advised to ensure that several appropriate people know the will exists and that copies are distributed, particularly to their doctor, lawyer, and family members. The will should be reviewed and updated regularly to ensure that it continues to reflect the person's current wishes.

The living will of the University of Toronto Centre for Bioethics, unlike most published to date, specifies many health situations that individuals could face. These include permanent coma, terminal illness, stroke, and dementia. Within each problem a mild, moderate, and severe state is defined. The life-sustaining options with respect to these conditions are outlined and explained with the lay person in mind, for example, cardiopulmonary resuscitation, respirators, dialysis, surgery, blood transfusions, antibiotics, and tube feeding. Space is included for the individual to provide further instructions with respect to other health care situations that might arise.

Ideally, individuals who complete a living will consult with physicians, nurses, and perhaps their lawyer or other persons, so that they fully anticipate the situations that might arise, and comprehend the treatments available to them. This helps them to make sound choices, and ensures that these are clearly expressed in the living will.

Organ Donation

The field of transplantation has grown tremendously in recent years. The long-term survival rates for lung, heart, kidney, and liver transplants have improved remarkably. Patients who would have died otherwise may live more than five years longer with good quality of life. Transplantation in general has become a proven, cost-effective alternative to other treatments, especially in the case of renal transplants.

In Canada, organ donation is generally viewed as morally justified when treatment alternatives to transplantation are not readily available, and respect for the autonomy of donors and their families is maintained through appropriate legislation and guidelines.

Ironically, recent successes of transplant programs have contributed to the problem of limited availability of organs. The supply of donor organs has not kept pace with the growing need. Furthermore, advances in the neurosciences, compliance with seat-belt legislation, and a reduction in drinking and driving have reduced the numbers of deaths where there is a potential for organ donation. This situation has led to efforts to maximize all potential donors. Strategies explored have included changes to the legislation regarding the consent process, donor incentives, education, and a further redefinition of death.

The ethical issues associated with organ donation include the determination of brain death, consent, and donor management. The organ donation process, if not managed properly, can be highly stressful for nurses as well as clients' families.

Nurses caring for a donor patient may experience moral conflict during the donation process. It is important that they understand all aspects of this process and the relevant ethical issues so that they can deal more effectively with the difficult transition from trying to save the life of a patient to managing that patient's organs for the benefit of others. Greater understanding, together with ethical management of the process by all members of the team, can make this an enriching experience for all involved.

The following case study illustrates some of these ethical and legal challenges.

CASE STUDY

A gift or an obligation?

Mr. R., a patient who has ingested a large quantity of barbiturates, is admitted to an Intensive Care Unit (ICU). The drugs have damaged his brain to such a degree that he has been declared brain-dead. He remains on a ventilator and is presently haemodynamically stable. In the same hospital, another patient, Mr. S., is dying as a result of a rejection episode following a heart transplant. Mr. S. has less than 24 h to live unless another suitable heart is found for retransplantation.

Mr. R. is judged by the ICU team to be a suitable donor for the urgently required heart. Further, a signed organ donor card was found in his wallet. As is the practice in most hospitals, and despite the existence of this card, the ICU team approaches Mr. R.'s parents and requests them to consent to donating their son's organs. The parents categorically refuse consent. They are not informed about Mr. S., for fear that this would constitute coercion. Mr. S. dies the next day.

Issues

1. What is the legal status of a signed organ donor card?
2. Is the consent of the donor's family required?
3. Could health professionals be more aggressive in encouraging the donor's family to give consent? Should family be told about the recipient in need?
4. Might further legislation in the area of consent help? How?

Discussion

The current approach to organ donation in Canada is a voluntary system of expressed consent. This is based on the principle of beneficence, doing good and avoiding harm. Because society does not oblige us to help others or to be altruistic, the system is based on the notion of voluntarism, and encourages organ donation through such mechanisms as providing individuals an opportunity to indicate on a driver's licence, health care card, or organ donor card their willingness to donate organs at the time of death. Supporters of this system argue that procurement built on voluntarism promotes socially desirable virtues such as altruism and, at the same time, protects the rights of persons who might refuse to donate.[92]

Certain problems have arisen in regard to this approach:

- Individuals may choose not to sign a donor card, even when they support the concept.
- The donor card is not always available to health professionals at the time of a patient's death.
- Regardless of whether a donor card is signed, families are approached and, in practice, their decision takes precedence.
- Health professionals are still reluctant to approach families or to initiate a complex and time-consuming donation process.[93]

The last point raises some ethical issues with respect to the role of the team (especially nurses) as participants in organ donation. Some health professionals cite the grieving process of the family as the reason for not approaching them with regard to organ donation. Others claim that the cultural or religious perspectives of some patients preclude organ donation. The problem here is that when we decide not to raise the issue with the family, or fail to look for a signed organ donor card, then we are in fact making the decision for them not to donate, and this is disrespectful of the individual's autonomy.

Furthermore, we cannot make assumptions about the views of various cultural and religious groups. In fact, most world religions support organ donation and transplantation. These include the Christian, Jewish, and Hindu religions. The Japanese Shinto religion and some sects of Tibetan Buddhism prohibit (or discourage) organ transplantation because of beliefs about the dead, taboos against injuring the body after death, and the extensive purifying rights required after death occurs.[94]

Nurses are in a good position to raise the issue of organ donation with patients' families. The nurse caring for the patient has the most opportunity to interact with the family throughout this difficult process. Nurses often develop a supportive relationship with family as they prepare them for the inevitable, and most have the communication skills to raise the issue of organ donation sensitively. Given the fact that families often forget about organ donation in the midst of crisis, it is important that nurses advocate to ensure that the issue is raised.

Regardless of the decision, the nurse has represented the interests and wishes of the patient and his or her family. Taking part in this process also eases the nurse's own transition from caring for the patient to maintaining that patient's organs for the benefit of future recipients. The relationship continues, as the nurse ensures that the patient's wish to give to others is fulfilled.

The declaration of brain death remains a controversial process that continues to create emotional tension for health professionals. It is difficult to accept that a patient is dead when the chest continues to rise and fall and skin colour and body temperature seem normal. Some health facilities use particular rituals to acknowledge the occurrence of a death. For example, some settings observe a moment of silence to respect the deceased and to acknowledge the feelings of family and staff. This observance can also ease the transition to the next phase of the donation process. Such rituals are an issue particularly for nurses in the Operating Room, who may be left alone with the patient after removal of the organs.[95] Hospitals should be sensitive to the needs of staff left in such a situation and endorse the means to support them.

Low donor rates in relation to the growing number of patients who need organ transplants have raised questions about whether alternative systems for organ donation should be considered. Following is a brief overview of some possible approaches.

Recorded Consideration

The recorded consideration approach attempts to deal with the issue of families' not being asked.[96] It requires that health care staff routinely consider and document the appropriateness of a dying or brain-dead patient for organ donation. If the patient's organs are appropriate, then the family is to be approached. If the organs are not appropriate, or if the family refuses consent, then staff are required to document this in the patient's chart. (This is required by law, for example, in Prince Edward Island.[97])

Required Request

With this system, all patients are asked about their position on organ donation when admitted to hospital or when they use the health system in any way. Concerns have been raised about whether such questions are unduly stressful for patients, who hope to have their health care needs met in the hospital and thus may not wish to entertain the possibility of imminent organ donation.[98]

Presumed Consent

This approach is commonly referred to as "opting out." The assumption is that the dying or brain-dead patient would have donated his or her organs, unless he or she expressed otherwise beforehand. Those who favour this method reason that it would make approaching the family easier and would result in more organs being made available. They argue that autonomy is respected, since individuals still have the right to refuse. Those who disagree with this approach say that consent, particularly of the bereaved, cannot be presumed, and that it undermines the notion of altruism. It has been noted that in countries where presumed consent is the law (e.g., France, Belgium, Singapore), organ donor rates improved for a while, then levelled off. This phenomenon was apparently related to the continuing reluctance of health professionals to approach families.[99]

Market Strategies

Some suggest that organ donor rates would improve if there were a financial incentive involved, ranging from a lump-sum payment to coverage of the deceased's funeral expenses. Again, concerns arise that this approach would not only undermine the notion of altruism, but might take advantage of those compromised by poverty. As well, a coercive element would be introduced into the process of consent.[100] In Canada at present, buying or selling human tissue or organs is prohibited by law in every province and territory. Penalties for breach of this prohibition vary from province to province, but they include steep fines and several months' imprisonment.

Education

Strategies to educate the public and health professionals have been encouraged. Further knowledge and better communication would ensure that the notion of brain death is understood, that individuals are aware of the donation options available to them, and that health professionals understand and accept their role in the organ donation process. It is not adequate to educate only health professionals working in hospitals. A significant role exists for nurses practising in the community to represent the interests of health care in general and to educate their clients about these specific issues.[101]

Redefining Death

Some health professionals have responded to the shortage of organs by suggesting that the definition of death be extended to include cortical death, as in the case of the anencephalic donor. This definition would include patients in a persistent vegetative state, who have no cortical activity although the brain stem is intact. Such persons can maintain their vital functions, and their body can live for years with appropriate nursing care. However, all that makes them a person—their ability to communicate, to relate to others, to remember—is gone. These patients may live for years, or may have treatment withdrawn and be allowed to die.

Those who seek to redefine death argue that we are losing a potential pool of organ donors who may have previously expressed, while competent, the wish to donate organs at the time of death. Those who argue against this redefinition suggest that we cannot redefine death whenever it is convenient to do so. Further, they argue that these questions should be raised not in the context of organ donation, but out of a duty and responsibility to the patient in the persistent vegetative state.[102] To do otherwise would be to treat individuals, as Kant would say, as means and not as ends in and of themselves.

Redefining death to include cortical death would present procedural problems. Would this redefinition apply universally, or only in cases of organ donation or with the families' permission? In any case, when would biological life be deemed to end? Would this happen immediately after cortical death is declared? Or would it end when convenient—for example, when a transplant recipient is in need?[103]

Legal Definition of Death

Removal of organ tissues from deceased donors is bound up with the legal and medical determination of death. Few jurisdictions in Canada or the United States provide a legislative definition of the moment of death. Historically, physicians have concurred that a person is dead when all vital signs (heartbeat, pulse, respiration) have ceased. In religious terms, death is seen as the moment when the soul leaves the body, generally at the time when the person's heart ceases to beat. Until well into the 20th century, the courts recognized that a person was legally dead when the "vital functions [have] ceased to operate. The heart [has] always been regarded as a vital organ" in this determination.[104]

In the last half century, sophisticated medical technology has allowed physicians to sustain the lives of seriously ill patients in situations where previously such persons would have died. A patient who can no longer breathe on his or her own or whose heart function has ceased can now be kept alive with the aid of respirators and other devices to sustain blood circulation. As well, advances in medical transplant technology have made possible the transplantation of viable organs from deceased donors into the bodies of living persons. We have also learned much more about the human brain, its role in controlling not only vital bodily systems, but also as the source of personality, intelligence, emotion, and a host of other human characteristics.

It has become apparent that the traditional medical criteria for determining the fact of death have become inadequate. The question now is: Can a person whose brain function has completely and irreversibly ceased, but whose other bodily functions remain active, still be considered a living human being?

In 1975, Manitoba became the first (and so far the only) province to enact a legal definition of the moment of death. The Manitoba *Vital Statistics Act* provides that, for all civil purposes (i.e., not for the purpose of criminal law), "the death of a person takes place at the time at which irreversible cessation of all that person's brain function occurs."[105] This definition conforms to the accepted definition of death within the modern medical community. In arriving at a new medical definition of death, a committee of the Harvard Medical School suggests that brain death is established with the cessation of all brain function, both cerebral and brain-stem, and that the cessation of such brain function must be irreversible.

With respect to human tissue donation, the laws of most of the provinces require that the death of a prospective donor be determined in this way.[106] Manitoba's legislation provides specifically that death must be determined according to the definition set out in the *Vital Statistics Act,* with bodily circulation still intact as necessary for the purposes of a successful transplant, and that such determination can only be made by at least two physicians.[107]

Further ethical and legal problems arise with respect to the removal of tissue and organs from the bodies of anencephalic neonates. Brain-stem anencephaly is demonstrated by the absence of the cerebrum, although the mid-brain cerebellum and brain stem are present and functioning. In such a newborn, there is enough lower brain function that the neonate can breathe and maintain a heartbeat for some time. It may be difficult to establish that all brain function has indeed ceased. Furthermore, because an infant's brain cells are resistant to damage, caution must be exercised in applying brain-death criteria to children under five years of age. Specific criteria do exist for children under five, but not for infants under two weeks of age.[108]

Eventually, an anencephalic child will stop breathing. Yet, he or she can be kept on a respirator to ensure that the organs are kept healthy and viable for transplantation. There is no question that such a child would ever be able to live a meaningful life, since anencephalics are not conscious and have no mental capacity. Such a child is doomed to live in a vegetative state for the rest of its brief life, a few days at most.

The question that arises in this situation is whether such a child should be considered legally dead so that its organs may be removed for transplant to save another child's life. Clearly, an anencephalic is alive even by modern medical criteria, since the lower brain is still functioning and is able to sustain breathing and circulation, to a degree. The definition of death based on irreversible cessation of all brain function is of no help in this situation.

Consequently, physicians and ethicists alike have recently argued for a revised definition of death that would address such a situation.

Some ethicists have argued that anencephalic donors ought to be deemed dead while respiration and circulation are maintained to keep the organs viable. Others opt for a special category of "brain absent" persons, such as anencephalics. This definition would permit removal of organs for transplant while the infant's brain is not yet dead. It is argued that this is a more utilitarian solution that preserves the donor child's humanity, spares it from further physical pain, saves the lives of recipients, prevents deterioration of the organs, and allows the parents the dignity and comfort of knowing that their child's condition and brief life were not in vain.

The Manitoba procedures for determining death in the *Human Tissue Act* address this situation in part by permitting circulation to be maintained to ensure a successful transplant. However, even that province still relies on the complete cessation of all brain function.

Human Tissue Legislation across Canada

All provinces and both territories have enacted legislation dealing with organ donation before and after the death of the donor.[109] This legislation is remarkably uniform across Canada. The various statutes basically provide a mechanism for obtaining the consent of the donor (or others, where the donor is unable to consent) to the removal of tissue from the donor's body for transplant into the body of another, for medical education, or for purposes of scientific research.

There are two primary situations contemplated by the statutes: one where the donor is living and has consented to the removal of non-regenerative tissue[110] from his or her body for therapeutic use, such as a transplant to another person's body. This is legally referred to as an inter vivos gift of tissue, from the Latin meaning "among the living"; that is, the donor gives the tissue during his or her lifetime. The other situation occurs where the donor (or another, if the donor has expressed no wishes on the matter) has directed that specified body parts be removed from his or her body for transplant into another living person after the donor's death. This is legally known as a post mortem gift of tissue, that is, the donor (or other person authorized to consent, if the donor has not expressed any wishes on the matter) gives the tissue after he or she has died.

Legislation in all provinces and territories except Manitoba and Quebec specifically excludes such regenerative tissue as bone, blood or its constituents, skin, or other tissue that is regenerated naturally by the human body. In each of these eight provinces, an adult who is mentally competent and makes a free and informed decision may legally donate such regenerative tissue under the common law. The human tissue legislation does not apply to such a donation. For example, a person donating bone marrow in one of these provinces or territories need only be of the age of majority and mentally competent and may orally consent to giving such tissue. (In practice, most health facilities require a signed consent for the mutual protection of all parties concerned.)

In contrast, the law in Manitoba excludes only blood or its constituents.[111] Thus, the *Human Tissue Act* of that province does not apply to a blood donation. Rather, the common law requires merely that the donor be an adult, be mentally competent, and be able to make a free and informed decision. On the other hand, a bone marrow donation, or a donation of skin for a skin graft, would have to comply with the requirements of the Act.

Similarly, the Quebec *Civil Code* allows any person in Quebec of the age of majority who is mentally capable to consent to the removal of tissue from his or her body while that person is living.[112] Since the *Civil Code* does not define "tissue," one can presume that it includes any tissue from the donor's body, including blood and other such regenerative tissue, as well as kidneys.

Consent to Transplant During Donor's Life

In a case of an inter vivos gift—for example, where the donor consents to giving a kidney for transplant into the body of a sibling—the consent is valid if it is in writing and is signed by the donor. Although the statutes are silent on this point, the consent can be revoked (cancelled) at any time thereafter, either in writing or orally.

In all provinces and territories except Ontario, Prince Edward Island, and Quebec, only a person who has reached the age of majority may legally consent to an inter vivos gift of tissue. Ontario and Prince Edward Island allow persons below the age of majority but who are at least 16 years old to give consent without the approval of a parent or guardian.[113] In Quebec, a minor (a person who has not yet reached the age of majority) may consent to an inter vivos donation of regenerative tissue only with consent of a parent or tutor (in Quebec, the equivalent of a child's legal guardian) and with permission of the court, provided that the procedure does not result in serious risk to the health of the minor.[114] The New Brunswick[115] and Northwest Territories[116] statutes are silent on inter vivos transfers. However, the common law would likely permit such transfers where the donor was an adult, mentally competent, and making a free and fully informed decision.

Apart from being of the requisite age, a person in Ontario, Nova Scotia, Alberta, British Columbia, Newfoundland, Saskatchewan, or the Yukon Territory must be mentally competent to consent and must make a free and informed decision.[117] A "free and informed decision" (as discussed in Chapter Six) follows the same common law requirements for fully informed consent to medical treatment as set out by the Supreme Court of Canada in *Reibl v. Hughes*.[118] The physician must inform the donor of all potential and material risks inherent in the procedure that would be reasonably likely to affect the donor's decision.

For their consent to be valid, Prince Edward Islanders must specifically be able to understand the consequences and nature of transplanting tissue from their body during their lifetime.[119] If there is any doubt on this point, an independent assessment must determine whether the transplant should be carried out.[120]

Mentally Incompetent Inter Vivos Donors and Minors

Situations in which the prospective donor is a minor, or is mentally incompetent, or otherwise unable to make an informed decision through not understanding the nature and consequences of the procedure, pose a special problem. Such a situation might arise, for example, where the health risk to the donor is perfectly acceptable and minimal, and the tissue is urgently required to save the life of that person's sibling. As mentioned above, the Prince Edward Island statute provides for an independent assessment in a situation where the donor appears not to understand the nature and consequences of the transplant and yet consents to it. The assessors must consider whether:

- the transplant is the treatment of choice;
- the donor has been coerced or induced to give consent;
- removal of the tissue will create a substantial health or other risk to the donor; and
- the Act and its regulations have been complied with.[121]

This requirement also applies in the case of a donor under 16, even if he or she understands the nature and consequences of the transplant.[122] In Prince Edward Island, in the case of a minor under 16, parental consent is required for an inter vivos gift of regenerative tissue (e.g., bone marrow). Finally, the independent assessment must indicate that the transplant should be carried out.

The same factors must be considered in the case of a donor under 16, with the additional requirement that all other members of the donor's family must be eliminated as potential donors for medical or other reasons. The assessors must give written reasons for their decision. The PEI statute further provides that a person may appeal the decision to the Supreme Court of Prince Edward Island within three days.[123] The Court may confirm, vary, or quash (cancel) the assessor's decision, or return the matter to the assessors for further action. Pending the decision of the appeal, the transplant cannot proceed.

Similarly, Manitoba's *Human Tissue Act* permits persons under 18 but at least 16 to consent to the transplant of tissue while living. However, a physician who is not and never has been associated with the proposed recipient must certify in writing that he or she believes such person is capable of understanding and does understand the nature and effect of the transplant. Further, a parent must consent, and the donor must be a member of the recipient's immediate family.[124] The physician who makes the certificate cannot participate in the transplant operation. This provision addresses concerns over potential conflicts of interest.

In Manitoba, persons under 16 may donate tissue only while living if these conditions are met:

- the proposed recipient must be a member of the donor's immediate family;
- only regenerative tissue may be given;
- the recipient would likely die without the tissue;
- the life and health risks to the donor must be minimal;
- the donor consents to the transplant;
- the donor's parent or legal guardian consents;
- the transplant is recommended by a physician who is not and never has been involved in any way with the recipient and will not be involved in the transplant; and finally,
- court approval must be obtained.

The term "immediate family" specifically includes the donor's mother, father, or step-father or step-mother, brother, sister, step-brother or step-sister, or half-brother or half-sister.[125]

Neither Ontario, Alberta, Nova Scotia, British Columbia, Newfoundland, Saskatchewan, nor the Yukon Territory provides for an assessment procedure in the case of a minor or mentally incompetent inter vivos donor. Ontario's *Health Care Consent Act, 1996,*[126] for instance, specifically states that its provisions do not affect the law with respect to, among other matters, the removal of regenerative or non-regenerative tissue for implantation in another person's body. PEI's *Consent to Treatment and Health Care Directives Act*[127] contains a similar provision.

The human tissue donation statutes of most of these provinces are virtually identical. However, they do provide that where the donor has given consent, and is a minor, or is mentally incompetent to consent, or is unable to give a free and informed decision, the consent is still legally valid, provided that the person acting on that consent (presumably, the physician who will perform the transplant) has no reason to believe that the donor is a minor, or is mentally incompetent, or is unable to make a free and informed decision. There is thus a requirement of good faith on the part of the person performing the transplant, and a duty upon him or her to ensure that a prospective donor is indeed a mentally competent adult who is giving a free and informed consent.

In most cases, this provision does not pose a problem. Most physicians and nurses are competent to assess the general mental capabilities of their patients. A careful review with the patient of all material risks inherent in the transplant, within the criteria stated in *Reibl v. Hughes,* would likely address the problem of a free and informed consent. The case of the minor poses a slightly different problem when that person appears much older than he or she actually is. The level of maturity disclosed in the conversation between the health professional and the minor is not conclusive. This provision of the statute protects health professionals acting in good faith in such a situation.

Apart from this, such prospective donors would presumably require some sort of court authorization according to common law. This has been the traditional route in jurisdictions lacking procedures such as those required in Prince Edward Island, or explicit provisions for court authorization such as those in the Quebec *Civil Code*. A court reviewing such a case would likely consider factors such as those mentioned in the PEI Act, and further, would consider the impact of the procedure on the donor.

In the case of a minor, some courts have relied on the "competent minor" rule. This rule holds that a person under the age of majority may be sufficiently mature to comprehend fully the nature and consequences of the transplant. Since in these cases, the donor is not receiving a direct health benefit from the transplant, the courts, in some American states, have considered that the infant donor still derives an emotional benefit from the survival of his or her sibling. The family is thus relieved from the potential stress of the death of one of its members, and can provide full emotional support to the donor. Further, especially in cases where the infant donor is old enough to have expressed even a rudimentary wish to help the sibling (though not fully comprehending the nature and consequences of the transplant), that child is spared the emotional guilt that may develop later in life from not having had an opportunity to save the sibling's life.[128]

Interestingly, Prince Edward Island's *Human Tissue Donation Act* deals expressly with the question of regenerative tissue donation by an infant sibling.[129] It provides that, with the consent of the infant donor's parents, and the approval of the independent assessors, bone marrow may be removed from such a child during the child's life for implantation into the child's biological sibling. Of course, the assessors will have eliminated all other eligible family members for medical or other reasons.

Post Mortem Donations

Consent to donation of tissue after the donor's death is somewhat different. The policy behind the law in such cases is to encourage the donation of organs after death, since there is always a large pool of recipients who urgently need them. Thus, the requirements for lawful consent are more relaxed and flexible.

In all provinces and both territories, a person over the age of majority (over 16 in Ontario and Prince Edward Island) may consent in writing to the removal of any and all tissue for either therapeutic, medical educational, or medical research purposes. Except in Quebec, the written document containing the consent may be part of a will or other testamentary instrument (e.g., organ donor card, driver's licence), regardless of whether such will is legally valid.

In Manitoba, persons under 18 but at least 16 years of age may consent to such removal, but only with the consent of the donor's parent or guardian, unless the parent or guardian is unavailable (e.g., dead, physically or mentally ill, or otherwise absent).[130] This provision permits flexibility and promotes the availability of organs.

Consent given by a person under 16 is deemed valid if the person who acted on it had no reason to believe that the donor was in fact under 16. This mirrors the provisions of inter vivos donations in most provinces, and imposes a requirement of good faith on the part of physicians acting upon the donor's directive.

In Quebec, a minor 14 years of age or older may authorize the removal of organs or tissue or give his or her body for medical or scientific purposes. A minor under 14 may also do so with the written consent of a parent or guardian.[131]

Most provinces allow the consent to be made orally by the donor in the presence of two witnesses during the donor's last illness. Manitoba and Prince Edward Island do not specify whether the consent must be written or may also be made orally. The statutes of those two provinces speak of the removal of tissue "as may be specified in the consent," which implies a requirement for written consent. However, in a case where a clear, unequivocal oral consent is given in the presence of two or more witnesses, it is possible that such consent would be permissible as clear evidence of the donor's last wishes. In all cases, the donor may revoke (cancel) his or her consent at any time prior to death. The law will respect the absolute final wishes of the donor and the right to change his or her mind, even at the last possible moment.

The consent is effective upon the donor's death. The determination of death can be problematic, as discussed above. All statutes across Canada require that, in cases where organs are to be removed, death must be determined by at least two physicians. Neither may be persons associated with the intended recipient such as might influence the physician's judgement. Conversely, no physician involved in determining the death of the donor may participate in the transplant. This is to avoid potential conflicts of interest.

A valid consent may not be acted upon if the person acting on it has reason to believe that the donor has not reached the age of consent, is not mentally competent, or is not able to make a free and informed consent. Thus, physicians and nurses involved in the transplant should be alert to any such indications. If there is no reason for such suspicions, the consent will be valid even if it later turns out that the donor was underage, was mentally incompetent, or was otherwise unable to make a free and informed consent.

The consent grants complete authority to use the body, and remove and use parts named in the consent for any purpose specified, unless the person acting on it has reason to believe that consent was withdrawn by the donor before death. This is consistent with the principle permitting the donor to change his or her mind at any time. The withdrawal can be made either orally to witnesses, or in writing, signed by the donor.

Post Mortem Donations Lacking Deceased's Consent

What of situations where the deceased expressed no wishes regarding donation of tissues or organs after death, or was incapable of giving consent? This
is different from specifically refusing consent, since the law requires that such
refusal, however unfortunate for the prospective recipient, be respected. Yet,
in such cases (e.g., the prospective donor has expressed no wishes, and death
is imminent in the opinion of a physician), organs or tissue may be urgently
needed to save the life of another. Here, the law in all jurisdictions allows
other specific persons to make the decision regarding the removal of tissue or
organs from the deceased's body.

There is a hierarchy of persons who may be approached to make this decision:

(1) first, the spouse of the donor;
(2) if there is no spouse, any of the donor's children over 18;
(3) if there are no children, either one of the donor's parents (or legal
    guardian, in some provinces);[132]
(4) any of the donor's siblings;
(5) the donor's next-of-kin; and finally, if no such persons are available,
(6) anyone who is in lawful possession of the body may give the required
    consent.

The statutes make clear that the sixth category excludes the coroner,
medical examiner, embalmer, and funeral director. It might conceivably
include the executor or administrator of the donor's estate, since such person
is responsible for the proper and respectful disposal of the deceased's
remains, either by burial or cremation.

Sometimes, relatives of the deceased will differ over permitting the
removal of organs or tissue. For example, the wife of a patient whose death
is imminent might refuse a physician's request for removal of the man's kidneys, whereas the patient's father may favour such a request. The law in most
provinces and both territories provides a resolution to such a conflict: no person may act on a consent given on behalf of a dying or deceased donor if such
person knows of an objection to it by anyone having the same or closer relationship to the donor than the one who gave the consent. Thus, in our case
study, Mr. R.'s wife's wishes would overrule those of the donor's parents.
Similarly, in a case where the donor's sister gave consent and the donor's
brother objected, that objection would void the consent and this would be
the end of the matter, unless another relative closer in relationship to the
donor consented.

Manitoba's legislation does not provide a mechanism for resolving such
disputes, but it is likely that a health professional in that province faced with
a similar conflict could resolve it in this manner. Quebec law allows the same
hierarchy of persons as in the other provinces; further, the *Civil Code* permits
the deceased's heirs or successors to give or refuse consent.[133] There is no
mechanism for conflict resolution in the *Civil Code*. However, a person qual-

ified to give consent to care of the donor (when living) may also consent to the removal of tissues or organs from the deceased's body.[134] In Quebec, a physician may proceed with the transplant of an organ or tissues from a deceased if two physicians certify that they were unable to obtain such consent in due time, and that the operation was urgently required to save a human life or significantly improve the quality of a life.[135]

Finally, the law, as always, respects the deceased or dying donor's wishes. If a health professional acting on the consent of a donor's spouse or other relative has reason to believe that the donor would object to the removal (or, in Manitoba,[136] that such removal would be contrary to the donor's religion), he or she cannot proceed on the basis of the consent. Similarly, if the health professional in charge of the case believes that the deceased's death occurred in circumstances requiring an inquest by a coroner or medical examiner, that professional cannot proceed on the basis of the consent unless the coroner or medical examiner agrees. This requirement preserves the evidentiary value of a post mortem examination of the body in cases where the deceased has not died of natural causes and an inquest into the cause of death is required.

Provincial Strategies to Promote Organ Retrieval

Manitoba has made an attempt, in its *Human Tissue Act,* to encourage physicians and other health professionals to identify potential organ donors. That Act requires the last physician who attended the deceased to consider, upon the death of one who has given no direction as to organ donation (or whose direction is invalid because the person was incompetent) whether it is appropriate to request permission of the donor's proxy or other relative to remove tissue or use the body for therapeutic purposes.[137] The physician must take into account the condition of the body and its tissues, the need for the use of these for therapeutic purposes, and the emotional and physical condition of the deceased's survivors. The Manitoba statute specifically provides for the removal of the pituitary gland and eyes (for corneal transplants).

Prince Edward Island requires a record to be made of whether any attending physician or other person discussed tissue donation with any of those authorized to provide consent on behalf of the patient to removal of organs or tissue. Such a case might arise in a hospital when a patient's death seems imminent. If no such discussion has taken place, the reason that it has not must be recorded.[138] This is as far as the PEI legislation goes. It does not demand that such consultation take place.

In contrast, Ontario's *Public Hospitals Act*[139] requires the board of every public hospital in the province to pass by-laws to establish procedures encouraging organ and tissue donation. Such procedures include identifying potential donors and making them and their families aware of the opportunities for organ and tissue donation.[140]

Application to Case Study

The misconceptions and misinformation surrounding organ tissue laws in Canada are regrettable, and have contributed to a low rate of organ retrieval across the country. The case study of Mr. R. and Mr. S. raises the issue of whether the ICU team ought to have been more persuasive with Mr. R.'s family. This would have been an appropriate role for the nurses in Mr. R.'s team. With the valid organ donor card, they could have proceeded despite the parents' wishes. However, in practice, most hospitals do not contravene the wishes of the deceased's next-of-kin, even with a valid consent from the deceased. This is unfortunate. The reason for this practice may be that attempting to persuade the deceased's family to consent might be deemed coercive. However, if the team approaches the family in a gentle, diplomatic, and sensitive way, the request need not be coercive; in fact, it might garner more support from such families. Many more lives could be saved if this situation were expressly addressed in each province's legislation.

Further, can it be said that Mr. R.'s family made a truly informed consent, as they were not given the complete facts of the situation—namely, Mr. S.'s need? Legislative reform might focus on the extent and nature of the information to be given to those authorized to make such decisions on behalf of donors. It may be within the rights and duties of the nurse to make such information known to those making a similar decision.

Foetal Tissue Transplantation

A recent and controversial area of transplantation involves the use of foetal tissue for the treatment of neurological disorders and, potentially, other diseases. The major focus to date is in the treatment of Parkinson's disease, where there is the potential not only for control of the disease, but also a cure. Other opportunities exist for the treatment of Alzheimer's disease, Huntington's chorea, multiple sclerosis, ALS, spinal cord injuries, acute leukemia, illnesses resulting from radiation accidents, and diabetes.[141,142] The controversy over the use of tissue is recent, though historically, foetal thymus and islet cells have been used for research into the treatment of thymus disease and diabetes and in the development of the polio vaccine.[143] Foetal tissue is highly suited to transplantation because of the lack of differentiation of the cells and, therefore, reduced risk for rejection. Unlike adult neural cells, which cannot be replaced, foetal neural tissue grows rapidly.[144]

The controversy over the use of foetal issue for research purposes and for treatment is fuelled by its link to elective abortions, the main source of tissue. Spontaneous miscarriages provide abnormal and unusable tissue, and in most instances, occur outside the clinical setting. Tissue can be used from ectopic pregnancies and stillbirths, but the numbers are too low to meet the need.[145]

Whether one is for or against abortion, a number of concerns have been raised about the use of foetal tissue. These include concern over the commercial use of tissue, the exploitation of pregnant women, and encouragement of abortion or pregnancy for the purpose of donation.[146,147]

The abortion debate is at the heart of the controversy over foetal transplantation. There are three views on the status of the foetus:[148]

- the foetus is simply tissue;
- the foetus has the potential for human life;
- the foetus is a human being.

Those who consider the foetus as simply tissue would have no serious moral concerns with foetal transplantation. They would consider that the tissue belongs to the pregnant woman, who may dispose of it in any way she chooses. Those who support the second and third perspectives believe that the foetus has some moral standing given its potential for life, or the belief that life already exists.[149] On the other hand, it is argued that it is also morally relevant that this potential can be fulfilled only through development within women's bodies.[150] If one objects to abortions, then it would follow that deriving gain from such a process would be inappropriate. Some with these views, however, might accept the concept of foetal transplantation, depending on the possibility of separating the act of abortion from the use of tissue from dead foetuses (i.e., the decision to abort is separate from the decision to donate). In this case, they would argue that foetal tissue should be afforded the same respect as cadaveric tissue from human donors.[151]

Guidelines associated with the use of foetal tissue have been recommended to address the concerns of those who oppose abortion, to reduce the chance that the opportunity for transplantation would influence a woman's choice to abort, and to eliminate the risk of financial incentives.

At present, there is a legislative void on the issue. The laws of most common law provinces would likely treat foetal tissue as any other human remains. In common law, there are no property rights attaching to a dead body. A deceased person's executor has a limited right to possession of the body for the purposes of arranging a funeral and burial, but this is clearly not applicable in cases involving foetal tissue. Although proposed amendments to the *Criminal Code* will regulate embryonic research and surrogacy, they are silent on the issue of foetal tissue transplantation.

Other problems have been identified relating to the distinct difference between the use of brain tissue versus the use of other organs or tissue for transplantation. The difference is that the brain is deemed a "defining organ of human behaviour and personality," responsible for cognition, the experience of pain and pleasure, consciousness, and sense of self.[152]

The problematic area of concern is that tissue may be taken from parts of the brain responsible for cognition or self-awareness, and then transplanted into parts of another brain responsible for cognition or self-awareness. If the amount of tissue were great, its placement in the recipient might alter cognition or self-awareness.[153] These concerns can be addressed, however, since the number of cells currently transplanted is small, and tissue is usually removed from lower parts of the cerebrum not responsible for cognition or self-awareness. Also, through the consent process, the recipient will have been made aware of potential risks as well as benefits.[154]

Further concerns associated with foetal transplantation relate to the process of consent. Similarly to discussion related to transplantation in general, the approach to consent could include expressed donation, presumed donation, or expropriation of tissue.[155] Other views suggest that this would be a case of abandonment in that the mother, in choosing abortion, has relinquished the right to make decisions about the tissue or product of the abortion.[156] Consent in this case, it is argued, is similar to the arguments supporting parental consent for children, in which the requirement is based on the assumption that parents have the best interests of their child in mind. When a pregnant woman chooses to abort, the validity of her consent is thus in question.[157,158]

There are a number of arguments in favour of the use of foetal tissue, particularly related to the potential benefits of treating and curing diseases that reduce lifespan and result in severe morbidity. There are perceived benefits associated with reduction in the cost of care, reduction of ongoing physical and psychological suffering, and ability to save lives.[159]

The area of foetal transplantation is in its early stages. New opportunities for its use will likely emerge, even as the controversy continues.

Summary

Nurses today belong to a health care culture that constantly strives to overcome the mysteries of life and death. This chapter has explored many difficult ethical and legal issues that nurses face in day-to-day practice.

Many advances in science and technology allow us to manipulate and control the process of reproduction, and the nature of the life that results. The availability of these resources raises legal and ethical questions. The technologies are expensive, and available only to those who can pay—raising troubling questions about equity. Further, the social consequences that arise out of these many approaches raise other legal and ethical dilemmas about the nature of family, truth-telling, and privacy.

The emphasis in medicine and health care on the principle of sanctity of life has driven the development of treatment modalities and technologies that can cure many previously terminal diseases and save lives, but that can also prolong the process of dying. People's fear of dying in isolation, and in pain and suffering, has driven society to seek other options to ensure that we are protected from this fate.

Nurses can play an important role in ensuring that clients' rights and dignity are respected throughout the process of dying. The ultimate goal of nursing should be that patients are made comfortable, are kept free of pain and suffering, and remain in control. For example, they should be able to make decisions about where they die, and the people with whom they wish to be at that time. As members of Canadian society, nurses share in the debate about the ethics of assisted suicide, euthanasia, and the like. At the least, their professional role should ensure that these measures will not be necessary for their clients.

The key points introduced in this chapter include:

- the extent of advances in reproductive science and technology
- the nature and influence of genetic technologies
- the legal, social, and ethical dimensions that arise from recent advances in the area of reproduction
- the legal and ethical issues surrounding death and the process of dying
- the legal definitions of death, euthanasia, and assisted suicide
- the legal and ethical implications of withdrawal of treatment
- the use and legality of advance directives (living wills)
- the legal and ethical issues surrounding tissue donation and organ transplantation
- some possible new definitions of death
- the ethical and legal issues respecting foetal tissue transplantation.

Critical Thinking

These case studies are for further reflection, discussion, and analysis. As you review each case, consider the following questions as well as those specific to the case.

1. Have the nurses in these cases violated any ethical or legal standards?
2. If so, what are these standards?
3. Is there risk of any civil or criminal liability?
4. How could these situations have been prevented?

CASE STUDY: IN WHOSE BEST INTERESTS?

Ian is a 29-year-old man who sustained a major head injury in a car accident seven years ago. He is presently in a long-term care facility. Ian cannot communicate in any way, requires total care, and is incontinent of urine and stool. He is likely in a persistent vegetative state, and his prognosis is thought by the team to be hopeless. He has a gastrostomy tube and receives regular feedings.

Ian's parents believe that their son would not wish to be maintained in this way and have requested that the feeding tube be removed. They have repeated this request several times in past years. However, the hospital's policy does not allow discontinuation of tubes. As tubes are replaced at regular intervals, Ian's family is now asking that their son's tube not be replaced in the event that it accidentally falls out.

QUESTIONS

1. What are your views on this hospital's policy regarding withdrawal of treatment?
2. As a nurse, how would you support this family?
3. Do you agree with the family's plan?
4. In this situation, what would be the legal requirements for organ donation in your home province?
5. What criteria does your hospital use for determining death?

CASE STUDY: WHOM DO I WANT BESIDE ME?

Saleem is a 74-year-old man who suffered a serious heart attack, causing a small hole in his ventricular septum. His condition is critical; his only option is to be placed on an intra-aortic balloon pump (to assist cardiac output) and undergo immediate surgery. He agrees to this treatment plan.

Saleem's wife and children remain in the ICU's waiting room during his surgery, which takes about six hours. They are relieved when he is wheeled into the ICU; they have been told they will be able to visit within a few minutes of his return. When this does not happen, they inquire and are told they will have to wait, as it is the change of shift and the nurses are giving report. A half-hour passes, and they ask again. This time, they are told that the nurses are still organizing Saleem's care; they must wait a bit longer. What is in fact happening is that Saleem is still bleeding from the surgery. The nurses are in the process of giving him blood; he is being assessed by the surgeon and a haematologist. An hour and a half later, the family has still not been allowed into his room. After asking again, they are allowed a five-minute visit.

QUESTIONS

1. What are the nurses' responsibilities to Saleem and his family? Did they meet these responsibilities?
2. What policies in hospitals and intensive care units might restrict nurses from meeting the needs of patients and families?
3. How might nurses and nursing leaders ensure that policies and rules reflect high ethical and professional standards?
4. Can you think of similar situations in your own practice?

CASE STUDY: CONFLICT IN VALUES

Gillian, a registered nurse, works on a busy gynaecology unit. One evening, two of her patients experience abortions. Sue, a 24-year-old single woman, has had a saline abortion, as she and her boyfriend decided late (at 16 weeks) that they did not wish to proceed with the pregnancy. The process was painful, and Sue found it disturbing to see the foetus. Afterward, she was tearful and unable to sleep.

Gillian's other patient, Linn, has spontaneously aborted at 24 weeks. She has just returned from having a D&C. Linn and her husband were part of the in vitro fertilization program at the hospital. This was her third pregnancy; she aborted each time. As there are no embryos left, they will have to begin the process again, and her obstetrician does not recommend this. Linn is also very upset and cannot sleep.

Gillian's time is limited. Now, she wonders which patient needs her most.

QUESTIONS

1. What would you do in Gillian's situation? What principles would guide your actions?
2. Should both these patients be on the same unit? Should both have been assigned to Gillian?
3. What responsibilities do nursing leaders have to ensure that hospital environments and structures minimize ethical conflicts for nursing staff?

CASE STUDY: CARE AFTER DEATH

Liz has just learned that her only brother Glen has been killed in a motor vehicle accident. Though his identity has been confirmed, Liz and her parents wish to see him. They are directed to the hospital's Emergency Department, where the nurses say little to them beyond indicating that they have called a supervisor.

When the supervisor arrives a quarter of an hour later, she offers condolences and tells them how hard the team worked to save Glen. When Liz expresses her need to see her brother, the family is taken to the hospital morgue. They are distressed to seem Glen wrapped in a plastic sheet, his hands bound and his face covered in blood.

QUESTIONS

1. What responsibility did the nurses in the Emergency Department have to this family? Was the morgue a suitable environment for viewing the body?
2. Does respect for the person extend beyond life, or do other factors (such how busy the unit may be) take precedence?
3. How do you think this experience will affect the family's experience of grief?

CASE STUDY: THE COST OF COMFORT

Carla, a case manager in the home care setting, is currently coordinating the care of a cancer patient dying at home. Darlene is expected to die within the next few days. Community nurses visit daily, but mainly her daughters and husband are caring for Darlene. Though she receives morphine on a regular basis she is still in great discomfort. Darlene is emaciated; the skin over her coccyx has broken down, and the cancer has metastasized to her bones. One daughter comments to Carla that during a recent hospital admission the nurses placed her mother on a special mattress that relieved her discomfort considerably. Carla explains that this mattress is not covered by home care, and instead offers special-duty nurses for the next few nights. Anticipating Darlene's imminent death, she is concerned that the family will need their rest. The family refuses the offer of nurses, since they want to remain with their mother and ensure they are with her when she dies. They make arrangements to rent the mattress themselves at their own cost.

QUESTIONS

1. What are Carla's responsibilities to ensure that Darlene's care needs are met?
2. Does it make sense that a less costly, more practical intervention be denied? How can nurses change agency policies in order to introduce guidelines that focus on individual needs? (Or, should all client be treated the same way?)

QUESTIONS FOR DISCUSSION

1. Identify the key arguments in favour of the new reproductive technologies. In your opinion, are these arguments valid? What are the opposing arguments?
2. How can exploitation of women be prevented as new reproductive technologies emerge? What concerns in this regard have been expressed by feminist thinkers?
3. What are your views on the legalization of euthanasia and assisted suicide? If euthanasia is legalized, what safeguards should be in place? What role should nurses play?
4. What guidelines are in place in your facility to ensure that a person has a peaceful and dignified death? Can these guidelines be improved?
5. Has your facility any policies or rules that limit family access to patients? Can these rules or policies be supported ethically?
6. Identify the key differences between organ/tissue donation and transplantation in general, and the new territory of foetal tissue transplantation. Can foetal transplantation be supported by those who oppose abortion?

References

1. Canadian Nurses Association (CNA). (1997). *Code of ethics for registered nurses* (pp. 13–14). Ottawa: Author.
2. Stanworth, M. (1987). Reproductive technologies and the deconstruction of motherhood. In M. Stanworth (Ed.), *Reproductive technologies: Gender, motherhood and medicine.* Minneapolis: University of Minnesota Press.
3. Ibid., p. 10.
4. Ibid., p. 11.
5. Ibid., p. 10.
6. Ibid., p. 21.
7. Robertson, J.A. (1995, November). Ethical and legal issues in human embryo donation. *Fertility and Sterility,* 885–894.
8. Fluker, M.R., & Tuffin, G.J. (1996). Assisted reproductive technologies: A primer for Canadian physicians. *Journal of SOGC.*
9. Ibid.
10. Government of Canada. (1996). *New reproductive and genetic technologies: Setting boundaries, enhancing health.* Ottawa: Author.
11. Ibid.
12. Schiedermayer, D.L. (1988, Fall). Babies made the American way: Ethics and interests of surrogate motherhood. *The Pharos,* 2–7.
13. Government of Canada, supra footnote 10.
14. Fluker & Tuffin, supra footnote 8; Government of Canada, supra footnote 10.
15. Government of Canada, supra footnote 10.
16. Fluker & Tuffin, supra footnote 8; Government of Canada, supra footnote 10.
17. Ibid.
18. Fluker & Tuffin, supra footnote 8.
19. Ibid.
20. Robertson, supra footnote 7.
21. Ibid.
22. Ibid.
23. Ibid.
24. Ibid.
25. Sherwin, S. (1992) *No longer patient: Feminist ethics and health care* (pp. 117–136). Philadelphia: Temple University Press.
26. Government of Canada, supra footnote 10, p. 12.
27. Ibid.
28. Ibid.
29. Ibid. p. 6.
30. Ibid. p. 5.
31. Ibid. p. 6.
32. Ibid. p. 7.
33. Bill C-47, 1996. House of Commons of Canada.
34. Sherwin, supra footnote 25, p. 118.
35. Ibid.
36. Ibid.
37. Ibid., p. 120; Overall, C. (1987). *Ethics and human reproduction* (pp. 5–116). Boston: Allen & Irwin; Oakley, A. (1987). From walking wombs to test-tube babies. In Stanworth, M. (Ed.). *Reproductive technologies: Gender, motherhood and medicine.* Minneapolis: University of Minnesota Press.
38. McIlroy, A. (1996). Ottawa to regulate baby trade. *Globe and Mail,* p. 1.
39. Government of Canada, supra footnote 10.
40. Sherwin, supra footnote 7.
41. Ibid.

42. Schiedermayer, supra footnote 12.

43. Government of Canada, supra footnote 10, p. 21.

44. Zipper, J., & Sevenhuijsen, S. (1987). Surrogacy and feminist notions of motherhood. In Stanworth M. (Ed.), *Reproductive technologies: Gender, motherhood and medicine.* Minneapolis: University of Minnesota Press.

45. Government of Canada, supra footnote 10.

46. Ibid.

47. Dickens, B.M., (1987) Artificial reproduction, infertility treatment and artificial conception. In G. Sharpe (Ed.), *The law and medicine in Canada* (2nd ed., p. 642). Toronto: Butterworths.

48. See In re Quinlan, 137 NJ Super. 227; 348 A.2d. 801 (Ch. Div. 1975), In re Quinlan, 70 NJ 10, 355 A.2d. 647 (SC 1976).

49. See *Rodriguez v. British Columbia (AG),* [1993] BCWLD 347; (1992), 18 WCB (2d) 279 (SC); aff'd. (1993), 76 BCLR (2d) 145; 22 BCAC 266; 38 WAC 266; 14 CRR (2d) 34; 79 CCC (3d) 1; [1993] 3 WWR 553; aff'd. [1993] 3 SCR 519.

50. *R v. Latimer,* [1997] 1 SCR 217; 152 Sask. R. 1 (SCC). Sentence following second trial order by Supreme Court of Canada: (1998), 121 CCC. (3d) 326.

51. See *Nancy B. v. Hôtel-Dieu de Québec et al.,* [1992] RJQ 361; (1992), 86 DLR (4th) 385; (1992) 69 CCC (3d) 450 (SC).

52. Government of Canada. (1995). *On life and death.* Report of the Special Senate Committee on Euthanasia and Assisted Suicide. Ottawa: Author.

53. Canadian Nurses Association (CNA). (1997). *Code of ethics for registered nurses* (p. 13).

54. Ibid., p. 14.

55. See Law Reform Commission of Canada (1980), *Medical treatment and criminal law* (p. 71). Working paper no. 26. Ottawa: Author.

56. *R v. Latimer,* supra footnote 50.

57. Caralis, P.V., & Hammond, J.S. (1992). Attitudes of medical students, house staff, and faculty physicians towards euthanasia and termination of life-sustaining treatment. *Critical Care Medicine, 20,* 683–690.

58. Genuis, S.J., Genuis, S.K., & Chang, W.C. (1994). Public attitudes toward the right to die. *Canadian Medical Association Journal, 150,* 701–708.

59. Supra footnote 49.

60. Ibid., per Lamer J. (dissenting), at pp. 530–531 (SCR).

61. *Charter of Rights and Freedoms,* Part I of the *Constitution Act, 1982,* being Schedule B of the *Canada Act, 1982 (UK),* 1982, c. 11, section 7.

62. Ibid., section 15(1).

63. Ibid., section 12.

64. The provision in the *Criminal Code of Canada* making it an offence to commit or attempt to commit suicide was repealed in 1972. See *Criminal Law Amendment Act,* SC 1972, c. 13, section 16.

65. Supra footnote 61, section 1.

66. Supra footnote 49, p. 592 (SCR).

67. Ibid., pp. 595–596.

68. [1993] 2 SCR 119. This case is discussed in detail in Chapter Six.

69. Supra footnote 51.

70. (1990), 72 OR (2d) 417 (CA). This case is discussed in detail in Chapter Six.

71. Supra footnote 49, p. 606 (SCR), citing a *Harvard Law Review* note: Physician-assisted suicide and the right to die with assistance, (1992) 105 *Harv. L. Rev.* 2021, at pp. 2030–2031.

72. Law Reform Commission of Canada. (1983). *Euthanasia, aiding suicide and cessation of treatment.* Report no. 20. Ottawa: Author.

73. Supra footnote 49, p. 603 (SCR).

74. Ibid., p. 608.

75. Ibid., per Lamer J. (dissenting), p. 544.

76. Ibid., per Lamer J. (dissenting), pp. 530–531; Fluker & Tuffin, supra footnote 8; Government of Canada, supra footnote 10.

77. Ibid., per Lamer J. (dissenting), p. 559.
78. Ibid., pp. 566–567.
79. Ibid., p. 579.
80. Ibid., per McLachlin J. (dissenting), L'Heureux-Dubé (concurring), p. 618.
81. RSM 1993, c. 33, CCSM, c. H27.
82. RSNS 1989, c. 279.
83. RSBC 1996, c. 6.
84. SO 1992, c. 30, as amended by SO 1994, c. 27, SO 1996, c. 2.
85. SA 1996, c. P-4.03.
86. 14 CED (Ont. 3d.), Title 72, section 177, citing an unpublished article.
87. Supra footnote 84, section 46(1).
88. Supra footnote 81.
89. Supra footnote 82.
90. Supra footnote 85.
91. RSBC 1996, c. 405 (not yet in force at time of writing).
92. Task Force on Presumed Consent. (1994). *Organ procurement strategies. A review of ethical issues and challenges* (p.7). Toronto: Multiple Organ Retrieval & Exchange Program of Ontario.
93. Ibid., p.6.
94. Ibid., pp. 10–11.
95. Youngner, S.J., et al. (1985, August 1). Psychosocial and ethical implications of organ retrieval. *New England Journal of Medicine,* 321–324.
96. Ibid., p. 17.
97. Infra footnote 109.
98. Youngner, et al., infra footnote 95, p. 18.
99. Ibid., pp. 21–25.
100. Ibid., pp. 13–17.
101. Ibid., pp. 12–13.
102. Keatings, M. (1989). The persistent vegetative state: Nursing perspectives. *Transplantation Proceedings.*
103. Ibid.
104. *R v. Kitching and Adams,* [1976] 6 WWR 697, at p. 711 (Man. CA), per O'Sullivan J.
105. RSM 1987, c. V60, section 2; CCSM, c. V60, section 2.
106. Alberta: infra footnote 109, section 7(1); British Columbia: infra footnote 109, section 7(1); Newfoundland: infra footnote 109, section 9(1); Nova Scotia: infra footnote 109, section 8(1); Prince Edward Island: infra footnote 109, section 11(1); Quebec: infra footnote 109, article 109; Saskatchewan: infra footnote 109, section 8(1); Yukon Territory: infra footnote 109, section 7(1).
107. Manitoba: infra footnote 109, section 8(1).
108. Capron, A.M. (1987). Anencephalic donors: Separate the dead from the dying. *Hastings Centre Report,* 17(1): 5–9.
109. See Alberta: *Human Tissue Gift Act,* RSA 1980, c. H-12, as amended; British Columbia: *Human Tissue Gift Act,* RSBC 1996, c. 211; Manitoba: *The Human Tissue Act,* SM 1987-88, c. 39, CCSM, c. 180, as amended; New Brunswick: *Human Tissue Act,* RSNB 1973, c. H-12, as amended; Newfoundland: *Human Tissue Act,* RSN 1990, c. H-15; Northwest Territories: *Human Tissue Act,* RSNWT 1988, c. H-6; Nova Scotia: *Human Tissue Gift Act,* RSNS 1989, c. 215, as amended; Ontario: *Human Tissue Gift Act,* RSO 1990, c. H.20; Prince Edward Island: *Human Tissue Donation Act,* SPEI 1992, c. 34; Quebec: *Civil Code,* articles 19, 23–25, 42–45; Saskatchewan: *Human Tissue Gift Act,* RSS 1978, c. H-15, as amended; Yukon Territory: *Human Tissue Gift Act,* RSYT 1986, c. 89.
110. This effectively means kidneys, and recently, liver lobectomies, since no person can live with the loss of any other non-regenerative organ.
111. Manitoba Act, supra footnote 109, section 1, "tissue" (c).
112. Quebec Civil Code, supra footnote 109, article 19, paragraph 1.
113. Ontario Act, supra footnote 109, section 3(1); Prince Edward Island Act, supra footnote 109, section 6(1).

114. Quebec *Civil Code*, supra footnote 109, article 19, paragraph 2.
115. New Brunswick Act, supra footnote 109, section 1. "Donor" speaks of consent that specified body part or parts be used after the donor's death.
116. Northwest Territories Act, supra footnote 109; sections 1(1) and (2) speak of specified body parts used after the donor's death.
117. Alberta Act, supra footnote 109, section 3(1); British Columbia Act, supra footnote 109, section 3(1); Newfoundland Act, supra footnote 109, section 4(1); Nova Scotia Act, supra footnote 109, section 4(1); Ontario Act, supra footnote 109, section 3(1); Saskatchewan Act, supra footnote 109, section 4(1); Yukon Territories Act, supra footnote 109, section 3(1).
118. [1980] 2 SCR 880; (1980) 14 CCLT 1; 114 DLR (3d) 1; 33 NR 361 (SCC).
119. Prince Edward Island Act, supra footnote 109, section 6(1).
120. Ibid., sections 6(2) and (8).
121. Ibid., section 8(6).
122. Ibid., sections 7(1) and (4).
123. Ibid., section 9(1).
124. Manitoba Act, supra footnote 108, sections 10(1) and (2).
125. Ibid., sections 10(4) and 11(3). This applies in both the case of a child donor under 16 and of a person between 16 and 18.
126. *Health Care Consent Act, 1996,* SO 1996, c. 2, Sched. A, section 6, paragraph 3.
127. SPEI 1996, c. 10, section 12(e).
128. This issue is more fully discussed in Sneiderman, B., Irvine, J.C., & Osborne, P.H. (1989), *Canadian medical law* (pp. 220-223). Toronto: Carswell.
129. Prince Edward Island Act, supra footnote 109, section 7(2).
130. Manitoba Act, supra footnote 109, sections 2(1) and (2).
131. Quebec *Civil Code*, supra footnote 109, article 43.
132. In Prince Edward Island, the person's guardian ranks above his or her spouse.
133. Quebec *Civil Code*, article 42.
134. Ibid., article 45, paragraph 1.
135. Ibid., article 45, paragraph 2.
136. Manitoba Act, supra footnote 109, section 4(3)(a).
137. Ibid., section 4(1).
138. Prince Edward Island Act, supra footnote 109, section 4.
139. RSO 1990, c. P.40.
140. O. Reg. 518/88, section 4(1), as amended by O. Reg. 34/90.
141. http://www.nhk.or.jp/forum/life/e/title/t-09htm
142. Childress, J.F. (1997). *Practical reasoning in bioethics* (p. 302). Bloomington: Indiana University Press.
143. Ibid.
144. Supra footnote 141.
145. Ibid.
146. Childress, supra footnote 142, p. 307.
147. Mahowald, M.B. (1997). The brain and the I: Neurodevelopment and personal identity (p. 1). http://ccme-mac4.bsd.uchicago.edu/CCMEFaculty/Mahowald/Brain.html
148. Childress, supra footnote 142, p. 304.
149. Ibid.
150. Mahowald, supra footnote 147, p. 4.
151. Childress, supra footnote 142, p. 305.
152. Mahowald, supra footnote 147, p. 6.
153. Ibid., p. 6.
154. Ibid.
155. Childress, supra footnote 142, p. 312.
156. Ibid., p. 316.
157. Ibid.
158. Mahowald, supra footnote 147, p. 5.
159. Ibid., p. 6.

CHAPTER Eight

Patient Rights

LEARNING OBJECTIVES

The purpose of this chapter is to enable you to:
- define the rights of patients and the obligations of health professionals
- appreciate patients' rights to confidentiality and the conditions under which disclosure is permitted
- understand patients' rights to information, respect, and discharge from a health facility.

Introduction

As we have seen in Chapters Four and Six, patients have the rights to respect, privacy, and confidentiality; to be told the truth; and to give or refuse informed consent. Further, as we discovered in Chapter Seven, they have the rights to refuse treatment (or to request that it be withdrawn) and to die with dignity. When an individual has a right, then others have an obligation to ensure that right is protected.

Nurses are obliged to ensure that patients' rights are respected and upheld. Further, to fulfil the role of caregiver, nurses must advocate on behalf of their patients and clients, especially when they are unable to speak for themselves. These obligations are clearly expressed throughout the CNA's *Code of Ethics for Registered Nurses,* for example:

> Nurses support and advocate a full continuum of health services including health promotion and disease prevention…, as well as diagnostic, restorative, rehabilitative and palliative care services.[1]
>
> Nurses respect the informed decisions of competent persons to refuse treatment and to choose to live at risk.[2]
>
> Nurses observe practices that protect the confidentiality of each client's health and health care information.[3]

Many agencies and health care institutions demonstrate their commitment to respect for patient rights by developing and publishing a bill of such rights, or they may express this commitment in their mission statement. Others state that they have adopted the values of a professional code such as the *Code of Ethics for Registered Nurses*.

In this chapter we will clarify the relationship between rights and obligations, and provide illustrations of the important rights of patients and clients within the health care system.

What Is a Right?

A **right** is a claim or privilege to which one is justly entitled, either legally or morally. Legal rights make explicit an individual's claim to such entitlement. For example, one explicit right under the Canadian *Charter of Rights and Freedoms* is the freedom or liberty of an individual to think, say, write, or otherwise act in accordance with his or her beliefs.[4] This suggests another aspect of rights, that is, autonomy, or the right to act on one's own, free of interference or control of the state or others. However, this right is not absolute. Our laws must also regulate the behaviour of citizens, and this somewhat limits the freedom of each citizen to do as he or she pleases.

A right carries a corresponding obligation. For example, in the context of health care, if someone has the right to care, then another person (or, more often, the state) has the corresponding obligation to provide that care. Otherwise, the right becomes meaningless.

The rights of patients are made explicit and clear through standards contained in professional codes of ethics. These impose an obligation on health professionals to provide adequate levels of safe and competent care to patients.

Legal rights are enforced by individuals through court action, that is, through the coercive power of the state to compel individuals to act or refrain from acting in particular ways. In Chapter Three, we described the basic legal and political rights and freedoms held by Canadians under the *Charter of Rights and Freedoms* and in various statutes of Parliament and the provincial legislatures.

Moral rights include the right to be treated with respect for one's autonomy, for example, to be treated courteously. In a health care context, patients have the moral right to be informed not only of the risks of treatment (for purposes of granting or refusing informed consent) but also to more general information as to what the facility and its caregivers can and cannot do. This might include information about the state of a patient's health, the treatment resources and alternatives available, the role of the facility's health professionals, the proposed treatment plan, and the plan of care after discharge. Of course, this also includes the patient's right to refuse or otherwise control the information he or she receives.

These rights are not all necessarily formally recognized in law, but they are acknowledged as societal norms of North American culture. They are based on the ethical principles of autonomy, beneficence, and non-maleficence (as discussed in Chapter Two). That is, the patient has the ultimate right to make any and all decisions respecting treatment. These rights are enforced, not necessarily through the courts, but through the maintenance of superior practice standards and the ethical values and rules practised by health professionals every day. If necessary, however, these rights could be enforced through court action in civil negligence or criminal proceedings, should their breach bring harm to the patient.

What Are Obligations?

We have noted that moral and legal rights carry corresponding **obligations** on others. An obligation is anything that a person must do or refrain from doing in order to permit the full exercise of the rights of another. For example, in order for a patient to exercise the right to make an informed consent, the health practitioner charged with that person's care is obliged to ensure that all relevant information has been provided, that the patient has been told of all relevant material risks and consequences inherent in the procedure, and that the patient's questions and concerns have been answered to the best of the health practitioner's ability.

The health practitioner must also ensure that he or she acts in a professional manner and observes all applicable standards of practice. These include the obligation to be informed and aware of the latest developments in his or her area of practice, to maintain up-to-date knowledge and competency, and to treat patients with respect, dignity, and courtesy.

Informed Consent

We have already discussed the right to informed consent in Chapter Six. This is not only a legal but also a moral right based on the ethical principles of autonomy, individual respect, respect for self-determination, and the right of individuals to make decisions about the course of their lives. In order to exercise these rights, patients must be fully informed regarding their health condition, prognosis, and treatment options, together with the consequences and risks. Lack of information, or the giving of incorrect or insufficient information, deprives the patient of the right to make a truly informed decision about the course of treatment. As we have seen in previous chapters, the giving of treatment without a fully informed consent can lead to legal liability for negligence—even battery, if no consent was given.

As discussed earlier, the *Code of Ethics for Registered Nurses* makes explicit the rights of patients to control their own care. Nurses have a responsibility to inform patients of the nursing care available to them and to welcome patients as active participants in their own care. The patient also has the right to know the extent of the assessment that the agency is performing.

A learner's right?

Ming has consented to have vaginal polyps removed. Her gynaecologist has explained the procedure in detail. Ming is also aware that while she is under the anaesthetic she will undergo a thorough pelvic exam. However, the gynaecologist has not told her specifically that there will be medical students present during the procedure. This is a teaching hospital, and all patients are expected to be informed, when they are admitted, of the role of students.

Third-year medical students are present during Ming's procedure. To give them experience in conducting pelvic exams, the gynaecologist allows three of them to undertake separate examinations. Robert, the circulating nurse, expresses his concerns about this to the gynaecologist. He tells Robert that Ming has consented to the examination and that there is nothing wrong with giving the students some experience. How else are they going to learn?

Issues

1. Who is right?
2. In the circumstances, is Ming's consent to this examination legally and morally valid?
3. Were any of Ming's rights violated?
4. What should Robert do?
5. What is the hospital's responsibility?
6. How may appropriate learning experiences for students be ensured?

Discussion

Chapter Six explored the elements and aspects of a truly informed consent. The consent must not only be informed; it must also be free of undue interference by others. There must be no coercion, inducement, or other pressure placed upon the patient to give the necessary consent, nor should the patient be forced to receive information that he or she does not wish to receive. Any fraud perpetrated on the patient to obtain consent would vitiate (negate) it.

As part of the obligation to provide general information the health care team should, upon a patient's admission to a health facility, provide him or her with an orientation to the roles of the caregivers, their functions, the physical layout of the unit, as well as the unit's routines, procedures, and schedules. This advice would include information about promoting health and preventing disease. Such information is usually provided by primary care nurses (in a clinical setting) and community nurses (such as those in public health).

In the case of teaching hospitals, patients should be made aware of the role of students within that facility and the nature of their relationships within the health care team. However, a general overview of the involvement of students (e.g., interns, residents, student nurses) does not fulfil the obligation to provide more explicit information in particular circumstances where patients are at risk, or if their privacy will be invaded. For example, patients should be aware when residents are to play a primary role during an operative procedure. In our case study, the gynaecologist had an obligation to inform Ming and to seek her consent to allow the students this learning opportunity. Teaching hospitals should ensure that processes are in place to fulfil this standard.

Right to Health Information and Teaching

Nurses across the system are expected to facilitate a smooth, safe, effective transition to the community for the patient and family (for example, to ensure that home care resources are available and initiated in a timely way). Further, nurses are required to provide discharged patients with the knowledge and skills to care for themselves (to the extent that they are able) after they are released from hospital. When the patient is not able to provide self-care, then family members or friends may be involved. Client teaching might include information on nutrition, the proper use and maintenance of any equipment at home, the proper administration of medication, and the changing of dressings. Clients should also be given any assistance they require in seeking further information.

Knowledge of how to gain access to the health care system is invaluable to all clients. Here, the nurse can provide a service by informing clients about the workings of the system, treatment alternatives and facilities, alternatives to traditional Western medical care, and so forth. For discharged or elderly patients, information as to available home care services is essential. Where incompetent patients are concerned, the nurse should discuss these matters and ensure a good working relationship with the substitute decision maker(s). This is important, as the nurse involved in the day-to-day care of such a patient will be intimately aware of all aspects of his or her treatment and progress—what is and is not working—and will be able to relate this information to the proxy decision maker. This, in turn, will enable the proxy to make better-informed treatment decisions in the patient's best interests.

One challenge that may arise is a patient's request to a nurse about the diagnosis. Here, the nurse must proceed carefully. In Ontario, for example, under the *Regulated Health Professions Act, 1991*,[5] "communicating to the individual or his or her personal representative a diagnosis identifying a disease or disorder as the cause of symptoms … in circumstances in which it is reasonably foreseeable that the individual or his or her personal representative will rely on the diagnosis" is a controlled act. The nurse would be permitted to make a diagnosis only if authorized to do so under the *Nursing Act, 1991*,[6] as the holder of an extended certificate (nurse practitioner), or if a physician delegated the making of the diagnosis to the nurse according to the rules and regulations governing the delegation of controlled acts. Ontario's *Nursing Act, 1991* now includes the communication of a diagnosis among those controlled acts that may lawfully be performed by nurses.[7] Other provinces may or may not legally restrict the making of a diagnosis, for example, in their medical professional statutes.

A special problem for the nurse arises when the patient's physician refuses to communicate a diagnosis. If the nurse is sufficiently experienced and knowledgeable to know the diagnosis, should he or she inform the patient, regardless of the physician's refusal? In such a case, the nurse should endeavour to change the physician's mind on this point and advocate for the patient, stressing his or her right to be informed. If this does not work, the nurse may have to turn to the physician's superiors or higher authorities in the health facility.

In most cases, an answer to the patient's question by the nurse need not entail the communication of a diagnosis, but simply the confirmation of what the patient sees as self-evident. For example, suppose that a female patient has previously been told that she may have breast cancer. Surgery is performed to explore the extent of the tumour and to remove it. The patient, once awake in the Recovery Room, asks the attending nurse whether a tumour was found and if so how much, if any, of her breast was removed. She already feels some pain from the incision and knows that her breast does not feel right. The patient's physician has left for the day without having a chance to talk to her about the results of the operation. Should the patient be left in suspense to await the physician's return? The nurse, by exercising common sense, could properly confirm the patient's suspicions with a few well-chosen words to ease her mind and lessen the emotional stress of not knowing. The nurse should be prudent, exercise judgement, and consider all the alternatives.

Cardiopulmonary Resuscitation

Special challenges are also posed by no-CPR (no cardiopulmonary resuscitation) and DNR (do not resuscitate) directions from a patient, which must be respected as part of the patient's autonomous right to refuse treatment.

A dignified death—whose choice?

Joe, an 18-year-old man, is dying of lymphoma. He has expressed his wish to die at home. All aggressive treatment attempted so far has failed, and for the past few weeks Joe has been receiving palliative care at home.

One night Joe experiences sudden shortness of breath. His family panics and calls 911. By the time the ambulance team arrives he has settled, but the attendants insist he be taken to the closest Emergency Department. Joe is admitted to a medical unit while the physician on call attempts to locate the primary physician.

Meanwhile, as two of the nurses are settling him into his room, Joe stops breathing. The nurses are faced with a dilemma. They are aware of his history. His family is outside in the waiting room. Since the nurses have not heard from the primary physician, they do not have a no-CPR order. They have two choices: they can call a code, or they can invite Joe's family into the room and give them some privacy.

Issues

1. What are Joe's rights in this situation?
2. How would the policy in your institution (if applicable) guide you in this scenario?
3. What is the role of policy in assisting nurses to make the right decision?
4. What is the right decision in this case, legally and ethically?

Discussion

A distinction should be made between "no CPR" and "DNR." The latter is a broader concept that includes any treatment given to sustain life (e.g., blood transfusions, artificial ventilation, dialysis, antibiotic therapy). CPR is limited to the technique of compressing the patient's chest without applying artificial ventilation. It is important to document carefully the precise nature of the patient's wishes (or those of the substitute decision maker) in this respect.[8] The order withholding CPR in no way limits the administration of other treatment to which the patient has not withheld consent.

Some caregivers may feel that honouring the patient's wishes regarding resuscitation conflicts with the principles of beneficence and non-maleficence, that is, to promote the patient's well-being and prevent harm. Certain guidelines have been developed to resolve such conflicts. These guidelines are similar to those followed in other treatment situations and outlined, for example, in Ontario's *Substitute Decisions Act, 1992*.[9]

First, the patient should be assessed to determine whether his or her life would likely be prolonged by the intervention of CPR. The results of the assessment should be disclosed to the patient when possible, and his or her wishes obtained and respected. The course of action to be followed, and any discussions held among caregivers, the patient, and the patient's family with respect to the decision, should be carefully documented in the patient's chart. Further, the reasons for the decision should be documented and communicated directly to the health care team. The no-CPR decision should be reviewed at regular intervals decided upon by the decision maker, either the patient or his or her substitute. It should also be communicated to the care team of any other unit to which the patient is subsequently transferred.

In cases where the patient is incompetent, his or her advance directive should be respected, subject to any changes expressed by the patient after making it. Such changes should be documented and made known to the attending physician. If there is no advance directive and no substitute decision maker appointed, the decision to implement or withhold CPR will be made by others on the basis of their knowledge of the patient's values and wishes.

In this case study, the information available to the nurses indicates that Joe and his family had accepted the inevitability of his death. Joe chose a course of action inconsistent with aggressive medical intervention. Clearly, he had chosen to die in his own environment, close to his family and friends. Policies are meant to guide action. Rigid adherance to "rules" in every circumstance may, in fact, contradict good judgement and conflict with individual choice.

Right to Confidentiality

In some circumstances, a patient's right to confidentiality may conflict with the health professional's broader obligations to provide care and to prevent harm.

CASE STUDY

Conflicting obligations

Jim is a 34-year-old man who is well known to the community health centre that he and his family have attended for several years. He is married and has two young children. His wife is eight months pregnant. He is a computer salesman and spends much time away from home travelling to clients across the country.

A few weeks ago, Jim presented to the clinic complaining of generalized fatigue and lethargy. He had recently lost five kilograms and had noticed some unusual lesions on his inner thighs. As part of the blood screening done at that time, an HIV test was undertaken. This turned out to be positive. Given his clinical picture, it was likely that he had already developed AIDS.

Jim's primary care nurse is present when his physician relays the bad news to Jim. Clearly distraught, Jim admits that he has had sexual intercourse with a number of women during his business trips, and on several occasions did not bother to use a condom. Fearful of the effects that this revelation would have on both his family and his business contacts, Jim pleads with his caregivers to keep this information, and his diagnosis, confidential. Given his wife's pregnancy, he feels this knowledge might cause her undue harm. He assures them that he and his wife have not had intercourse since her pregnancy. He refuses any treatment for his AIDS-related symptoms, since this would make the diagnosis obvious to everyone. Instead, he asks that his family, including his wife, be told that he has terminal and incurable cancer. Jim's physician (who is also his friend) says that he will respect Jim's wishes for now.

Issues

1. Did the clinic have the right to test Jim for HIV without his knowledge or consent?
2. Should the health care team keep Jim's diagnosis confidential from his wife?
3. Should the fact that Jim's wife is also the clinic's patient influence their actions and decisions?
4. Does the team have an obligation to follow Jim's instructions and misrepresent his diagnosis to others?
5. If the primary nurse disagrees with the decision of the physician, what can she do?

Discussion

The patient has the right to know the extent of the assessment that the agency is performing. In some provinces, public health laws require that a health care agency obtain consent for HIV testing.

The primary legal rule with respect to any information that the health practitioner obtains from the patient during the course of their professional relationship is that such information is confidential and may not be disclosed to anyone who has no valid purpose for requesting it. There are exceptions to this rule, both in the common law and as provided by statute. But in many provinces, the improper disclosure of confidential information respecting a patient constitutes professional misconduct.[10]

For example, it may be necessary for one health professional to share with another selected information contained in the patient's medical records for consultative purposes. Or, a health practitioner who has become involved in a patient's treatment may need to know what treatment has been provided thus far, and the progress of the patient's recovery. This is a normal part of obtaining a history, which the patient should expect upon being admitted to health facility. No specific consent need be obtained in such a case, since it is clearly implied that all persons involved in the patient's treatment have a valid reason for inspecting that patient's records. Nevertheless, the patient always has the right to expect that any information divulged to a nurse or other health practitioner will remain confidential until and unless another professional has a valid need for it.

In our case study, the nurse and the physician are faced with a challenge to the patient–professional relationship. They should consult with and support Jim, giving him time to digest and understand his situation, and clarify why his wife should be involved. If necessary, they should support him in disclosing this information to her. Because there is still the potential for harm to Jim's wife and their unborn child, the team has a moral and professional obligation to inform her of Jim's infection. Certainly, the clinic owes Jim's wife an equal duty of care, since she too is their patient. Further, the nurse and physician must tell Jim that, given the high risk of infection with HIV, they have a legal obligation to inform the local medical officer of health of his infection. This is required by law in all provinces and territories.

The nurse should discuss these points carefully with the physician. If he still refuses to manage this situation as required, it would be appropriate for the nurse to appeal to the next level of authority until she is satisfied that action is taken. The nurse should not simply let the matter drop.

Statutory Duty of Disclosure

In many provinces, statute law requires certain patient information and conditions to be disclosed. For example, many public health laws require health practitioners to disclose the identity of anyone diagnosed with certain communicable diseases or sexually transmitted diseases (such as gonorrhoea and HIV/AIDS, among others) to the local medical officer of health. This is especially important with respect to HIV/AIDS.[11]

In most provinces, the identity of the patient and the nature of the disease must be reported to the local medical officer of health (usually employed in the municipality by a local board of health or other such authority). In this way, the potential spread of such diseases can be controlled to some extent. The virulence and seriousness of these illnesses are deemed sufficient to justify the infringement on the patient's right to confidentiality. For example, in the case study, it would be unlawful for the physician at the clinic not to divulge the fact that Jim was HIV positive (and may, in fact, have full-blown AIDS) to the local medical officer of health.

Similarly, there may arise instances when a patient tells a nurse that he or she intends to hurt or kill another person. Such a remark may be a manifestation of the patient's illness; nevertheless, if the patient has a history of violent behaviour through which others have been hurt or killed, or if the patient seems likely to harm himself or herself or others, such a statement should be reported to the authorities in the institution and to the police.

The nurse's duty of confidentiality towards the patient is somewhat analogous to a lawyer's towards a client; however, there are situations when the law requires the nurse to disclose certain information about a patient. A lawyer is under a continuous duty to ensure that any information that a client discloses during the course of their professional relationship must remain confidential. For example, the lawyer may not divulge the fact that the client told the lawyer that he or she committed a crime. Such disclosure is unethical and may constitute professional misconduct.

The law has not recognized a corresponding privilege of confidentiality among other client–professional relationships such as doctors, psychiatrists, nurses, counsellors, accountants, or clergy. Legally, there is no obligation on a health professional to aid police in their investigations. However, where a patient poses a threat to others, there is an ethical obligation to report this.

However, the right to confidentiality may be limited in cases where there is a legal obligation to divulge the information, such as in a disciplinary hearing of the health professional, a civil or criminal trial, or a coroner's inquest or other government-authorized inquiry. The right is also limited when the information must be disclosed to avoid harm to the patient or to a third party. In practice, however, most courts will not readily violate the client–professional relationship without a strong or compelling reason to do so.[12] For example, if required by a court, the health professional must answer any and all questions put to him or her. Failure to do so would place the practitioner in danger of being found in contempt of court and liable to a heavy fine or possible imprisonment.

A confession of prior illegal activity made to a health practitioner may not have to be disclosed. But, it is possible that at some point a court may compel the practitioner to disclose such a fact. The only professional who would be exempt from disclosing such facts would be a lawyer (yet even a lawyer would have to guard against being an accessory to the client's crime). Although the health practitioner is under no obligation to aid police, concealing the whereabouts of a fugitive could be construed as aiding and abetting such a person. This is especially likely in light of the *Criminal Code* offence of being an accessory to a crime after the fact.[13] One is an accessory when one "knowing that a person has been a party to the offence, receives, comforts or assists that person for the purpose of enabling that person to escape."[14] By not divulging the information with the intent that the patient should avoid detection by the police, the health practitioner may be subject to criminal charges.

There are instances where provincial law requires disclosure, such as information concerning those having a communicable or sexually transmitted disease, or in cases of suspected child abuse. Many provinces have set up child abuse registries. The laws that establish these are intended to encourage the reporting of situations in which a child has been sexually or physically abused. Indeed, these laws require child care workers, physicians, nurses, and other health practitioners to report suspected cases of child abuse, either to the police or to the local Children's Aid Society for further action. In most cases, it is an offence punishable by fine or prison for a health practitioner to fail to report an instance of suspected child abuse that he or she encounters in the course of practice.

We have discussed, in Chapter Five, the obligation of the health practitioner in Ontario and some other provinces to disclose incidents of sexual abuse of patients by other health practitioners. Indeed, even in provinces where there is no such explicit requirement with respect to abuse by health professionals, such behaviour is a reportable criminal offence and constitutes professional misconduct.

Disclosure of Information in Workers' Compensation Matters

Some nurses are employed as case managers by various Workers' Compensation Boards across Canada. All information gathered on employers and workers by such boards in the course of their investigations remain strictly confidential. Indeed, in British Columbia, the Northwest Territories, Ontario, Manitoba, and Saskatchewan, it is an offence to disclose such information without proper authority. The laws in these jurisdictions include substantial fines for contravention. The remaining provinces also impose sanctions and penalties for improperly divulged information. In some provinces, nurses employed by such boards may be required to take an oath of confidentiality as a condition of employment.

Ontario and British Columbia provide a full right, through their freedom of information and privacy protection Acts, to access by a worker to his or her file. Generally, workers, their dependents in the case of death, the worker's personal representative (such as a guardian or attorney for personal care), and the employer may have access to information respecting the worker. Access by employers to health information in Ontario respecting a worker is restricted to only those details related to the specific injury and its treatment. The worker must be notified by the Board of its intention to divulge health information to his or her employer.

The Boards also generally have the right to health information and records from a worker's health practitioner that are relevant to the injury or illness in the claim. A worker who files a claim for benefits is deemed to consent to the release of such information by the practitioner on request. Delays associated with such release can harm the worker in that payment of benefits is often conditional on the Board's receiving this information.

Disclosure of Confidential Information in Court Testimony

There will be occasions, such as in a medical malpractice action, or an inquest into a death, when the nurse must disclose information in court testimony. Most provincial nursing statutes and regulations permit such disclosure. However, the nurse should be careful even when lawfully disclosing patient information. Only those details that are relevant to the issues in the hearing, trial, or inquiry should be disclosed. The nurse should not give a "blanket" disclosure of all possible information, which may not be relevant to the issues under inquiry. Here, the nurse must use discretion and common sense.

Ensuring Confidentiality in the Treatment Setting

A nurse may inadvertently disclose confidential information in casual conversations with colleagues, friends, or relatives who have no valid interest in such details. Thus, nurses must take care at all times not to divulge confidential patient information when engaged in casual conversation in social settings unconnected to their work and duties.

Likewise, the old saying "the walls have ears" applies to hospitals and other health facilities. For example, care should be taken when discussing details of a patient's condition in hallways, stairways, and elevators. Even when discussing a case with a colleague, only such disclosure should be made as is absolutely necessary for that person's participation in the patient's care and treatment. This requires great caution and discretion on the part of the nurse.

There are other instances where confidential information may inadvertently be disclosed. For example, when a patient is being seen by a nurse in an Emergency Room in the presence of other people, the nurse should speak in a low voice in discussing the problem so as to avoid being overheard. The best way to prevent such a situation is to segregate the patient in a private room or area where privacy can be assured. Often, simply closing a door or drawing a curtain around the patient's bed will suffice.

Computer Records and Confidentiality

Many hospitals and other health facilities now use a computerized system to maintain patient and other records. Consequently, there is wider access to a great deal of information by a potentially greater number of people. Access in most cases is controlled by means of magnetized cards and passwords. It is important for nurses to use their own passwords and not to use others' means of access since, in many cases, the use of the password and card is the nurse's electronic signature. Thus, if a nurse were to share his or her access code with another care provider, then any action or documentation undertaken on the system would be attributed to the nurse who "owns" the code.

Many computer systems document the fact that a particular person gained access to a particular patient's record. The date and time of such access will also be noted in the computer record. In a few cases, hospital nursing staff have been disciplined for using their access cards for improper and unwarranted access to patient files simply to satisfy their own curiosity.

Automated records provide many benefits for patient care and for improving the nurse's efficiency. Some of the positive aspects include greater accuracy and validity of documentation, timeliness of recording, and ready access to important information—across the system—about that patient's episode of care, previous admissions, and treatment.

Right to Privacy

The right to privacy goes hand in hand with the right to confidentiality; one cannot have one without the other. As we have seen in the context of consent to treatment, this implies a right to be free from control of the state or others as to the course of treatment to be followed.

But the right to privacy carries with it more practical aspects with respect to nursing. For example, when a patient is bathing, and to the extent that it is safe to leave the patient alone, he or she should be ensured complete privacy. This right extends to treatment situations and examinations. Thus, care should be taken when examining a patient to ensure that the room is not fitted with mirrored windows, that unauthorized persons are not permitted into the room, or that pictures not be taken without the patient's permission, even if this is done for educational purposes.

Similarly, in instances where the nurse feels that a consultation with clergy or a social worker may benefit the patient, the nurse may request such a consultation on his or her behalf. Nevertheless, the patient may refuse such help, in which case the patient's privacy must be respected.

Right to Respect

Health professionals have an obligation to treat all clients with respect and dignity. Disregard for privacy, or failure to involve clients in decisions relevant to them, violates nurses' ethical responsibility to those in their care.

CASE STUDY
Who advocates for the patient?

Alan underwent emergency coronary artery by-pass surgery 10 days ago, and since then, his condition has remained critical. He has never completely regained consciousness. Owing to a lung infection, he remains on a ventilator under heavy sedation. In the past week he has developed one complication after another—total body sepsis, a life-threatening arrythmia, hypotension, and some liver failure—for which he has received a number of drugs. Now he is in kidney failure and requires dialysis.

His family have been at the hospital since Alan's ordeal began. They have been allowed only short visits once or twice per shift. The nurse and doctor now inform them of the kidney failure, and leave them alone to discuss whether they should consent to dialysis.

Alan's family knows his prognosis is poor. They also know he would not wish his life to be extended in this way. They believe he has suffered enough, and decide to refuse the dialysis, knowing he will die. They request a meeting with the team to communicate their decision.

While visiting Alan a short while later, his wife notices that he is still receiving drugs to maintain his blood pressure, as well as the antibiotics that so far have not improved his condition. Further, the nurse informs her that because Alan's potassium is elevated, he will be given calcium polystyrene enemas in an attempt to bring it down.

The family is distraught. Together, they gather the courage to tell Alan's nurse that they do not wish to subject him to these enemas which, if effective in the short term, will only prolong his dying. Further, they insist that the drugs be discontinued, and that they be allowed to remain with him in privacy.

Alan's nurse supports the family's position and communicates their wishes to the physician on call. The family is permitted to stay with Alan until he dies peacefully a short time later.

Issues

1. How did this case evolve to the point where Alan's family needed to advocate on his behalf?
2. How could this situation have been avoided? What process would have resulted in a better outcome for everybody?
3. What rights did Alan and his family have? Where these rights respected?
4. Identify the contradictions in this story.

Discussion

The right to respect includes the right to be treated courteously, to privacy, to be addressed by one's preferred name or title, and the corresponding obligation of the nurse to introduce himself or herself by name to the patient. It is important for the nurse to listen carefully, to focus on the patient's perceptions and needs, to respect his or her culture, religion, values, and relationships with friends and family. For example, talking about the patient as if he or she were not present diminishes that person's humanity and is disrespectful, as is administering needless medical treatment that will do nothing to improve the patient's welfare and will cause more pain and suffering. This is especially important when caring for patients who are dying.

Dying is a significant process for patients, families, and caregivers. It is a time that requires all the nurse's powers of empathy. Providing as dignified a death as possible means being concerned about the patient's pain and symptom control, respecting the patient's privacy, and knowing when he or she wishes to be left alone or with family and friends. It also means being concerned with where the patient wants to die. Some patients may wish to remain in hospital or to be referred to a palliative care facility. Others may prefer to be at home, yet may not be aware of the resources available to make this choice possible. Rarely does anyone want to die alone.

As much as possible, nurses should keep the patient's family and friends informed of the patient's status so that they will be available when necessary. When the patient's condition deteriorates, the family should be informed promptly. The nurse does not need permission to telephone a family member to let that person know what is happening and that his or her presence may be necessary.

Unfortunately, many patients in hospitals die during the process of cardio-pulmonary resuscitation. It is common that, during this procedure, families are removed from the patient's room. This limits the patient's right to have a caring family member or friend present when death is imminent. Caregivers are uncomfortable with the idea of family members witnessing what is often a distressing experience. Nevertheless, this is the patient's right and the family's choice. When it appears to be their wish, a full description of the arrest procedure should be explained to family members, who have the right to choose whether to be present. On occasion, loved ones have been present at arrests, sitting quietly and stroking the patient's face, apparently oblivious to the resuscitation efforts. As part of their role in patient advocacy and leadership, nurses might attempt to change systems and processes within their facility to ensure that this can happen more frequently.

Certain aspects of the right to respect find formal recognition in the law. For example, all patients have the right to equal access to health care resources and facilities without regard to sex, colour, mental or physical disabilities, ethnicity, creed, or religion. These rights are enshrined in various provincial human rights codes.

Right to Be Discharged from a Health Care Facility

Discharge from Hospital

Can a patient be prevented from being discharged from a hospital? In many cases, a patient who wishes to leave a hospital or other health facility against medical advice must sign a waiver acknowledging that he or she has been advised that leaving is not desirable at this time. If the patient refuses to sign the waiver, the fact that he or she is leaving against medical advice (AMA) should be carefully documented in the chart. Ultimately, there is nothing hospital staff can do to prevent a patient from leaving. A hospital is not a prison.

In cases involving psychiatric patients of unsound mind, the mental health statutes of most provinces may permit such persons to be prevented from leaving if they pose a threat or danger to themselves or to others.

When a patient is discharged, the hospital has an obligation to ensure that he or she arrives home safely. For example, in cases involving same-day surgery, a patient should not be sent home if the sedative has not yet worn off. Such a patient may have to be sent home by taxi or other means, as he or she would not be in a condition to drive. There have been reported cases in which patients still under the effect of sedatives have subsequently driven home and have been charged with impaired driving. In many hospitals and health agencies, patients who have been sedated are required to wait a specified period of time and to be accompanied by another person when they leave the institution.

Discharge from a Mental Health Facility

Most provinces have legislation governing admission to and discharge from a mental institution.[15] As a rule, if a person's state of mental health is such that he or she poses a threat either to self or to others, such a person may be committed to a mental health facility for treatment upon the order of an examining physician. The determination that such a state of mind exists must be made by a physician.[16] In Newfoundland, a person may be detained in such a treatment facility only if two physicians certify that the patient is a danger to self or others by reason of a mental disorder.[17]

Generally, there are two categories under which a patient is admitted to a mental institution. The first comprises persons who may suffer from some mental disorder but who are not thereby a threat to themselves or others. These are usually voluntary patients. They cannot be detained without their consent.

Violent patients who do pose a threat to their own or others' safety generally may be admitted to an institution on an involuntary basis and may be detained without their consent. The matter does not end there, however. There are certain procedural safeguards in place to provide for a review of the detention of involuntary patients and to ensure they are not arbitrarily detained or detained without proper grounds. If they cease to pose a danger to themselves or others, the law generally requires that they be released when they wish.

In the Yukon Territory, the recently passed *Mental Health Act* articulates the rights of mental patients. As in many provinces, only minimal physical restraints may be used on such patients—that is, only what is reasonable and necessary, considering the person's physical and mental condition.[18]

Other rights in the Yukon include the right to receive and make phone calls;[19] to have reasonable access to visitors;[20] to have access at any time to the patient's legal representative, guardian, or other authorized person;[21] to send and receive correspondence; to vote; to wear clothing of the person's choice; to security of his or her person; to confidentiality;[22] and to be informed (if detained) of the reasons for detention.[23] In other jurisdictions, similar rights exist in common law, if they are not expressed in statute.

Summary

This chapter has dealt with the rights of patients and clients within the health care system, and the obligations of health professionals to ensure that these rights are respected. A health professional's obligations to respect patients' rights are not always clear; in fact, they may conflict with equal obligations to respect the rights of others. These rights and obligations evolve from the ethical theories and principles described in earlier chapters.

Nurses are obliged to ensure that patient rights are respected and upheld. The pressures of downsizing, heavy workloads, and other factors in today's health care setting can lead us to overlook, in day-to-day practice, even such basic patient rights as privacy and dignity. Professional codes of ethics, and patient bills of rights, help to ensure that our clients are informed of their rights and our obligations to protect them.

The key points introduced in this chapter include:

- the rights of patients and the obligations of health professionals
- patients' right to confidentiality and the conditions under which disclosure is permitted
- patients' rights to information, respect, and discharge from a health care facility.

Critical Thinking

These case studies are for further reflection, discussion, and analysis. As you review each case, consider the following questions as well as those specific to the case.

1. Have the nurses in these cases violated any ethical or legal standards?
2. If so, what are these standards?
3. Is there risk of any civil or criminal liability?
4. How could these situations have been prevented?

CASE STUDY: TO INTERVENE OR NOT?

Margaret, a registered nurse, is visiting her mother, a patient in a long-term care facility. Upon hearing raised voices in the next room, Margaret leaves her mother's bedside to investigate. She witnesses a nurse shouting at a patient that he wasn't doing enough to help her move him. When the nurse leaves the room obviously frustrated, Margaret goes in to see if the patient is all right.

This patient is a 60-year-old man with Guillain-Barré syndrome. Most of his body is paralyzed, but he does have minimal function in his upper body.

He tells Margaret that "everything is okay." He does not want her to discuss the event with anyone on the unit. He says, "It's easier this way. I'm totally dependent on the staff here, and the nurse didn't hurt me. She's just over-worked."

QUESTIONS

1. What should Margaret do?
2. What are the patient's rights in this situation? Are there conflicting rights here?
3. Does Margaret have any obligation, since she is not an employee of this facility?

CASE STUDY: A CONFIDENCE SHARED

Charlene is an occupational health nurse in a large manufacturing company. She is managing the case of an employee, Earl, who fractured his wrist when a heavy piece of equipment fell on him. Earl has had problems in the workplace; his manager has often spoken to him about his tendency to become distracted. This is a concern because of the safety risk to Earl and his co-workers.

Now Earl's wrist has healed and he is functionally able to return to work. However, he confides to Charlene that he is currently under great personal stress: his wife is dying of cancer, and he is so depressed that he can think about nothing else. Charlene recognizes that this stress may have contributed to Earl's injury and that, unless addressed, it might cause him further harm. However, Earl asks Charlene to keep this information confidential. He does not want his manager to know anything about his personal life. He simply wants to return to work.

QUESTIONS

1. Does Earl have the right to ask Charlene to keep this information confidential?
2. What other rights does Earl have that Charlene must respect?
3. Does the company, its managers, and other employees have any rights here?
4. What should Charlene do?

CASE STUDY: ACCESS AND DISCLOSURE

Karen is a registered nurse in the Emergency Department of a local community hospital. One evening, a neighbour, Louise, presents at the ED with abdominal pain of unknown origin. Karen is on duty when Louise is admitted to a surgical unit.

Some days later, another neighbour asks Karen how Louise is doing. At work, Karen accesses her chart via the hospital's computer system and discovers that Louise has been diagnosed with advanced liver cancer and further, that this information has been kept from her. The surgeon caring for Louise is well known for his paternalistic attitude. Karen recognizes that she must not share this information with anyone. However, she is unsettled to discover that Louise has been kept ignorant of her diagnosis and prognosis.

QUESTIONS

1. As an employee of the hospital, did Karen have the right to access Louise's chart?
2. Should the hospital have a policy to ensure privacy with the use of computerized information systems? What should this policy say?
3. In the circumstances, can Karen ensure that Louise's right to information is respected?

QUESTIONS FOR DISCUSSION

1. Does your setting have a bill of rights for patients/clients? How is this statement communicated? Do you believe it is the nurse's responsibility to ensure that patients know their rights?
2. Can you think of situations in which the rights discussed in this chapter might potentially conflict with the rights of the institution? Of the nurse? Of other patients and families? How do we balance these rights?
3. How do visiting hours in your facility support the rights of patients/clients? What processes are in place to support families of the terminally or seriously ill?
4. What procedures and policies need to be in place to guard against sexual harassment of patients by staff?

References

1. Canadian Nurses Association (CNA). (1997). *Code of ethics for registered nurses* (p. 8). Ottawa: Author.
2. Ibid., p. 11.
3. Ibid., p. 15.
4. Canadian *Charter of Rights and Freedoms,* Part I of the *Constitution Act, 1982,* being Schedule B of the *Canada Act 1982 (UK),* 1982, c. 11.
5. SO 1991, c. 18, section 27(2), paragraph 1.
6. SO 1991, c. 32.
7. *The Expanded Nursing Services for Patients Act, 1997,* SO 1997, c. 9, as amended the *Nursing Act* to allow nurse practitioners to make a diagnosis.
8. These guidelines and procedures are taken from the *Toronto Hospital Policy and Procedure Manual,* Policy #2.1.160, "No Cardiopulmonary Resuscitation Order" (pp. 1–3).
9. SO 1992, c. 30.
10. See Alberta: *Nursing Profession Code of Ethics,* Alta. Reg. 456/83, section 2(3); Manitoba:

Registered Nurses Act, RSM 1987, c. R40, CCSM, c. R40, section 46(2); New Brunswick: *Nurses Act*, SNB 1984, c. 71, section 42(1); Northwest Territories: *Nursing Profession Act*, RSNWT 1988, c. N-4, section 22(e); Ontario: O. Reg. 799/93, section 1, paragraph 10; Saskatchewan: *Registered Nurses Act, 1988*, SS 1988, c. R-12.2, section 26(2)(h).

11. See, e.g., Alberta: Alta. Reg. 238/85, schedule 4 "AIDS," amended by Alta. Reg. 357/88; British Columbia: *Health Act* Communicable Disease Regulation, B.C. Reg. 4/83, Schedule a; Manitoba: Man. Reg. P210-R2, amended by Man. Reg. 338/88R; New Brunswick: N.B. Reg. 86-66, section 94(1)(s); Newfoundland: Nfld. Reg. 60/87; Nova Scotia: Regulation in respect of communicable diseases, N.S. Reg. 171/85; Ontario: RRO 1990, Reg. 557, as amended; Prince Edward Island: Notifiable and Communicable Diseases Regulation, E.C. 330/85; Quebec: Regulations respecting the application of the *Public Health Protection Act*, RSQ c. P-35, regulation 1; Saskatchewan: Sask. Reg. 307/69, amended by Sask. Reg. 2/88.

12. See, e.g., *A.G. v. Mulholland*, [1963] 2 QB 477; *Slavytych v. Baker*, [1975] 4 WWR 620 (SCC).

13. *Criminal Code of Canada*, RSC 1985, c. C-46, section 23(1), as amended.

14. Ibid.

15. See British Columbia: *Mental Health Act*, RSBC 1996, c.288, as amended; Alberta: *Mental Health Act*, SA 1988, c. M-13.1; Yukon Territory: *Mental Health Act*, SYT 1989–90, c. 28; Northwest Territories: *Mental Health Act*, RSNWT 1988, c. M-10; Saskatchewan: *Mental Health Services Act*, SS 1984–85–86, c. M-13.1, as amended; Manitoba: *Mental Health Act*, RSM 1986, c. M110, CCSM, c. M110, as amended; Ontario: *Mental Health Act*, RSO 1990, c. M.7, as amended; Quebec: *Mental Patients Protection Act*, RSQ 1977, c. P-41, as amended; New Brunswick: *Mental Health Act*, RSNB 1973, c. M-10,. as amended; Nova Scotia: *Hospitals Act*, RSNS 1989, c. 208, as amended; Prince Edward Island: RSPEI 1988, c. M-6, as amended; Newfoundland: *Mental Health Act*, RSN 1990, c. M-9.

16. Ontario Act, ibid., section 15(1).

17. Newfoundland Act, supra footnote 14, section 5(2).

18. Yukon Act, supra footnote 14, section 18(1).

19. Ibid., section 40(2)(a).

20. Ibid., section 40(2)(b).

21. Ibid., section 40(2)(c).

22. Ibid., subsections 40(3), (4) and (5), and section 42.

23. Ibid., section 41.

CHAPTER Nine

Nursing Documentation

LEARNING OBJECTIVES

The purpose of this chapter is to enable you to:
- clarify the legal requirements of proper nursing documentation
- appreciate the importance of accurate and complete documentation in ensuring safe and effective nursing care
- establish guidelines for timely and accurate documentation, and apply them to hypothetical case studies and real case law
- appreciate the role of nursing assessments and their importance in the nursing notes
- explain the use and significance of incident reports
- clarify how nursing notes may be used in a legal proceeding
- explain the role of expert witnesses in interpreting nursing documentation.

Introduction

Careful and accurate documentation is a key component of professional nursing practice. The nurse's assessment and progress notes monitor, on a continuing basis, the course of treatment and the effect of interventions. From this record, a clearer picture emerges of the patient's or client's progress towards the stated goals and outcomes; also, any impending complications can be identified before they become problematic.

As we have seen in the case of *Bergen v. Sturgeon General Hospital et al.* (Chapter Three), failure to document specific acts or treatment accurately and contemporaneously can have dire consequences for the health practitioner in a negligence action. Inadequate documentation, or failure to review client information and history, negatively influences the quality of care.

Because nurses need to understand the rationale behind most organizations' focus on the assessment and progress notes, this chapter will examine the legal and practical aspects of proper documentation.

C A S E   S T U D Y

Documenting—is it enough?

An eight-month-old boy is brought into a hospital Emergency Department late one evening presenting with vomiting and diarrhoea and a history of toxoplasmosis. On arrival, his pulse rate is 120; his respiration rate 24. He is seen by the physician on duty in the Emergency Department and then by the hospital paediatrician, who admits the child and writes treatment orders for an IV, as well as tests for haemoglobin and BUN electrolytes.

While in hospital, the child's condition deteriorates. The nurses monitoring him over the next four to five hours note that his heart rate has increased to 164 and that his respiration is 64. Nurse H., who is looking after the boy, is concerned. She speaks to the charge nurse, who confirms her concerns, then phones the child's physician at his home.

It is now the middle of the night. Nurse H. informs the physician of the child's condition, pulse rate, respiration, and of the results of the tests for haemoglobin and BUN electrolytes, which were also abnormal. In particular, the CO_2 level was at 10.9 instead of the normal range of 22 to 32. The physician replies: "Well, that's fine; just continue doing what you've been doing."

Nurse H. is not satisfied with the doctor's response. After her telephone conversation with him, she again speaks to the charge nurse, who says: "Well, you're not the doctor; he is. Whatever he says, that's fine; don't worry about it."

All these abnormal results and readings are duly recorded by Nurse H. in the boy's chart. Also noted is the conversation with the charge nurse and the boy's physician, and the times at which these took place. The boy dies the next morning at 06:00 h.

Issues

1. What should the charge nurse have done when Nurse H. consulted her after phoning the boy's physician?
2. Should Nurse H. have taken her concerns about the boy's poor test results to a higher authority?
3. What steps should have been taken with respect to documenting the boy's vital signs and fluid intake, both in the Emergency Department and in Paediatrics?
4. Should Nurse H. have called the physician back to confirm his instructions? In speaking with the doctor, should she have placed greater emphasis on the boy's abnormal vital signs and test results?

Discussion

In this case study, the critical issue is that the charge nurse should have assisted Nurse H. in getting the help of the physician. Firstly, Nurse H. should have attempted to contact the physician a second time to impress upon him the urgency of the situation, especially if he'd been roused from a deep sleep that might have clouded his judgement.

Secondly, Nurse H. obviously realized the seriousness of the boy's condition from the vital signs that she observed. The standard of care in this case demanded that Nurse H. by-pass her non-supportive charge nurse and find a higher authority for instructions. Lack of support from a supervisor, even if accurately documented in the patient's chart, would not protect a nurse from liability.

Further, a nurse, having determined the high risks of inaction, must act and cannot hide behind the excuse that "the doctor said..." The nurse cannot avoid liability for inaction by simply documenting the doctor's instructions. There is also a corresponding duty to protect the patient from harm. In this case, the appropriate standard of care demanded that the nurses should have known and understood the severe consequences of inaction when the boy was in this condition. The conduct of both nurses in this case study clearly fell below the required standard of care.

In the real-life situation on which this case study is based,[1] a coroner's inquest was called to investigate the boy's death. (For a discussion of the coroner's function and role, see Chapter Five.) One of the issues that arose at the inquest was related to documentation of the fluid balance, particularly in the Emergency Department. It had not been totalled accurately, and it was difficult to determine how much fluid the patient had been given, both in the Emergency Department and in the Paediatrics Ward.

At the inquest, the boy's physician denied that the nurse had reported the patient's vital signs. The doctor further denied that he'd been given the results of the electrolyte tests (specifically, the CO_2 level). There were no other nurses on the floor that evening who witnessed what was going on, and thus no one to corroborate the nurse's telephone conversation with the physician. The doctor claimed he'd been roused from a deep sleep, that he had been up all the night before, that he was very tired, and that if the nurse had really had such a pressing concern, she should have phoned him back to confirm his instructions and make sure he realized the severity of the situation. In such a case, he said, he certainly would have taken the appropriate action. It was obvious that, regardless of which version of events was the correct one, the child died because of a serious breakdown in communication.

The coroner's jury found that the nurse should have documented her concerns in greater detail, and that this record should ideally have been witnessed by another nurse. She should have called the doctor back to repeat her concerns and had another nurse present to attest that she did so. Secondly, the hospital should have had procedures in place to by-pass the physician's instructions and to seek another doctor in the hospital to ensure that proper instructions were provided in the treatment of this child.

The cause of death, as determined in the autopsy, was dehydration. The IV that had been administered to the child was wholly inadequate. The inquest determined that the boy's fluid intake should have been checked more frequently and recorded systematically. In particular, the levels might have been checked and recorded by nursing staff just prior to the child's leaving the Emergency Department, and then again by the nurses in Paediatrics, immediately upon his transfer to that ward.

The jury did not accept the physician's excuse in this case, and he was found negligent for having given improper instructions. He was subsequently reported to the College of Physicians and Surgeons of Ontario and severely disciplined.

The Need for, and Uses of, Documentation

In most cases, the patient's chart, nurses' progress notes, and other documentation constitute the only written evidence of what care a patient has received. This record is vital during the course of treatment in that it facilitates communication between nurses and other health professionals actively involved in the patient's care. Without it, effective, safe, and proper care would be impossible. In this case, as the fluid balance was inaccurately recorded, the standard of accurate and complete documentation was not met.

The record is also a useful tool in planning the course of treatment. It encourages an accurate tracing of the patient's vital signs and condition. This promotes quality control of nursing and medical care, and permits caregivers to assess which interventions should be altered and which left in place. Thus, assessments must be complete and comprehensive. The documentation should also reflect the nurse's judgements, including identification of any problems and the focus of the action to be taken. This, in turn, permits others to follow through and to follow up on the efficacy of any action taken.

For example, suppose that an assessment of a patient notes that she is in severe pain. How adequate is such a description? Was this pain reported to the patient's physician? Was any medication given, or some other intervention tried? Did such medication or intervention work? Or, as another example, if the patient is agitated, what is the source of the agitation? Was there a review of the previous documentation? What was done before, and did it work? Accurate documentation aids in addressing such issues and in ensuring a consistent standard of care.

Further, a good patient record will contain information on any allergies (including allergies to medications) to which that patient may be susceptible, and some information about whom to contact in an emergency. This is especially important in cases where the patient is not capable and a substitute decision maker has been appointed to make treatment decisions on the patient's behalf. Equally important, the record should contain all previous treatment orders for the patient, plus any notes concerning follow-up of those orders.

Finally, the record is important in that it is evidence of the adequacy of any treatment that is administered, the appropriateness of care, and the quality of care received. This is especially important for audit purposes, in any disciplinary proceedings for alleged improper or unprofessional conduct, and in any negligence actions, criminal proceedings, or coroner's inquests in the event of the patient's death under circumstances requiring investigation.

Accuracy of Documentation

The documentation must be an accurate record of what was done, what medication was administered, and what the patient's condition was at the time the action was taken.

In the case of *Meyer v. Gordon,*[2] the parents of a newborn infant, who suffered severe brain damage and ensuing cerebral palsy as a result of a negligent delivery, brought an action for negligence against two of the participating nurses, the hospital, and the attending physician. In all, three nurses were involved in the delivery. The plaintiff had previously had a very fast labour, her first child having been born within four hours of the onset of labour. The plaintiff's doctor knew this, but had not advised the nursing or hospital staff that this might be a fast delivery when he had his patient admitted to the hospital on the morning when her labour began. Ascertaining the patient's birth history would be a normal and standard part of any labour assessment to be performed by a nurse. The plaintiff was admitted at approximately 11:30 h.

The first nurse who examined the plaintiff, Nurse W., did not ascertain whether this was her first or second birth, and in fact failed to obtain any obstetrical history. It was clear at the trial that, had she done so, the history would have indicated that this patient should be closely watched. As well, there was evidence that the charting done by the two nurses who attended the plaintiff was inaccurate and incomplete. As a result, the nurses' notes were rejected by the trial judge as unreliable. Nurse W.'s failure to ascertain the obstetrical history of the mother in this case shows a marked departure from acceptable standards of practice in Canada.

At approximately 11:30 h, Nurse W. performed the first examination of the plaintiff and ascertained that she was in the early stages of labour. She did not record this, however, and was imprecise as to the position of the foetus at that time, noting the position only as "mid." Neither did the nurse record the duration of the contractions during her first, and only, vaginal examination. At this point, she ascertained that dilation was three centimetres, but the character of the cervix (an important indication of the progress of labour) was not recorded accurately.

A second nurse, Nurse M., assisted Nurse W. in these examinations. Neither nurse appears to have recognized the danger of leaving the mother lying on her back, in which position she remained until delivery. The court found, among other things, that permitting the plaintiff to remain in this position contributed greatly to foetal distress and constituted a marked departure from the standard of care at that hospital, which was known for excellence in obstetrics. The mother should clearly have been repositioned on her side.

The foetal heart rate was checked at 11:50 h and again at 12:00. However, this information does not appear to have been recorded until much later. At noon, the patient's doctor prescribed an injection of Demerol and Gravol to ease her pain and nausea. Although this was not explicitly stated by the court or in the evidence as reported, the giving of Demerol would no doubt have had a sedative effect not only on the mother, but also on the foetus. This could have contributed to the onset of foetal distress. He did not instruct Nurse M. to conduct a vaginal examination prior to administering the Demerol and, in fact, none was conducted before the drug was given at 12:05 h. This was also against generally accepted practice.

From the time the Demerol was given until the child was born at 12:32 h, the plaintiff was left lying on her back, alone and completely unattended despite her excruciating and rapid labour pains and despite Nurse W.'s opinion that the foetal heart rate ought to have been checked every 15 min at that point. The court noted that, although the obstetrical ward appeared to have been extremely busy that day, the plaintiff did not appear to have been anyone's patient in particular from that point on.

At 12:15 h, the plaintiff's husband, distressed by his wife's extreme pain, sought out Nurse W. He told her that he believed his wife was about to give birth and needed assistance. The evidence at trial indicates that Nurse W. may have brushed off his concern, dismissing him as a nervous husband. The court found it deplorable that there was no nursing care available to the plaintiff when her husband sought it.[3]

At approximately 12:30 h, the plaintiff's husband again sought out a nurse, saying that his wife was giving birth. A third nurse (Nurse T.) responded and went to the plaintiff. She found the baby's head already born with a very large amount of meconium around it. She completed the delivery; however, as Nurse M. (who assisted her) had failed to include a suction bulb in the emergency bundle, Nurse T. was unable to suction the meconium from the baby's nose and mouth. This was also deemed a serious oversight by the expert physicians who testified at trial.

It is clear that the baby was not breathing when she was born. Nurse T. described the baby as "very flaccid and limp." Further time was lost in bringing the baby to the case room for resuscitation. Another doctor was involved in resuscitation using initial suctioning, positive pressure ventilation, and oxygen with endotracheal suctioning. As the court noted later, all these factors contributed to the risk of brain damage as a result of foetal distress. The resuscitation efforts continued for some time with the assistance of two other physicians and were ultimately successful. The child was moved to the hospital's Intensive Care Nursery. It was soon discovered, however, that she had suffered brain damage as a result of foetal distress and resulting asphyxia in conjunction with meconium aspiration.[4]

The plaintiffs sued the mother's doctor, the doctors involved in the resuscitation efforts and, more importantly, the nurses and hospital that had provided the nursing care. The court dismissed the suit against the doctors (except the plaintiffs' own doctor, whom it found 25% liable on the basis that he had failed to instruct Nurse M. to conduct a vaginal examination of the plaintiff prior to administering the Demerol). The hospital was found 75% responsible for the baby's brain damage, as a result of its negligence in failing to provide adequate and proper nursing care.

The court noted that both nurses had gone back and altered the chart some hours after the delivery to make the record appear more complete than it actually was. These facts meant that the court was unable to rely upon the nurses' notes as an accurate account of what had happened. Much was made of the fact that the nurses' notes were inaccurate and inadequate. For example, the time of the plaintiff's arrival at the hospital was not recorded.[5] Upon her initial examination of the patient, Nurse W. noted that the foetal heart rate was "normal," that the plaintiff's labour was "good," and that her cervix had dilated three centimetres, with "strong" contractions every two minutes.[6] The duration of the contractions was not recorded, as it should have been. Nurse W. also noted that the position of the foetus was at "mid" station.

The court found that the description of the labour as "good" did not indicate the fact (later brought out in Nurse W.'s testimony) that the plaintiff was also in active labour, which would normally have required a foetal heart rate check every 15 min.[7] The court was equally critical of the inexact description of the foetus' position as "mid" and of the lack of record as to the character or effacement of the cervix. This inaccuracy contributed to a poor appreciation of the extent and advanced stage of the plaintiff's labour.

In most court cases, failure to document a particular act during the course of treatment may mean that the court will assume the act was not done. Such failure seriously undermines the "weight" of the evidence, that is, how probative it is (how much the testimony proves, or how convincing it is that the act was actually done). If the record is sketchy and incomplete, it may not be accorded much weight by the court.

In assessing the quality and accuracy of Nurse W.'s recorded observations, the court relied on the expert evidence of two nurses (presumably, with obstetrical experience) who stated that an obstetrical nurse, when assessing foetal position, looks for the height of the presenting part of the foetus in relation to the ischial spines of the mother's pelvis. One of the experts, when asked about Nurse W.'s assessment of the foetal position as "mid," commented that such a notation was not specific enough to aid in the evaluation of the labour. The other expert stated that the expression "mid" used in the record had no meaning.[8] This case thus illustrates the importance of accurate and precise observations when documenting details of patient care and treatment.

Other Standards of Documentation

There are agency and government regulations that govern how records ought to be made and organized. For example, the Canadian Council on Health Services Accreditation (CCHSA) has set standards, as has each provincial regulatory body. As well, the particular health care agency's nursing department will likely have standards and policies governing proper patient documentation, for example, charting by exception. In this practice, a problem or condition is documented only if it deviates significantly from what one would normally expect in such circumstances. Otherwise, no notation is made.

Another practice is that of recording facts by means of defined checklists. For example, nurses may initial beside a listed procedure. This may mean (according to the policy manual on documentation) that the procedure was completed with no problems. If problems or changes in the patient's condition had occurred, the policy would require further documentation in the progress notes.

Whatever standards are in use, these will be backed by policies of the institution and definitions of those standards. When these standards, definitions, and policies exist, such documentation falls within legally acceptable standards.

Guidelines for Proper Documentation

Some rules of thumb have evolved to ensure timely and accurate recording, from both a legal and a practice perspective, of various details of a patient's care, condition, and treatment from hour to hour.

Record Contemporaneously

The record should be made at the time of occurrence of the event or action that is recorded. If not, the record or note should be made as soon as possible after the event. This makes the record more accurate and reliable, ensures safer care, and affords the record greater weight in any legal proceedings.

It is not always possible to record items, events, or actions at the time they occur, especially during emergencies. The longer the delay in documenting a fact, the more likely it is that the accuracy of the observation or detail will be questioned later, especially in a court trial. For example, in *Meyer v. Gordon*,[9] the nurses who treated the plaintiff had recorded some of their observations a considerable time after the fact, and further, had altered the record to make it appear that the observations had been recorded contemporaneously. Thus, the nurses' notes were deemed unreliable as an evidentiary source.

Another reason for contemporaneous documentation is that memory fades with time. A fact is more likely to be recorded accurately and completely soonest after the occurrence. Documentation of treatment is vital in court proceedings, as it is often the only source of evidence on what occurred. As considerable time may pass before a trial or hearing is convened, a well-constructed and well-maintained record serves to refresh the memory of the person who made it.

If it was not possible to record the act or event when it occurred (e.g., the nurse had other pressing obligations, or simply forgot), the late entry should still be recorded, to the nurse's best recollection, and noted as a late entry, thus:

> 12:30 h, patient regurgitated reddish coffee-ground fluid; recorded at 13:30 h because called away on emergency to assist in another patient's resuscitation. [*Signed*, etc.]

A late entry is clearly better than no entry at all. The nurses in the Meyer case attempted to cover up the fact that some of their entries had been made late rather than contemporaneously. This practice is strongly discouraged.

Record Only Your Own Actions

The nurse should record only his or her own actions. Since the notes may form the basis of testimony in any ensuing legal criminal or civil proceedings, the nurse will be permitted to testify only as to his or her own actions.

In particular, care should be taken when documenting a fact or detail on computer. The nurse should use only his or her own password or access card when gaining access to the computer record. This ensures that the computer log will accurately reflect the fact that a particular nurse made the entry.

Record in Chronological Order

All entries should be made in chronological order. Otherwise, a confused record would result, which could have serious repercussions in the course of treatment, especially with respect to the administration of medication. It would also make the record of limited use in any litigation and undermine the nurse's testimony.

Record Clearly and Concisely

Entries should be clear, concise, factual, and as objective as possible. Any evidence that leads the nurse to draw a particular conclusion should be carefully documented. A subjective entry potentially creates problems in patient care, and might leave the nurse's testimony open to challenge in a court proceeding.

Make Regular Entries

The nurse should make sure that the record contains regular entries throughout. If there are significant gaps in the record, the benefits of continuous monitoring of the patient are lost. Further, a lengthy gap in the record would be questioned in court (e.g., a gap of a number of hours prior to a patient's cardiac or respiratory arrest, pulmonary edema or, in a psychiatric setting, a psychotic event or suicide attempt).

Record Corrections Clearly

Any alterations, corrections, or deletions to the record should be carefully documented, dated (including the hour), and initialled by the nurse who makes the change. Otherwise, the nurse's credibility could be undermined in a court proceeding. No attempt should be made to cover up one's mistakes by surreptitiously altering the record to make it look complete.

In cases where a coroner's investigation is begun, the coroner usually quickly seizes nursing notes and other patient records in order to ascertain the circumstances of the patient's treatment or condition in the moments prior to death. This is especially so with the advent of computerized records. An entry in the computer is dated with the computer signature of the person making it. Because this can never be altered in most computer systems, the recorded act is "etched in time." Yet, there have been situations where nurses have attempted to alter the record upon learning of a coroner's inquest, only to learn later that the coroner had already seized the record and made copies of it. The coroner thus had an accurate version of the record at the moment of the patient's death, as well as evidence that the nurses attempted to alter the record afterward. Such situations are embarrassing. It is best to avoid them by making clear that one is documenting a fact some time after it has occurred, or that one is correcting a previous inaccuracy.

Record Accurately

Vague terms should be avoided. For example, rather than describing the foetal position as "mid," the nurse in the Meyer case should have documented the height of the foetus' presenting part relative to the ischial spines of the mother's pelvis.

Nursing assessments are key to care planning. The initial assessment when a patient enters the care process is crucial, and should therefore be thorough and comprehensive. Most agencies and hospitals require that initial assessments be made within a specified period from the time of admission. Inaccurate or incomplete assessments can affect the outcomes of care and raise serious questions in any ensuing legal proceedings.

The frequency of repeat assessments is based on patient need, complexity of care, and agency protocols. For example, in some settings, the initial assessment determines whether a patient is fall-prone. If so, this would necessitate reassessment on a regular basis. If this part of the assessment were omitted, and the patient subsequently fell, a negligence suit against the nurses and hospital could result. The trial would question why the assessment was incomplete, and would likely conclude that hospital staff were negligent in (a) failing to foresee that the plaintiff was prone to falling, and (b) failing to take appropriate precautions to prevent this.

Key aspects of the initial assessment are: the name of the person to contact in an emergency; the name of the patient's proxy (if any); any decision made by the patient or proxy regarding CPR (see Chapter Seven); and whether the patient has made an advance directive. All details from the initial assessment should be recorded in the patient's chart. Any reassessment should likewise be documented to ensure a complete record.

Thus, a notation in the patient's record: "Slept well, had a good day" is of limited use. In a court trial, the nurse who made the note could well be asked detailed questions about what he or she meant by "a good day" (e.g., any pain felt by the patient, symptoms, vital signs) in an attempt to pinpoint the patient's condition at the time when the notation was made. The nurse would probably be unable to answer such questions helpfully, as the original meaning of "had a good day" would have been forgotten.

For example, it is far better to document: "Patient reported sharp pains in chest radiating down the left arm of 10 min duration, relieved with rest," rather than: "Patient reported chest pain." The latter notation would not bear scrutiny in a legal proceeding. More importantly, it would be of limited use in an attempt to diagnose the patient's ailment accurately.

File Incident Reports

Sometimes a patient falls, or a mistake is made in administering medication. In such cases, a report should be prepared that documents and describes the incident, all relevant facts, any injuries sustained by the patient, and any remedial action.

Accident reports do not form a part of the medical record. They are used, firstly, to document occurrences out of the ordinary, for investigative or quality assurance purposes. For example, an insurance company might investigate a claim made against a hospital's general liability insurance policy; or, a hospital may be monitoring or auditing the rate of occurrence of certain types of incident over a specified period. Thus, such reports can contribute to the hospital's risk management by identifying possible problem areas in systems or procedures. The information gained can be used to educate staff to prevent similar occurrences in future.

Finally, in the event that a negligence action is brought against the hospital arising out of an incident, the incident report can form part of the evidentiary record at trial and assist the court in understanding the cause of the incident. Such a report is usually introduced along with the testimony of the health care provider(s) who made it.

Record Legibly

The records, and any corrections, should be legible. This is especially important given the speed with which nurses sometimes are required to perform their duties. Illegible entries may be misinterpreted in a way that was never intended by the maker. This can have disastrous results.

Nursing Theories and Conceptual Frameworks

Many hospitals and agencies base their standards for nursing documentation on a nursing theory or conceptual framework. Theories and frameworks drive and guide the clinical processes used by nurses when deciding patient care. Thus, the chart should document the patient's plan of care. This would include assessment, analysis, nursing diagnosis, problems or outcome identification, nursing interventions, orders, and evaluation. Standards of care require that these processes be charted, not only to provide evidence that the plan was developed and implemented, but also to ensure effective communication among those providers involved in the patient's care.

Computerized Documentation Systems

Today, many organizations use computerized systems for documentation. The same legal and ethical standards apply as with manual documentation. The benefits of computerized systems include greater legibility, reduction in documentation errors, decreased time spent documenting, improved and timely communication across the team, timely and efficient retrieval of data or information, and greater opportunities for monitoring and improving quality of care. Further, integrated systems allow for shared data bases and interfaces with other departments, such as Laboratories and Radiology. Computers allow for one-time data capture (for example, if one enters a laboratory value, it would automatically appear in all the components of the system where that value should be documented).[10]

Issues of concern that arise with automated systems relate to security and confidentiality and the legality of the electronic signature. Health care systems usually identify who is doing the documenting through access cards and passwords or a double password system. This becomes the caregiver's electronic signature. When nurses share their access with another caregiver, they are effectively allowing that person to use their signature; this could present legal liability at a future date.

To address the issue of confidentiality, most health care computer systems are designed to restrict access points (for example, a technician in the laboratory may not be able to access all components of the record, only that information relevant to the test being conducted), limit access through the use of security codes and passwords, and monitor access of information. For example, programs are in place to monitor the extent to which patients' charts are accessed by those not involved in their care.[11] In many facilities, access is monitored on a regular basis. Breaches of confidentiality are taken very seriously. It is up to each facility to ensure that safeguards (e.g., standards, guidelines, quality review) are in place to protect clients' privacy.

Computer documentation systems have the further advantage of ensuring greater accountability for documentation in terms of timeliness and accuracy.[12] For example, in on-line systems it is difficult to tamper with or erase previous documentation. It is also impossible to document later and attribute the documentation to an earlier time.

As information technologies emerge, nurses have the obligation to keep their computer skills up to date. This will enable them to utilize their facility's system to the standards necessary to achieve all the potential benefits.

Telephone Advice

As new roles emerge for nurses, especially in the areas of home and community care, and case management in Workers' Compensation, insurance and rehabilitation settings, there is increased likelihood that nurses may manage clients primarily over the phone. This practice poses particular challenges in conducting assessments, giving appropriate advice, and developing a therapeutic relationship with the client.

A nurse should be very careful when giving advice over the telephone; but this does not mean that nurses should refrain from giving appropriate information and referrals, when necessary. When in doubt about a client's condition or safety, a referral to the appropriate caregiver, or a request to meet directly, should be undertaken. Here, accurate and complete documentation of the patient's name, address, phone number, and symptoms is crucial. As well, any advice given to a patient over the telephone should be carefully noted, as well as the date and time of the call. Patients who seem to be experiencing a serious medical problem should be told to attend at the nearest Emergency Department without delay.

Use of Documentation in Legal Proceedings

Evidentiary Use

In many medical malpractice cases, the trial of the action will often occur several years after the events leading up to and including the negligent acts.

Memories fade with time, and the evidence given by witnesses, such as nurses and physicians, will often be hazy or incomplete. Therefore, the notes and records prepared by the health care team assume added value and significance, as these are often the only documentation of what occurred.

The courts wish to obtain the truth. Often, the truth lies in the health care records. Courts are impressed by meticulous, clear, legible, and well-organized records. These not only help the court (i.e., the judge and, in some cases, the jury) to determine the exact sequence of events and the circumstances of treatment; they also improve the credibility of the witnesses who made them. Thus, with a well-constructed health care record, the nurses and other caregivers who made the notes will be able to impart their testimony more forcefully, and that testimony will be accorded greater weight than would be the case with an inadequate record.

The court will be interested in all aspects of the record, including nursing progress notes, care plan, checklists, flow charts, hospital policies in force at the time, and so forth. These will provide a more complete picture of events. In many cases, the record will also document the thought processes and frame of mind of the health professionals at the time. For example, the patient's chart may reveal that a certain treatment or intervention was or was not warranted under the circumstances and given that patient's condition. This is a further reason for ensuring that records are made and kept according to the highest possible standards.

Expert Witnesses

Assessing the conduct of nurses in a particular case in relation to the appropriate standard of care often involves drawing upon expert testimony. The court calls upon experts because the judges trying a case rarely possess the necessary expertise to make valid conclusions and draw inferences from technical data. A nursing expert, on the other hand, can interpret the health care record and assist the court in reconstructing the events and drawing inferences. Experts can also be used by the parties to a lawsuit either to support the plaintiff's position and interpretation of the evidence, or to refute these for the defence, and perhaps suggest another cause for the injury. Although such inferences are properly the function of the judge or jury, the expert, because of his or her unique knowledge and experience, is permitted to formulate and express an opinion. This is an exception to the general evidentiary rule that a witness's opinion on a matter in issue is inadmissible.

More importantly, the nurse, as an expert witness, is able to describe the appropriate standard of care in a particular case. The nurse expert is often called upon to review the health care record, and in particular, the nursing notes, in order to give an opinion on whether proper documentation and nursing procedures were followed.

Prior to giving testimony, the nurse must be qualified before the court as an expert. This means the lawyer for the party wishing to rely on the nurse's evidence must first ask the nurse questions about his or her education, experience, nursing background, and continuing education. The purpose here is to establish in the trial record that the witness has the necessary qualifications to give such testimony or opinion.

In some cases, the expert testimony may also be elicited as part of the nurse's own involvement in the care of the plaintiff. Here, the nurse may be asked questions on his or her notations in the patient's record. It is important that the nurse answer such questions truthfully and as accurately as possible. As well, it is important that he or she ensure accuracy, clarity, and objectivity when compiling those notes in the first place.

Problems may arise with respect to alterations, deletions, or additions made to the nursing notes some time after the original entries. As a rule of evidence, the nurse or other person recording the note or observation will be allowed to use those notes to refresh his or her memory when testifying in court. However, the court must first be satisfied that:

(1) the notes were indeed made by that person;
(2) it was part of that nurse's duty to make such notes;
(3) the notes were made contemporaneously (or reasonably so) with the event or act that they record; and
(4) there have been no alterations, additions, or deletions to those notes since they were made.

Usually, items 1 and 2 pose no problem, as the nurse witness will have been involved in the patient's care, and will have been the one who made the notes in the first place as part of his or her normal duty.

Item 3 can pose a problem. For example, in the case of *Kolesar v. Jeffries*,[13] the court commented upon the documentation practices in the surgical unit where the plaintiff was placed post-operatively. The plaintiff was returned to the Recovery Room shortly after 12:00 h, sedated and unconscious, secured in a supine position to a Stryker frame following surgery on his spinal column. Although the standard of care in such a case would include rousing the patient at frequent and regular intervals to cough to keep his lungs clear, the plaintiff was permitted to sleep undisturbed by an overworked staff who made one round at midnight with flashlights. At 05:00 h the next morning, one of the nurses discovered the plaintiff dead. He had suffered pulmonary edema and haemorrhage secondary to the aspiration of gastric juices.

The court heard evidence that no nursing notes were made over a period of seven hours. Indeed, it was the practice in that nursing unit to record vital signs and any other observations as to the patients' condition on scraps of paper during the shift. Afterwards, the nurses would get together, and with the aid of these scraps of paper, they would reconstruct the record for each patient over the last few hours. The nurses would assist "each other to recall and record the events of the evening." This practice does not fulfil the requirements of contemporaneous recording.

Upon discovering that no entries had been made on the plaintiff from 22:00 h until 05:00 h the next day, the assistant director of nursing asked one of the nurses on duty that night to write up a report of the events. Here, the court noted:

> One is always suspicious of records made after the event, and if any credence is to be attached to [the nurse's report], it shows that at all times the patient was quite pale, very pale, and was allowed to sleep soundly to his death.[14]

Thus, the absence of adequate nursing records served only to reinforce the court's opinion that the standard of nursing practised in this patient's care had been wholly inadequate. If efforts had been made to rouse the patient regularly in order to note and record his condition and vital signs, his death could have been avoided.

In *Meyer v. Gordon*,[15] the alteration of the records prompted Mr. Justice Legg to remark:

> The hospital chart contains alterations and additions which compel me to view with suspicion the accuracy of many of the observations which are recorded. The chart also contains at least one entry which was discovered during this trial [in May 1980] to have been made after the fact. That also casts suspicion on the reliability of those who made the entries and undermines the accuracy of medical opinions based upon these entries and observations.[16]

Thus, any attempt to conceal an alteration of the health care record can effectively cast doubt on the witness' evidence, as well as any other evidence based on the entries and observations contained in the altered record.

Legal Requirement to Keep Records

In all provinces, hospitals and other health facilities are required to keep and maintain records on all the patients they treat. For example, in Ontario, a record of admission, diagnosis, consent forms, treatment, care plan, nursing notes, and so forth must be kept on each patient.[17] Physicians' orders should be in writing and signed or authenticated by the physician who made the order. All entries in the patient record made by nurses and other health professionals must be initialled or signed and dated, and the exact time of the entry noted. Late entries should also be indicated.

As well, most provinces impose an obligation to obtain and record a diagnosis on an admitted patient within a specified period of time. Also, records must be kept for a specified time, for example, 10 years in Ontario.[18]

Summary

We have demonstrated in this chapter why full and accurate documentation is a key component of professional nursing. The nursing notes provide a continuous record of the patient's assessment and treatment, and the effect of interventions. From this record, the patient's progress towards stated goals and outcomes may be evaluated, and any impending complications can be identified before they become problematic.

As the health care system moves towards computerized records there is greater demand for accurate, timely documentation. Once information is documented on line, it cannot be changed, nor can the computerized signature of the caregiver be erased.

Standards of documentation are intended not only as a means of defending the nurse's actions and interventions in legal proceedings; in fact, they are the main means of ongoing communication about a client's care and progress. Nurses are required not only to meet standards of documentation but also to review this documentation on a regular basis. Thus, they will be in a position to provide safe and competent care to clients.

The key points introduced in this chapter include:

- the legal requirements of proper nursing documentation
- the importance of accurate and complete documentation in ensuring safe and effective nursing care
- guidelines for timely and accurate documentation, and their application to hypothetical case studies and real case law
- the role of nursing assessments and their importance in the nursing notes
- the use and significance of incident reports
- the use of nursing notes in a legal proceeding
- the role of expert witnesses in interpreting nursing documentation.

Critical Thinking

These case studies are for further reflection, discussion, and analysis. As you review each case, consider the following questions as well as those specific to the case.

1. Have the nurses in these cases violated any ethical or legal standards?
2. If so, what are these standards?
3. Is there risk of any civil or criminal liability?
4. How could these situations have been prevented?

CASE STUDY: KNOWING THE PATIENT'S STORY

Sylvana was admitted to hospital with anemia and a high fever. Preliminary investigations revealed that she also had a hydronephrosis of the left kidney caused by a stricture of the ureter. This was a result of chronic infection related to an ileal conduit she had had for about 30 years.

Because Sylvana's creatinine was also very high, it was decided that her left ureter must be dilated immediately. This procedure was extremely painful; afterward, Sylvana became septic and was seriously ill for about two weeks. The episode was appropriately documented in the medical record. A few weeks later, just as Sylvana was improving, a nurse accidentally removed the stent (in place to ensure the ureter remained dilated), and the dilation had to be repeated.

Sylvana's daughter Teresa accompanied her during the procedure. Both were concerned that she would become septic again. Teresa also knew the importance of monitoring her mother's vital signs, in particular her temperature, blood pressure, and urine output. The women's concern increased when, two hours post-procedure, Sylvana's nurse had not yet come to assess her.

Teresa approached Sylvana's nurse, who told her that this procedure was unusual on this unit (a medical unit), and that she had not known the protocol. Clearly, the nurse had not reviewed Sylvana's file, otherwise she would have appreciated the risks associated with this procedure.

QUESTIONS

1. Did the nurse in this scenario meet the standards of practice with respect to documentation? What other professional standards were not fulfilled in this case?
2. Would the facts that this procedure was rarely practised on this unit, or that this nurse had never cared for a patient needing this procedure, be an excuse?

CASE STUDY: A MODERN DILEMMA

Kim works in a busy Emergency Department. In this hospital, most of the patients' documentation is completed on a computerized system.

One of the residents arrives to assess a patient presenting with severe abdominal pain. This resident has forgotten to bring along the access card that allows him to review his patients' health care information on line.

Kim, aware of the urgency of this review (the patient's condition is rapidly deteriorating), lends the resident her access badge. She knows this is against the confidentiality policy she signed when she received her access card. Nonetheless, while reviewing the data on line, the resident notes abnormal findings that require immediate action, and orders further tests (via the system).

QUESTIONS

1. What dilemmas were facing the nurse in this scenario?
2. Can Kim's actions be justified, given the circumstances?
3. What action should Kim take now?

QUESTIONS FOR DISCUSSION

1. Identify the most important reasons for good documentation. Beyond meeting standards, how does good documentation ensure high-quality care?
2. Identify the ethical principles that support good documentation.
3. How are documentation standards evaluated in your facility?
4. Would the quality of your documentation meet the standard during a legal proceeding? Why or why not?
5. What are the key differences between manual and computerized documentation systems? What are the advantages of each approach?
6. In the case of *Kolesar v. Jeffries* described in the chapter, the nurses would assist one another in reconstructing the record of treatment over their previous shift by means of notes jotted on scraps of paper. How might a nurse's testimony based on such a method be challenged in a subsequent negligence action?
7. What are the risks inherent in using imprecise language when describing and documenting a patient's condition over time? How can you improve the precision of the language you use in your charting?

References

1. This case study is closely based upon a real situation related by Dr. Jim Cairns, Deputy Chief Coroner of Ontario, in a talk on the medical and legal aspects of charting for nurses, given at The Toronto Hospital on May 26, 1994.
2. (1981), 17 CCLT 1 (BCSC).
3. Ibid., p. 15.
4. Ibid., p. 9.
5. Ibid., p. 7.
6. Ibid.
7. Ibid., p. 12.
8. Ibid.
9. Ibid.
10. Fischbach, F.T. (1996). *Documenting care: Communication, the nursing process and documentation standards* (pp. 28–29). Philadelphia: F.A. Davis.
11. Ibid., pp. 535–536.
12. Ibid., pp. 251–254.
13. (1976), 9 OR (2d) 41 (HCJ); varied (1977), 12 OR (2d) 142 (CA); aff'd. (1977), 2 CCLT 170 (SCC).
14. Ibid., p. 48.
15. Supra footnote 2.
16. Ibid., p. 15.
17. See, e.g., RRO 1990, Reg. 965, as amended, made under the *Public Hospitals Act,* RSO 1990, c. P.42.
18. Ibid.

CHAPTER Ten

Caregiver Rights

LEARNING OBJECTIVES

The purpose of this chapter is to enable you to:
- understand the rights of Canadian nurses as citizens, professionals, and employees
- clarify when the right to a conscientious objection can be invoked
- clarify the responsibilities of nurses as employees to employers
- know the position of the law with respect to discrimination and sexual or physical abuse
- appreciate the role of labour relations and collective bargaining with respect to nursing
- understand the standards associated with occupational health and safety.

Introduction

Although most of this book focusses on the rights of patients and clients within the health care system, the nurses caring for these people also have rights. Along with all other Canadians, under the *Charter of Rights and Freedoms* nurses have the right to privacy and respect, and to freedom of expression—the right to think, say, write, or otherwise act in accordance with their beliefs. However, this right is not absolute. For nurses, professional rules and regulations, and ethical responsibilities to patients, may limit individual freedom. For example, when caring for a patient whose values and religious beliefs differ from the nurse's, it is not professionally or ethically appropriate to attempt to influence the patient towards the nurse's perspective.

Nurses are entitled to respect from one another, from other professionals, and from patients and clients. As individuals, they are entitled to freedom from any form of discrimination, harassment (sexual or otherwise), and physical or sexual abuse. As employees, nurses have the right to have their values respected, and to function within a work environment in which risks and harm are minimized. Also, nurses have the right to collective bargaining. This chapter explores some of these rights.

Right to be Protected from Harm

Many nurses work with seriously ill patients whose illnesses may, at times, cause them to become violent and lash out at their caregivers. Or, a nurse may encounter a patient who, owing to his or her personality, inflicts physical or verbal abuse as a means of self-assertion. The law affords nurses protection against these situations.

When faced with patients who are confused, agitated, or mentally ill, nurses recognize that these behaviours often result from illness and fear. Thus, nurses need good communication and management skills to defuse potentially violent or abusive situations.

Nurses need to be educated to identify and manage violence in confused and agitated patients. They require the skills to assess those clients who are medically or psychiatrically predisposed to violence. Then, they must be able to devise and initiate appropriate strategies for preventive management.

The nurse visiting patients in their home may seem especially vulnerable owing to isolation. Yet, abuse of nurses is more prevalent in psychiatric and emergency departments. Employers have the responsibility to minimize the risk of harm to nurses regardless of where they work, and especially in high-risk environments.

Safeguards and protections to reduce the risk of harm include maintaining reasonable staffing quotas and ensuring that restraints are available (as a last resort, and as appropriate). Further, nurses should not be sent into unsafe areas alone. Nurses working in high-risk environments should be given instruction in self-defence. Many institutions now offer such training, and have implemented violence response teams for emergencies.

Abuse from mentally competent patients may afford grounds for assault charges. In such cases, there is no question that the assault is intentional insofar as the patient/client or family member intends to harm the nurse. The matter can then proceed as a criminal prosecution.

Conscientious Objection

As employees, nurses are under a contractual obligation to provide adequate and competent care. There are times, however, when the duty to provide care may conflict with the nurse's personal values, for example, having to participate in a procedure that he or she finds objectionable on moral or religious grounds. Is the nurse still required to provide care in these circumstances?

Most such situations will not be emergencies. In an emergency, the nurse's foremost ethical obligation is to do good and not to do harm to the patient. Refusing to act would go against these ethical principles; therefore, in an emergency, the nurse is bound to act, until alternative care is available.

C A S E   S T U D Y

A conscientious objection?

Frances, a registered nurse of five years' standing, works in the Obstetrics Department of a secular public hospital in a large urban centre. She is religious and deeply opposed to abortion. Frances accepted her position with the understanding that no therapeutic abortions were performed in Obstetrics. In this hospital, abortions are usually performed in the Gynaecological Department; some such procedures involve saline injections. Frances would never be asked or required to work in this unit.

Recent cutbacks in funding to the hospital have meant staff reductions and bed closures. Consequently, when beds are tight, an abortion might occasionally be performed in Obstetrics. One afternoon, Frances discovers that she has been scheduled to assist in a second-trimester saline abortion which is to take place in the Obstetrics unit later that day. Angry and upset, she accosts her manager: "There's no way I'm going to assist with this! Find another nurse!"

Issues

1. What are the hospital's ethical and legal obligations to Frances and to the patient seeking the abortion?
2. How can the conflict between these interests be resolved?

Discussion

Whenever possible, employers are obliged to respect the conscientious objections of employees who decline to participate in certain actions on moral or religious grounds. Here, we are not speaking of discrimination or indulging the employee's prejudices. Ethically, the employee has the right not to be compelled to engage in actions to which he or she objects. In this case study, the treatment in which Frances is being asked to participate is not an emergency. If it were, she would be ethically bound to render any and all assistance needed of her. This priority would override her conscientious objections.

For example, it would be Frances's duty to render assistance if the patient were suffering complications as a result of an abortion, such as internal bleeding following a saline injection, regardless of her personal opinion of the patient's actions. While Frances could refuse to participate in the abortion, she might be compelled to render emergency life-saving treatment after the fact.

Further, a nurse working in a Palliative Care Unit in which there was an AIDS patient could not ethically refuse to treat him on the grounds that he

might be a homosexual or a drug abuser. This would be a clear case of preju-
dice, which an employer is not obliged to indulge.

Problems relating to conscientious objection are best avoided by informing
the prospective nursing employee, prior to employment, of his or her expected functions, roles, duties, and responsibilities. The nurse should be advised
that, once employment is accepted, he or she will have no option but to provide the care required. Thus, if a prospective nursing employee applies for a
position in the Gynaecological Department of a secular hospital, he or she
should understand that the duties may include assisting during abortions. The
nurse then has the opportunity to decline such employment without the difficulties of having to do so later.

However, if the nature of the nurse's job changes after he or she has begun
employment, the agency or hospital is obligated to reassign that nurse to areas
where the objectionable activities are not performed. Yet, there are no guaran-
tees, since in emergencies, nurses are ethically obliged to provide care. They
may withdraw from such situations only when it is safe to do so, or when others are available to provide the required care. In very small facilities it may not
be possible to reassign nurses, or to guarantee exemption from involvement. In
these cases, the nurse may face the difficult choice of seeking employment
elsewhere.

The ethical principles that apply here are justice (the patient's right to be
treated fairly and equitably), beneficence (the nurse's obligation to do good for
the patient), and non-maleficence (the nurse's duty to do the patient no harm).
For example, if a nurse were to withdraw his or her services arbitrarily because
of an objection that placed the patient in danger, that nurse would be violating the principle of non-maleficence.

As stated in the CNA's *Code of Ethics for Registered Nurses,* nurses are not
obliged to act on the wishes of a client when those actions pose a serious moral
conflict for the nurse. However, the nurse is obliged to ensure that other
arrangements are available to a patient/client when the care required conflicts
with the nurse's beliefs but is legally acceptable.

Discrimination Issues in Employment

The case study above also raises an employment law issue and illustrates the
competing interests of employees' and employers' rights. Legally, the matter
involves the application of provincial human rights legislation. This legislation is virtually identical from province to province and is essentially
designed to prohibit discrimination against persons on the basis of race, sex,
sexual orientation, creed, religion, physical or mental disability, nationality,
or ethnic origin. The thrust of the legislation is that employers are obliged, to

the greatest extent possible, to structure work conditions and requirements so as to cause the least possible interference with the religious or cultural views, or physical or mental handicaps, of their employees. For example, employers must accommodate work conditions such that no employee is unduly inconvenienced by reason only of his or her sex, as in the case of providing adequate washroom facilities.

In the case study, Frances's religious views conflict with her employer's work requirements. If we alter the circumstances and say that she was reassigned to the unit by a supervisor who held her religious views in contempt and merely wanted to harass her by requiring her to work in a setting to which she strongly objected, she would have valid grounds for a complaint before the provincial Human Rights Commission. If her rights have been infringed, Frances may be awarded compensation, depending on the laws of her province or territory. She should not be forced to work in a setting to which she objects on moral or religious grounds, subject, of course, to the ethical rules and legal considerations reviewed above.

Professional vs. Employee Responsibility

Nurses are accountable to their profession, their regulatory body, their patients or clients, and their employers. These multiple accountabilities can at times pose dilemmas or conflicts for the nurse. In many settings, another dimension is added to these complex relationships when nurses are also members of a union or collective bargaining unit.

A situation that occurred in Toronto in the mid-1970s illustrates the conflict that can arise between nurses' rights as employees and union members under a collective agreement, and their duties and responsibilities as professionals. In *Re Mount Sinai Hospital and the Ontario Nurses Association*,[1] the staff of the Mount Sinai Intensive Care Unit (ICU) was informed one evening of the urgent need to admit a patient with cardiac problems from the Emergency Department. This occurred during the night shift, when the ICU was already working at maximum capacity. The nurses informed the Admitting Department that they could not handle another patient. They claimed, further, that they were not obliged to take such an additional patient under the terms of the union's collective agreement with the hospital. The medical staff, despite the nurses' refusal to help, brought the patient to the unit. None of the nurses on the night shift agreed to render assistance to the admitting resident, who was required to care for this very ill patient by himself for the duration of the night.

As a result of their refusal to care for the additional patient, the nurses were disciplined and suspended for three tours of duty. They grieved the matter (see Grievance Procedures, page 314), and the issue was passed on to an arbitrator. The arbitrator ruled in favour of the hospital and found the nurses guilty of insubordination, as they had refused a direct order by their supervisor to provide care. They were not entitled, under the collective agreement, to refuse such an order.

Quite apart from the labour aspect, this case raises interesting ethical issues. For example, the nurses had not reassessed their workload and staffing, nor had they tried to determine whether some patients in their unit could be discharged to make room for the new admission. As they had not even tried to restructure their assignments to accommodate the patient, they violated the principles of beneficence and non-maleficence. Further, they had not accorded the patient justice, fairness, or equity.

The rule that evolved from this case is now termed the "obey and grieve" rule. It provides that, even if a nurse employee has a legitimate grievance under the terms of a collective agreement, or with respect to workload or working conditions, the nurse must obey the orders of the supervisor and provide needed care, then grieve the matter to the union if he or she feels there is a legitimate complaint. There is plenty of opportunity for such complaints to be heard and adjudicated upon at a more appropriate time, using the collective agreement's grievance procedures. In the present moment, however, the rights and needs of the patient must come first, and the fact that a nurse has a complaint must not be permitted to interfere with proper patient care.

The employee is the servant of the employer and, during regular hours of work, is under the employer's control. There are ample mechanisms to protect the employee's rights should these be violated by the employer, but the patient's care is paramount, especially given the fact (as seen in Chapter Five) that the health facility is under a legal duty to provide competent and proper nursing care once a patient is admitted. This implies a corresponding right of the employer to discipline the employee, and even to terminate the employment of a nurse who repeatedly fails to work to proper nursing standards. The corresponding right of the employee in this situation is to grieve or, if not unionized, to have recourse to the courts in an action for wrongful dismissal.

Labour Relations and Collective Bargaining

Many nurses in Canada work in public hospitals and other health facilities in which the employees are unionized. It is thus helpful for nurses to have a basic understanding of such labour relations concepts as union formation, the collective bargaining process, grievance procedures, arbitration, and the right to strike, since they will likely come across these matters at some point in their practice. An exhaustive study of labour law and labour relations is beyond the scope of this book. However, a brief review of these basic concepts and some of the related procedures follows, in order to provide a general understanding of this subject.

Similarly, the field of occupational health and safety (OH&S) has grown widely in the last 30 years. Many provinces have enacted stringent OH&S statutes in an effort to ensure that working conditions of all employees (whether unionized or not) are made as safe and healthy as possible. This impetus has arisen from growing technology and a better understanding of how the human body reacts to its environment and the hazards posed by toxic or dangerous substances or activities in the workplace. This legislation also will be briefly reviewed in this chapter as it relates to the nursing profession.

Union Formation and Certification

Union Organization

The recognition of labour unions in Canada, as in the rest of the industrialized world, came about as a result of a long struggle fraught with social unrest, strikes, and violence throughout the late 19th and early 20th centuries. Gradually, unions and the principle of collective bargaining came to be seen as valid means to equalize the bargaining power of employees with that of the often large, wealthy, and powerful corporations who employed them. Unions were recognized as protectors of workers' interests, who ensured that they would receive fair wages and achieve better and safer working conditions. The right to unionize was constitutionally enshrined in 1982 in the *Canadian Charter of Rights and Freedoms*,[2] although such a right was recognized in law well before that time in Canada.

A **union** is a provincially certified group of employees, in most cases having a common employer. Unionized employees often work in common or related activities in the businesses or undertakings of these employers. The object of uniting is to provide bargaining influence, power, and leverage, by force of numbers, in negotiations pertaining to the terms of employment (e.g., wages, hours of work, benefits, work scheduling, layoff and termination, disciplinary matters and procedures, seniority and job security) affecting each member. Thus, by their common interest in terms of their employment, the employees, through their union, negotiate the terms and conditions of the employment contract collectively for the benefit of all employees. Each employee and member thus benefits by receiving the same terms and conditions of employment as other colleagues, and is better able to obtain these than if he or she were negotiating as an individual.

Most aspects of union certification and labour relations are governed by the provinces by virtue of the jurisdiction given to them by the Constitution (see Chapter Three). All provinces have passed labour relations legislation dealing with union certification, procedures for collective bargaining, procedures for strike votes (in some cases), definition of unfair labour practices, and prohibition of strike breaking, as well as the establishment of labour relations boards, their duties and powers.[3] The federal government has also passed labour legislation to deal with labour relations issues arising from industries or activities that fall under federal legislative jurisdiction.[4] Examples of federally regulated industries include certain airline employees, postal and telecommunications workers, since these activities come under federal constitutional jurisdiction. Similarly, civil servants at both the provincial and federal levels are usually covered by separate legislation specifically applicable to such government employees.

Before it can be certified, the union must be formed. Where there is no existing union willing to apply for certification on behalf of a group of employees, those employees may themselves form a union. The question as to whether a union is properly constituted usually arises during certification proceedings before a provincial Labour Relations Board. This body is charged, as part of its overall duties under the labour statute, with reviewing the union's application for certification and ensuring that all procedural formalities have been met.

An overview of the formalities necessary to the formation of a union was provided by the Ontario Labour Relations Board (OLRB) in one of its decisions in 1977.[5] Similar considerations would apply in other provinces. The OLRB laid down the following requirements:

(1) A constitution must be drafted wherein the purpose of the union (including the conduct of labour relations) must be stated and procedures for electing officers (i.e., president, secretary, treasurer) and calling meetings of the union must be set out.
(2) A meeting of the employees (in whose interest the union is being formed) must be held for the purposes of discussing and approving the proposed constitution.
(3) The employees attending such a meeting must be admitted as members of the union. (Here, membership cards may be issued to members.)
(4) A vote of the members at this meeting must be taken to ratify (approve) the proposed constitution.
(5) The new officers of the union should then be elected according to the procedures laid out in the newly approved constitution.

At this point, an application for certification can be filed with the labour board.

Certification

All provinces and the federal government have some form of **certification** process that must be passed before a union can represent the employees of a particular employer. The size and membership of the group of employees will usually be examined by the particular provincial labour board in order to determine whether it is appropriate for collective bargaining, that is, whether its members are truly employees and the group is of an appropriate size. Some provinces require that a specific percentage of all employees of an employer be members of the union. Others do not impose this requirement. In some provinces, a representation vote may have to be taken to determine the union's level of support among the employees of the employer.

Once certified, the union becomes the exclusive bargaining agent for its employees. That union alone is then authorized to negotiate a collective agreement on behalf of the employees in the bargaining unit (the specific group of employees of a specific employer or group of employers whom it was certified to represent).

The labour relations statutes do not apply to managerial employees, who are seen to represent employers. To allow managers to participate in union formation, membership, and activities would create a conflict of interest, because managers are usually charged with executing the employer's administrative, disciplinary, and evaluative policies; in many cases, they negotiate the terms of a collective agreement with the unions as the representatives of the employer. These activities are regarded as being inconsistent with the interests of workers in collective bargaining.

For example, a nurse manager whose duties are primarily administrative and managerial will not be covered by the collective bargaining scheme and provisions of the provincial labour relations statute. Such a nurse manager is not permitted to participate in the formation of the union, nor to be listed on the certification application as a union member and thus one of the employees represented. In the certification process, the provincial Labour Relations Board may determine that nurse managers are ineligible for inclusion in the quorum of employees who will constitute the bargaining unit.

Some provinces allow employees to refuse to join a union or to refuse to pay dues to a union on religious grounds. In such cases, the statutes provide that an amount equal to the union dues be paid by the dissenter to a charitable institution mutually agreed upon by the parties. In Manitoba, Saskatchewan, Ontario, and Quebec, an employee who is eligible for membership but is not in fact a member must still pay dues to the union. Such dues are usually deducted by the employer from the employee's paycheque and paid to the union.

In some provinces, closed shops are permitted. A **closed shop** is a place of employment that requires all employees to be members of the union as a condition of employment. This stipulation will appear among the terms of the collective agreement. Or, the contract may simply provide that, while union membership is not mandatory (that is, the place of employment is an **open shop**), preference in hiring will be given to union members over non-members.

In some provinces, certification may be automatic upon the union's demonstrating that it has achieved a certain level of membership. Not all employees of an employer need be members of the union seeking certification. But if a large majority of them are, this may be sufficient, in some provinces, for automatic certification. In Ontario, for example, it is possible for an employer to recognize a union as the bargaining agent for a group of employees without the need for certification.

Decertification

A union may also lose its right to act as bargaining agent for a group of workers, or it may be dissolved. This is usually referred to as **decertification.** For example, a union can lose its rights by failing to negotiate a collective agreement in good faith within a certain period of time. A group of the union's members can then apply for a declaration from the provincial Labour Relations Board that the union no longer represents, and thus can no longer negotiate for, the employees in a given bargaining unit.

In some provinces, a minimum number of employees may have to consent to such declaration before the board may decertify the union. The union may also lose its certification if it fails to give the employer notice within a certain period of time of its desire to begin negotiations for a new collective agreement or to renew an existing agreement.

It is important for nurses who are members of labour unions to know that in all cases, their employers are not free to give them individual advice if they are dissatisfied with the manner in which their union is representing them. At all times, nurses in such a situation have the right to consult with a labour lawyer. A legal professional can best advise the nurse or nurses on all appropriate courses of action and their legal rights.

Collective Bargaining

Collective bargaining is a process whereby workers, through their union representatives, meet with their employers in order to negotiate the terms and conditions of employment applicable to each worker. It is a right that was not recognized historically in common law and was even prohibited in past times as a conspiracy of persons in restraint of trade. Today, collective bargaining is fully recognized and promoted in the various labour relations statutes, both federal and provincial.

Under the laws of all provinces and the federal government, the parties to an expired collective agreement are obliged to negotiate a new contract when one of the parties serves the other with a notice to bargain for a new agreement (or, where there is no prior agreement and a union is newly certified, the first collective agreement). The notice begins the process of collective bargaining. In some provinces, a union can lose its certification and authorization to bargain for a specific bargaining unit if it does not serve such a notice and begin negotiation within a specified period of time. This will usually result in another union's being certified to represent the employees in the bargaining unit in place of the first union.

In collective bargaining, each side puts forth its desired terms and conditions for a new employment contract. Such matters may include wages, hours of work, work schedules, vacation pay, sick leave, pensions and other employee benefits, mechanisms for settling disputes that arise from the application, administration, interpretation, or alleged violation of the collective agreement (called grievance procedures), and perhaps representation on the joint OH&S committee set up for the workplace between the employer and employees.

Often, negotiations become mired in disagreement over one or more terms. These disputes, if not settled promptly, can lead to strike action by employees or a lockout of employees by an employer. Thus, the labour relations statutes contain procedures for appointing conciliators and mediators to assist the parties in resolving such disagreements and to negotiate a contract. A **conciliator** may be appointed at the request of either party to resolve outstanding issues, or, in some cases, the provincial minister of labour may choose to appoint a conciliator or mediator.

In all provinces, once a notice to bargain has been given, the employer cannot change the existing terms or conditions of employment, including wages, unless it has the permission of its board of directors and the union, or the provisions of the collective agreement permit it.

The Collective Agreement

The contract that emerges from the collective bargaining negotiations is called a **collective agreement.** In all provinces and at the federal level, the agreement must be for a minimum duration of one year. The agreement must be in writing, but need not be embodied in a single document. For example, an exchange of letters, notes, and memoranda may constitute the collective agreement if the parties set out the agreed-upon terms.

If the collective agreement expires before a new one is in place, the terms and conditions of the old agreement usually continue to apply provided that there is no evidence that the parties intended otherwise. Some contracts specify that they will continue after the expiry date until and unless either party notifies the other of its desire to terminate the agreement. In all provinces except Quebec and Nova Scotia, no employee is permitted to strike, nor may any employer lock out its employees, during the life of the contract. The reason for this is to preserve labour peace and maintain peaceful industrial relations. This condition applies even after the agreement has expired and until a specified period has elapsed from the time a conciliator is appointed by the minister of labour (or other authorized person) to the time a conciliator's report is released to the parties. This is colloquially known as a **cooling-off period.**

Grievance Procedures and Arbitration

Since workers are not permitted to strike during the currency of a collective agreement, nor employers to lock out workers, there must be a means of resolving disputes arising from the application, administration, interpretation, or alleged violation of the terms of the agreement. If not, labour tensions might build to an explosive point. The violence of past labour disputes has shown the necessity and desirability of having effective and timely dispute resolution procedures in place before matters get out of hand. Indeed, all provincial labour statutes except Saskatchewan's require collective agreements to contain procedures for settling management–labour disputes. If they do not, the legislation deems certain provisions to be part of the agreement.

Such grievance procedures will be negotiated as part of the terms of the collective agreement. Many agreements provide relatively informal mechanisms for the presentation of a grievance. As well, many workplaces have grievance committees with employee representatives.

For example, suppose a nurse is asked by her supervisor to work an additional hour beyond what the contract requires. The request may possibly result from a misinterpretation of the terms of the collective agreement. The nurse refuses to work and is disciplined. She may then choose to file a grievance with that supervisor.

Some hospitals have hospital association committees comprising members of the hospital's management and non-managerial nurse employees. They meet on a regular basis to review any grievances in an attempt to resolve them in an informal, cooperative setting before they become adversarial, and part of a formal grievance process. If informal mechanisms fail, however, grievance procedures are implemented.

The following grievance procedures are not necessarily followed across Canada, but are fairly common in many labour relations settings. They usually involve a progressive three-step process.

Step 1: Written Submission

In the event that the nurse's grievance is not settled satisfactorily after bringing it to the supervisor's attention, then, within a specified time, the grievance must be submitted in writing to the immediate supervisor for a response. Failing a settlement, it then must be filed within a specified time to the director of nursing for resolution. If it is still not settled, the procedure provides that it be submitted to the hospital administrator or other authorized hospital official within a set period of time for a meeting.

Step 2: Meeting with the Grievance Committee

The meeting is held among the administrator, the person who filed the grievance, the grievance committee, and a representative of the union. A decision by the hospital resulting from the discussions at the meeting must be made within a specified time. Thus, the procedure provides for the grievance's being submitted to a progressively higher and higher authority as long as it is not settled. (In many hospitals, this is managed through the Human Resources Department.) The collective agreement will also provide that if a settlement is reached under these procedures, then it is binding on the parties.

Step 3: Binding Arbitration

If the decision rendered by the hospital administrator does not settle the issue, then the matter is submitted to binding arbitration. If there is consensus, the collective agreement usually provides that the settlement is binding on the parties.

As we have said above, binding arbitration is a procedure mandated by the labour relations statutes of many provinces. Usually, one of the parties notifies the other within a specified time from the rendering of the hospital administrator's decision that that party wishes the matter to be submitted to binding arbitration. At the same time, it will nominate a person to be part of a three-member arbitration board.

The party to whom the notice is given then has a specified time in which to nominate a second person to that board. If a nomination is not forthcoming, the party who served the first notice may request that the minister of labour nominate a second person.

No person who has been involved in attempting to negotiate or settle the grievance prior to its submission to arbitration may sit on the arbitration board. These two persons, in turn, choose a third person to chair and complete the board. If they cannot agree, then the minister appoints a chair.

In recent years, certain issues have arisen in Ontario with respect to disputes over workloads and the right of nurses to refuse to provide services once the number of patients placed in their care exceeds their ability to provide adequate care. We have already mentioned *Re Mount Sinai Hospital and the Ontario Nurses Association,* in which case nurses refused to care for an additional patient assigned to their unit. The nurses were disciplined, and the disciplinary measures were upheld upon arbitration under the collective agreement. The arbitration board felt that the nurses had not had just cause under the circumstances to refuse to care for the additional patient. Such a situation is now dealt with by means of the professional responsibility clause of the collective agreement.

Earlier in this chapter, we mentioned the "obey and grieve" rule. Under this provision, a nurse who believes that he or she is being given a workload so large as to preclude proper patient care may file a complaint in writing to the hospital association committee within a certain period of time. The complaint, if unresolved, proceeds to an assessment committee hearing, whose members are chosen by both the hospital and the nurses' union. The committee then investigates the matter and holds a hearing to determine whether or not the complaint is well founded. It then reports its findings to the parties to the hearing and presumably makes recommendations in an attempt to resolve the situation. In this way, the professional integrity of nurses is maintained, and they are permitted some control over their workload and the number of patients under their care. Thus, their ability to deliver effective, efficient, and proper nursing care is maintained.

A matter may be submitted to arbitration only after all preliminary grievance procedures have been exhausted. A majority of the provincial Labour Relations Board determines the issue. All time limits for the giving of notice must be strictly observed; if notice that a party wishes the matter submitted to binding arbitration is not given within a specified time, the grievance is deemed to have been abandoned. Alternatively, the parties may agree that the matter be settled by a single arbitrator.

Thus, through arbitration, every attempt is made to resolve disputes arising out of the collective agreement. This procedure has been referred to as the *quid pro quo,* that is, something in return for the fact that the right to strike or to lock out is suspended during the life of the agreement.

There are a number of cases involving nurses disciplined for unprofessional conduct. In many of these, the nurse grieved the matter pursuant to the union's collective agreement.

In *Re Ontario Cancer Institute and Ontario Nurses' Association (Priestley),*[6] a nurse was discharged after striking a terminally ill patient. The nurse, through her union, brought a grievance against the hospital employer for unjust discharge. The union argued that the patient had provoked the nurse. Although there were no witnesses to the incident, the nurse had admitted the act to two colleagues and said that "... it felt good."[7]

The evidence presented at the hearing suggested that patient load had been very heavy in the unit for some months and that stress levels among staff were high. The patient struck by the nurse required the most attention in the unit, and was very demanding of the nurses' time and attention. He had a tracheotomy and was often confused, restless, and incontinent. The nurse admitted to striking the patient hard across the legs because she became frustrated with his restless behaviour the night before. In finding that the nurse's discharge was justified, the arbitrator stated, in part:

> I heard much evidence about what a difficult and heavy care patient [the patient] was. I accept that evidence.... However, the actions of a patient who is terminally ill and not in control of his mental or physical faculties cannot constitute provocation that would excuse a health care professional's physical retaliation.[8]

The arbitrator declined to interfere with the hospital's decision to discharge the nurse.

Similarly, in *Vancouver General Hospital (Health and Labour Relations Assn.) and British Columbia Nurses Union,*[9] a nurse was discharged for continuing to feed a patient in an inappropriate manner despite having been shown the correct way by an occupational therapist. She had previously been suspended for improperly responding to a patient's seizure because she was in a hurry to go home. In the second incident, which led to her dismissal, the nurse attempted to feed milk to a patient who was improperly positioned and already had food in her mouth. There was great risk to the patient of aspiration. Moreover, the patient was drowsy following surgery and insufficiently alert to be fed orally. The arbitrator held that the hospital had just cause for disciplinary action, given the nurse's record.

Right to Strike

Traditionally, the common law did not recognize the right of employees to refuse to work. Today's statutes usually distinguish between a lawful and an unlawful strike. The same distinction applies to a **lockout,** a practice whereby an employer shuts out or refuses to continue to employ union employees as a means to pressure and influence them during negotiations for a collective agreement. It, like the strike, is a coercive tactic.

In most provinces, during the life of a collective agreement, employees may not strike, nor may an employer lock out employees. Even after the expiration of the agreement, employees and employers must wait for the passage of the cooling-off period before a lawful strike or lockout can occur.

Once the collective agreement has expired, its terms can be continued while the parties negotiate a new agreement. However, if no agreement is reached, in some provinces, the provincial minister of labour may be requested or may decide to appoint a conciliation board in an attempt to settle outstanding issues and to effect a new collective agreement. Such board or conciliator (if one person is appointed) must file a report on the results (or lack thereof) of any conciliation efforts to the minister of labour, who then releases the report to the parties.

Once a specified period has elapsed after the report's release, or (if no conciliator has been appointed) after the minister has notified the parties that he or she considers it inappropriate to appoint a conciliator, the union may then lawfully call a strike. Similarly, the employer may lawfully lock out employees.

Certain activities during the life of the collective agreement may or may not constitute a strike according to the applicable labour relations statute. Employees may vote to work to rule (i.e., to work only as much as is demanded by the terms of their employment) as a form of protest; for example, they may refuse to work overtime when requested to do so. If such conduct has the effect of stopping all work in order to pressure an employer to accede to union demands, it may be deemed a strike by the provincial Labour Relations Board. However, a refusal to work because of hazardous working conditions would likely not be deemed a strike, as it is not intended to affect collective bargaining but rather to avoid potentially serious injury to workers.

In most provinces, nurses and other hospital employees are not legally permitted to strike. While this provision may not affect nurses who are not employed at hospitals (which are defined in detail in the statutes), any nurse working at an institution that falls within the definition of a hospital would be prevented from going on strike.[10] Similarly, hospitals are not permitted to lock out their employees at any time. These provisions are designed to ensure that vital hospital services are not compromised, nor services to the public diminished, as a result of labour disputes. This is not to say that nurses are not permitted to form unions and to bargain collectively; however, different dispute resolution procedures may apply, and employees will not be permitted to strike to enforce collective bargaining rights.

Strike breaking, that is, the use of strong-arm, threatening, or other such tactics by an employer in an effort to pressure striking employees to abandon a lawful strike or to yield in contract negotiations, is prohibited in all provinces.

Depending on the province, a strike vote among employees may be required before a strike can begin. If a strike vote is held, all employees in the bargaining unit may vote. Voting is usually by secret ballot. A vote may also be held to ratify an agreement concluded between management and the union's negotiators.

Unfair Labour Practices

All provinces have prohibited unfair management tactics, which in previous times were used by employers to pressure workers into returning to work or to induce employees to accept certain terms and conditions of employment.

For example, it is illegal for an employer to discipline a worker for taking part in a lawful strike or in lawful union activities, such as encouraging new members to join the union. Similarly, employers are prohibited from participating in or funding the creation of a union. Such prohibition is intended to avoid conflict of interest.

It is likewise illegal for an employer to discriminate in any way against employees because they either are or are not members of a union; to discipline them for exercising their rights under a labour relations statute; to use any form of intimidation against them for participating in union activity; or to induce them to join a particular union. Another illegal labour practice is the "yellow dog" contract, by which it is made a condition of a person's employment that he or she will not join a union or participate in any union activities.

If an employee alleges that an employer has engaged in an unfair labour practice, the employee can bring the matter to the attention of the union representative. The matter may be taken up as a grievance by the union or, if it is serious enough, it may be reported to a labour inspector appointed by the provincial Labour Relations Board. The labour boards of most provinces are given wide powers to order employers to cease and desist from engaging in such practices.

Occupational Health and Safety

In an effort to ensure that working conditions are as safe and healthy as possible, all provinces have enacted occupational health and safety (OH&S) legislation.[11] These statutes mandate the establishment of health and safety committees comprising representatives of non-managerial employees and management itself. The object of these committees is to identify and recommend solutions to potentially hazardous conditions in the workplace. Further, many provinces' statutes provide for the selection of OH&S representatives to inquire into and inspect hazardous working conditions, materials, substances, or unsafe equipment.

In some provinces, workers have the right to refuse to work under unsafe or unhealthy conditions. Other provinces exempt nurses from this right. As we saw with the "obey and grieve" rule, nurses, who must often work in potentially dangerous situations, are exempt at the outset from the right to refuse to work. Yet, it would not be unethical for a nurse to refuse to work under unsafe working conditions. Nurses may or may not have legal protection, however, if they are disciplined for refusing such work.

Many OH&S statutes also include obligations on employers to label hazardous substances present in the workplace and to provide safety equipment and instructions to employees on the proper use of such equipment. Further, they include regulations for the handling of hazardous waste and other toxic or harmful substances. This is especially important in a health care setting, with the ever-present dangers posed by biomedical waste. Nurses, as any other health professionals working with or around such materials, have the right to learn of any and all applicable handling procedures and methods as well as the right to maximum safety in the workplace. Employers have a corresponding obligation to provide a safe and healthy workplace.

Summary

This chapter has explored the rights of nurses as professionals, individuals, and employees. The varied work situations in which nurses perform their duties can lead to ethical and legal dilemmas that have an impact on their values, beliefs, and well-being. While nurses have the right to respect, and should be able carry out their duties in a safe work environment free from harm, harassment, or abuse, the reality is that some will face such difficult situations.

Employers have an obligation to represent the interests and rights of nurses. When this obligation is not fulfilled, then the collective agreement and collective bargaining rights of nurses who are unionized may provide protection and a mechanism for dealing with some of these situations. In other cases, the advice of a competent legal professional may be required.

Nurses should be aware of their rights, and the responsibilities and obligations of their employers, with respect to working conditions. The nurse has the right to a safe working environment and to the employer's assistance when making claims for benefits and compensation in work-related injuries. If nurses' rights are not protected in an environment based on mutual respect, then they will be unable to deliver high-quality care to clients consistent with the standards of their profession.

The key points introduced in this chapter include:

- the rights of Canadian nurses as citizens, professionals, and employees
- the right to conscientious objection, and when it can be invoked
- the responsibilities of nurses as employees to employers
- the position of the law with respect to discrimination and sexual or physical abuse
- the role of labour relations and collective bargaining with respect to nursing
- the standards associated with occupational health and safety.

Critical Thinking

These case studies are for further reflection, discussion, and analysis. As you review each case, consider the following questions as well as those specific to the case.

1. Have the nurses in these cases violated any ethical or legal standards?
2. If so, what are these standards?
3. Is there risk of any civil or criminal liability?
4. How could these situations have been prevented?

CASE STUDY: RIGHT OR PRIVILEGE?

Carmen, a nurse in a busy Critical Care Unit, is scheduled to work nights one weekend when she is invited to attend an informal university class reunion. She knows that it is too late to ask for the weekend off, and that few of her colleagues would willingly switch shifts with her on such short notice. As she has taken little sick leave, she decides to call in sick. Carmen believes that she is entitled to this time, and that this is a legitimate reason to take the weekend off.

That night a number of emergency patients are admitted to the unit. Owing to Carmen's absence, the nurses on duty that night must take a double assignment of patients. One of the nurses, aware of Carmen's reason for calling in sick, is so upset that the following Monday, she discloses this information to the nurse manager.

QUESTIONS

1. Is Carmen entitled to take this time off? If not, what disciplinary action may ensue?
2. If the manager chooses to discipline Carmen, can Carmen grieve the matter?
3. What ethical principles, if any, did Carmen breach?

C A S E   S T U D Y :   SAFETY IN THE WORKPLACE?

Connie, a public health nurse, is assigned to a young single mother, Sheryl, and her eight-month-old son, Sean. This family receives welfare and lives in a subsidized housing unit.

During one of Connie's regular visits, Sheryl's estranged boyfriend arrives. He has been drinking and becomes belligerent towards Sheryl. When Connie—concerned about her clients' safety—intervenes, the boyfriend turns his aggression on her, hitting her on the head. Connie falls and strikes her head on the edge of a coffee table, sustaining a serious injury.

Although Connie recovers physically, her mental capacity is such that she can never practise nursing again.

QUESTIONS

1. What obligations did Connie's employer have to ensure a safe working environment?
2. What responsibilities does the employer have with respect to Connie's permanent disability?
3. What charges can be laid against the boyfriend?
4. What obligations did Connie's employer have to educate her with respect to such potentially violent and dangerous situations?

C A S E   S T U D Y :   RIGHT TO STRIKE?

Andrew is an RN in a long-term care facility. Recently, contract discussions between his union and the facility have broken down. Neither side is willing to compromise, and staff have voted to strike. A plan is in place to provide assistance only for emergencies.

Andrew is concerned about the strike decision. He worries about his patients in the Geriatric Unit. Knowing how difficult and confusing the strike will be for them, he decides to cross the picket line and go to work. As he enters the building, Andrew is heckled by some of his colleagues.

QUESTIONS

1. What are Andrew's rights and responsibilities in this situation?
2. Is the behaviour of the nurses on the picket line justifiable?
3. What would you do in Andrew's place?

QUESTIONS FOR DISCUSSION

1. As a nurse, do you have rights that may supersede those of your patients/clients? What rights may at times be in conflict?
2. Do nurses give up certain rights when they assume their professional role?
3. What role should unions play in establishing rules that govern professional practice and conduct?
4. What mechanisms are in place in your facility to ensure the appropriate balance between caregiver and patient rights?

References

1. (1978), 17 LAC (2d) 242 (Ont. Arb.).
2. *Charter of Rights and Freedoms*, Part I of the *Constitution Act, 1982*, being Schedule B of the *Canada Act 1982 (UK)*, 1982, c. 11, section 2(d).
3. See British Columbia: *Labour Relations Code*, RSBC 1996, c. 244; Alberta: *Labour Relations Code*, SA 1988, c. L-12, as amended; Saskatchewan: *Trade Union Act*, RSS 1978, c. T-17, as amended; Manitoba: *Labour Relations Act*, RSM 1987, c. L10, as amended; Ontario: *Labour Relations Act, 1995*, SO 1995, c.1, Sched. A, as amended; Quebec: *Labour Code*, RSQ c. C-27, as amended; New Brunswick: *Industrial Relations Act*, RSNB 1973, c. I-4, as amended; Nova Scotia: *Trade Union Act*, RSNS 1989, c. 475, as amended; Prince Edward Island: *Labour Act*, RSPEI 1988, c. L-1, as amended; Newfoundland: *Labour Relations Act*, RSN 1990, c. L-1, as amended.
4. See *Canada Labour Code*, RSC 1985, c. L-2, as amended.
5. *Local 199 UAW Building Corp.*, [1977] OLRB Rep. July, 472, at p. 473.
6. (1993), 35 LAC (4th) 129 (Ont.).
7. Ibid., p. 129.
8. Ibid., pp. 135–136.
9. (1993), 32 LAC (4th) 231 (B.C.).
10. See, e.g., Ontario: *Hospital Labour Disputes Arbitration Act*, RSO 1990, c. H.14, section 11(1), as amended; Alberta: *Hospitals Act*, RSA 1980, c. H-11.
11. See Alberta: *Occupational Health and Safety Act*, RSA 1980, c. O-2, as amended; British Columbia: *Workplace Act*, SBC 1985, c. 34, as amended; Manitoba: *Workplace Safety and Health Act*, RSM 1987, c. W210, CCSM, c. W210, as amended; New Brunswick: *Occupational Health and Safety Act*, SNB 1983, c. O-0.2, as amended; Newfoundland: *Occupational Health and Safety Act*, RSN 1990, c. O-3, as amended; Northwest Territories: *Safety Act*, RSNWT 1988, c. S-1, as amended; Nova Scotia: *Occupational Health and Safety Act*, RSNS 1989, c. 320, as amended; Ontario: *Occupational Health and Safety Act*, RSO 1990, c. O.1, as amended; Prince Edward Island: *Occupational Health and Safety Act*, RSPEI 1988, c. O-1; Quebec: *Occupational Health and Safety Act*, RSQ c. S-2.1, as amended; Saskatchewan: *Occupational Health and Safety Act, 1993*, SS 1993, c. O-1.1.

Canadian Nurses Association Code of Ethics for Registered Nurses§

Preamble

The *Code of Ethics for Registered Nurses* gives guidance for decision-making concerning ethical matters, serves as a means for self-evaluation and reflection regarding ethical nursing practice, and provides a basis for peer review initiatives. The code not only educates nurses* about their ethical responsibilities, but also informs other health care professionals and members of the public about the moral commitments expected of nurses.

The Canadian Nurses Association (CNA) periodically revises its code to address changing societal needs, values, and conditions that challenge the ability of nurses to practise ethically. Examples of such factors are: the consequences of economic constraints; increasing use of technology in health care; and, changing ways of delivering nursing services, such as the move to care outside the institutional setting. This revised *Code of Ethics for Registered Nurses* provides nurses with direction for ethical decision-making and practice in everyday situations as they are influenced by current trends and conditions. It applies to nurses in all practice settings, whatever their position and area of responsibility.

Ethical problems and concerns, as well as ethical distress at the individual level, can be the result of decisions made at the institutional, regional, provincial and federal levels. Differing responsibilities, capabilities and ways of working toward change also exist at the client,[1] institutional and societal

§Reprinted with permission from the Canadian Nurses Association.

*In this document *nurse* means *Registered Nurse.*

1. In this document *client* means the individual persons, and groups of persons such as families and communities with whom the nurse in engaged in a professional relationship.

levels. For all contexts the code offers guidance on providing care that conforms with ethical practice, and on actively influencing and participating in policy development, review and revision.

The complex issues in nursing practice have both legal and ethical dimensions. The laws and ethics of health care overlap, as both are concerned that the conduct of health professionals show respect for the well-being, dignity and liberty of clients. An ideal system of law would be compatible with ethics, in that adherence to the law ought never require the violation of ethics. Still, the domains of law and ethics remain distinct, and the code addresses ethical responsibilities only.

Elements of the Code

A value is something that is prized or held dear; something that is deeply cared about. This code is organized around seven primary values that are central to ethical nursing practice:

- Health and well-being
- Choice
- Confidentiality
- Fairness
- Accountability
- Practice environments that are conducive to safe, competent and ethical care.

Each value is articulated by responsibility statements that clarify its application and provide more direct guidance. Where it is clear that an action or inaction would involve an *ethical violation* (i.e., the neglect of a moral obligation), the level of guidance is prescriptive. The statement is intended to tell the nurse and others what is ethically acceptable and what is not. Where the situation involves an *ethical problem*[2] or dilemma, guidance is advisory. No ready-made answers can be offered and thoughtful consideration is required to increase the quality of decision-making. Where the situation provokes feelings of guilt, concern, or distaste, it is a situation of ethical distress. In instances of *ethical distress* the level of guidance is more limited but there remains a responsibility for the nurse to examine the situation in light of the provisions of the code. Decisions will be influenced by the particular circumstances of the situation. Ethical reflection and judgement are required to determine how a particular value or responsibility applies in a particular nursing context.

There is room within the profession for disagreement among nurses about the relative weight of different ethical values and principles. More than one proposed intervention may be ethical and reflective of good practice.

2. Ethical problems arise when ethical reasons both for and against one or more courses of action are present and choices must be made. Disagreement about the type and amount of information needed for each an ethically acceptable decision may further complicate efforts to reach agreement on the appropriate course(s) of action.

Discussion is extremely helpful in the resolution of ethical issues. As appropriate, clients, colleagues in nursing and other disciplines, professional nurses' associations and other experts are included in discussions about ethical problems. In addition to this code, legislation, and the standards of practice, policies, and guidelines of professional nurses' associations may also assist in problem-solving.[3]

The values articulated in this code are grounded in the professional nursing relationship with clients and indicate what nurses care about in that relationship. For example, to identify health and well-being as a value is to say that nurses care for and about the health and well-being of their clients. The nurse–client relationship presupposes a certain measure of trust on the part of the client. Care and trust complement one another in professional nursing relationships. Both hinge on the values identified in the code. By upholding these values in practice, nurses earn and maintain the trust of those in their care. For each of the values, the scope of responsibilities identified extends beyond individuals to include families, communities and society.

Values

Health and well-being
Nurses value health and well-being and assist persons to achieve their optimum level of health in situations of normal health, illness, injury, or in the process of dying.

Choice
Nurses respect and promote the autonomy of clients and help them to express their health needs and values, and to obtain appropriate information and services.

Dignity
Nurses value and advocate the dignity and self-respect of human beings.

Confidentiality
Nurses safeguard the trust of clients that information learned in the context of a professional relationship is shared outside the health care team only with the client's permission or as legally required.

Fairness
Nurses apply and promote principles of equity and fairness to assist clients in receiving unbiased treatment and a share of health services and resources proportionate to their needs.

---

3. The CNA and its member associations publish policy statements and guidelines on a variety of issues, e.g., advance directives, resuscitative interventions, boundary violations, the use of technology in health care, quality of nurses' worklife, support for safe nursing care, etc.

Accountability

Nurses act in a manner consistent with their professional responsibilities and standards of practice.

Practice environments conducive to safe, competent and ethical care

Nurses advocate practice environments that have the organizational and human support systems, and the resource allocations necessary for safe, competent and ethical nursing care.

Health and Well-being

Nurses value health and well-being and assist persons to achieve their optimum level of health in situations of normal health, illness, injury, or in the process of dying.

1. Nurses provide care directed first and foremost toward the health and well-being of the client.
2. Nurses recognize that health is more than the absence of disease or infirmity and assist clients to achieve the maximum level of health and well-being possible.
3. Nurses recognize that health status is influenced by a variety of factors. In ways that are consistent with their professional role and responsibilities, nurses are accountable for addressing institutional, social, and political factors influencing health and health care.
4. Nurses support and advocate a full continuum of health services including health promotion and disease prevention initiatives, as well as diagnostic, restorative, rehabilitative and palliative care services.
5. Nurses respect and value the knowledge and skills other health care providers bring to the health care team and actively seek to support and collaborate with others so that maximum benefits to clients can be realized.
6. Nurses foster well-being when life can no longer be sustained, by alleviating suffering and supporting a dignified and peaceful death.
7. Nurses provide the best care circumstances permit even when the need arises in an emergency outside the employment situation.
8. Nurses participate, to the best of their abilities, in research and other activities that contribute to the ongoing development of nursing knowledge. Nurses participating in research observe the nursing profession's guidelines, as well as other guidelines, for ethical research.

Choice

Nurses respect and promote the autonomy of clients and help them to express their health needs and values, and to obtain appropriate information and services.

1. Nurses seek to involve clients in health planning and health care decision-making.

2. Nurses provide the information and support required so that clients, to the best of their ability, are able to act on their own behalf in meeting their health and health care needs. Information given is complete, accurate, truthful, and understandable, When they are unable to provide the required information, nurses assist clients in obtaining it from other appropriate sources.

3. Nurses demonstrate sensitivity to the willingness/readiness of clients to receive information about their health condition and care options. Nurses respect the wishes of those who refuse, or are not ready, to receive information about their health condition.

4. Nurses practise within relevant legislation governing consent or choice. Nurses seek to ensure that nursing care is authorized by informed choice, and are guided by this ideal when participating in the consent process in cooperation with other members of the health team.

5. Nurses respect the informed decisions of competent persons to refuse treatment and to choose to live at risk. However, nurses are not obliged to comply with clients' wishes when doing so would require action contrary to the law. If the care requested is contrary to the nurse's moral beliefs, appropriate care is provided until alternative care arrangements are in place to meet the client's needs.

6. Nurses are sensitive to their position of relative power in professional relationships with clients and take care to foster self-determination on the part of their clients. Nurses are sufficiently clear about personal values to recognize and deal appropriately with potential value conflicts.

7. Nurses respect decisions and lawful directives, written or verbal, about present and future health care choices affirmed by a client prior to becoming incompetent.

8. Nurses seek to involve clients of diminished competence in decision-making to the extent that those clients are capable. Nurses continue to value autonomy when illness or other factors reduce the capacity for self-determination, such as by providing opportunities for clients to make choices about aspects of their lives for which they maintain the capacity to make decisions.

9. Nurses seek to obtain consent for nursing care from a substitute decision-maker when clients lack the capacity to make decisions about their care, did not make their wishes known prior to becoming incompetent, or for any reason it is unclear what the client would have wanted in a particular circumstance. When prior wishes of an incompetent client are not known or are unclear, care decisions must be in the best interest of the client and based on what the client would want, as far as is known.

Dignity

Nurses value and advocate the dignity and self-respect of human beings.

1. Nurses relate to all persons receiving care as persons worthy of respect

and endeavour in all their actions to preserve and demonstrate respect for each individual.

2. Nurses exhibit sensitivity to the client's individual needs, values, and choices. Nursing care is designed to accommodate the biological, psychological, social, cultural, and spiritual needs of clients. Nurses do not exploit clients' vulnerabilities for their own interests or gain, whether this be sexual, emotional, social, political, or financial.
3. Nurses respect the privacy of clients when care is given.
4. Nurses treat human life as precious and worthy of respect. Respect includes seeking out and honouring clients' wishes regarding quality of life. Decision-making about life-sustaining treatment carefully balances these considerations.
5. Nurses intervene if others fail to respect the dignity of clients.
6. Nurses advocate the dignity of clients in the use of technology in the health care setting.
7. Nurses advocate health and social conditions that allow persons to live with dignity throughout their lives and in the process of dying. They do so in ways that are consistent with their professional role and responsibilities.

Confidentiality

Nurses safeguard the trust of clients that information learned in the context of a professional relationship is shared outside the health care team only with the client's permission or as legally required.

1. Nurses observe practices that protect the confidentiality of each client's health and health care information.
2. Nurses intervene if other participants in the health care delivery system fail to respect client confidentiality.
3. Nurses disclose confidential information only as authorized by the client, unless there is substantial risk of serious harm to the client or other persons, or a legal obligation to disclose. Where disclosure is warranted, both the amount of information disclosed and the number of people informed is restricted to the minimum necessary.
4. Nurses, whenever possible, inform their clients about the boundaries of professional confidentiality at the onset of care, including the circumstances under which confidential information might be disclosed without consent. If feasible, when disclosure becomes necessary, nurses inform clients what information will be disclosed, to whom, and for what reasons.
5. Nurses advocate policies and safeguards to protect and preserve client confidentiality and intervene if the security of confidential information is jeopardized because of a weakness in the provisions of the system, e.g., inadequate safeguarding guidelines and procedures for the use of computer databases.

Fairness

Nurses apply and promote principles of equity and fairness to assist clients in receiving unbiased treatment and a share of health services and resources proportionate to their needs.

1. Nurses provide care in response to need regardless of such factors as race, ethnicity, culture, spiritual beliefs, social or marital status, gender, sexual orientation, age, health status, lifestyle or the physical attributes of the client.
2. Nurses are justified in using reasonable means to protect against violence when they anticipate acts of violence toward themselves, others or property with good reason.
3. Nurses strive to be fair in making decisions about the allocation of services and goods that they provide, when the distribution of these is within their control.
4. Nurses put forward, and advocate, the interests of all persons in their care. This includes helping individuals and groups gain access to appropriate health care that is of their choosing.
5. Nurses promote appropriate and ethical care at the institutional/agency and community levels by participating, to the extent possible, in the development, implementation, and ongoing review of policies and procedures designed to make the best use of available resources and of current knowledge and research.
6. Nurses advocate, in ways that are consistent with their role and responsibilities, health policies and decision-making procedures that are fair and comprehensive, and that promote fairness and inclusiveness in health resource allocation.

Accountability

Nurses act in a manner consistent with their professional responsibilities and standards of practice.

1. Nurses comply with the values and responsibilities in this *Code of Ethics for Registered Nurses* as well as with the professional standards and laws pertaining to their practice.
2. Nurses conduct themselves with honesty and integrity.
3. Nurses, whether they are engaged in clinical, administrative, research, or educational endeavours, have professional responsibilities and accountabilities toward safeguarding the quality of nursing care clients receive. these responsibilities vary but are all oriented to the expected outcome of safe, competent and ethical nursing practice.
4. Nurses, individually or in partnership with others, take preventive as well as corrective action to protect clients from unsafe, incompetent or unethical care.
5. Nurses base their practice on relevant knowledge, and acquire new skills

and knowledge in their area of practice on a continuing basis, as necessary for the provision of safe, competent and ethical nursing care.

6. Nurses, whether engaged in clinical practice, administration, research or education, provide timely and accurate feedback to other nurses about their practice, so as to support safe and competent care and contribute to ongoing learning. By so doing, they also acknowledge excellence in practice.

7. Nurses practise within their own level of competence. They seek additional information or knowledge; seek the help, and/or supervision and help, of a competent practitioner; and/or request a different work assignment, when aspects of the care required are beyond their level of competence. In the meantime, nurses provide care within the level of their skill and experience.

8. Nurses give primary consideration to the welfare of clients and any possibility of harm in future care situations when they suspect unethical conduct or incompetent or unsafe care. When nurses have reasonable grounds for concern about the behaviour of colleagues in this regard, or about the safety of conditions in the care setting, they carefully review the situation and take steps, individually or in partnership with others, to resolve the problem.

9. Nurses support other nurses who act in good faith to protect clients from incompetent, unethical or unsafe care, and advocate work environments in which nurses are treated with respect when they intervene.

10. Nurses speaking on nursing and health-related matters in a public forum or a court provide accurate and relevant information.

Practice Environments Conducive to Safe, Competent and Ethical Care

Nurses advocate practice environments that have the organizational and human support systems and the resource allocations necessary for safe, competent and ethical nursing care.

1. Nurses collaborate with nursing colleagues and other members of the health team to advocate health care environments that are conducive to ethical practice and to the health and well-being of clients and others in the setting. They do this in ways that are consistent with their professional role and responsibilities.

2. Nurses share their nursing knowledge with other members of the health team for the benefit of clients. To the best of their abilities, nurses provide mentorship and guidance for the professional development of students of nursing and other nurses.

3. Nurses seeking professional employment accurately state their area(s) of competence and seek reasonable assurance that employment conditions will permit care consistent with the values and responsibilities of the code, as well as with their personal ethical beliefs.

4. Nurses practise ethically by striving for the best care achievable in the circumstances. They also make the effort, individually or in partnership with others, to improve practice environments by advocating on behalf of their clients as possible.

5. Nurses planning to participate in job action, or who practise in environments where job action occurs, take steps to safeguard the health and safety of clients during the course of the action.

References

Canadian Health Care Association/Canadian Medical Association/Canadian Nurses Association/Catholic Health Association of Canada/in association with the Canadian Bar Association. (1995). *Joint statement on resuscitative interventions*. Ottawa: Authors.

Canadian Home Care Association/Canadian Hospital Association/Canadian Long Term Care Association/Canadian Nurses Association/Canadian Public Health Association/Home Support Canada. (1994). *Joint statement on advance directives*. Ottawa: Authors.

Canadian Nurses Association. (1994). *A question of respect: Nurses and end of life treatment dilemmas*. Ottawa: Author.

Canadian Nurses Association. (1994). *Ethical guidelines for nurses in research involving human participants*. (2nd rev. ed.). Ottawa: Author.

Canadian Nurses Association. (1996). *Necessary support for safe nursing care*. Ottawa: Author.

Canadian Nurses Association. (1992). *The role of the nurse in the use of health care technology*. Ottawa: Author.

Canadian Nurses Protective Society. (1993, September). Confidentiality of health information: Your clients' rights. *Info Law, 1*(2). Ottawa: Author.

Canadian Nurses Protective Society. (1994, December). Consent to treatment: The role of the nurse. *Info Law, 3*(2). Ottawa: Author.

Some Suggestions for Application of the Code in Selected Circumstances

Steps to address incompetent, unsafe and unethical care
- Gather the facts about the situation and ascertain the risks;
- Review relevant legislation and policies, guidelines and procedures for reporting incidents or suspected incompetent or unethical care and report, as required, an legally reportable offence;
- Seek relevant information directly from the colleague whose behaviour or practice has raised concerns, when this is feasible;
- Consult as appropriate with colleagues, other members of the team, professional nurses' associations, or others able to assist in resolving the problem;

- Undertake to resolve the problem as directly as possible consistent with the good of all parties;
- Advise the appropriate parties regarding unresolved concerns and, when feasible, inform the colleague in question of the reasons for your action;
- Refuse to participate in efforts to deceive or mislead clients about the cause of alleged harm or injury resulting from unethical or incompetent conduct.

Nurse managers, professional associations and client safety
- Nurse managers seek to ensure that available resources and competencies of personnel are used efficiently;
- Nurse managers intervene to minimize the present danger and to prevent future harm when client safety is threatened due to inadequate resources or for some other reason;
- Professional nurses' associations support individual nurses and groups of nurses in promoting fairness and inclusiveness in health resource allocation. They do so in ways that are consistent with their role and functions.

Considerations in student–teacher–client relationships
- Student–teacher and student–client encounters are essential elements of nursing education and are conducted in accordance with ethical nursing practices;
- Clients are informed of the student status of the care giver and consent for care is obtained in compliance with accepted standards;
- Students of nursing are treated with respect and honesty by nurses and are given appropriate guidance for the development of nursing competencies;
- Students are acquainted with and comply with the provisions of the code.

Considerations in taking job action
- Job action by nurses is often directed toward securing conditions of employment that enable safe and ethical care of current and future clients. However, action directed toward such improvements could work to the detriment of clients in the short term;
- Individual nurses and groups of nurses safeguard clients in planning and implementing any job action;
- Individuals and groups of nurses participating in job actions, or affected by job actions, share the ethical commitment to client safety. Their particular responsibilities may lead them to express this commitment in different but equally appropriate ways;
- Clients whose safety requires ongoing or emergency nursing care are entitled to have those needs satisfied throughout any job action;
- Members of the public are entitled to information about the steps taken to ensure the safety of clients during any job action.

A Code of Ethics History

1954   CNA adopts the ICN Code as its first Code of Ethics

1980   CNA moves to adopt its own code entitled, *CNA Code of Ethics: An Ethical Basis for Nursing in Canada*

1985   CNA adopts new code called, *Code of Ethics for Nursing*

1991   *Code of Ethics for Nursing* revised

1997   *Code of Ethics for Registered Nurses* adopted as updated code for CNA

University of Toronto Joint Centre for Bioethics Living Will§

What Is a Living Will?

A living will, sometimes called an "advance directive," is a document containing your wishes about your future health or personal care. You make a living will when you are able to understand treatment choices and appreciate their consequences (i.e., when you are "capable"). A living will only takes effect when you can no longer understand and appreciate treatment choices (i.e., when you are "incapable"). Living wills that meet certain technical legal requirements are also called "health care directives," "advance health care directives," "representation agreements," "mandates," "authorizations," "personal directives," and "powers of attorney for personal care," depending upon the province in which you live. There are two parts to this living will: a *proxy directive* and an *instruction directive*. Because proxy and instruction directives are complementary, your living will should, if possible, contain both of these directives.

What Is a Proxy Directive?

A *proxy directive* specifies *who* you want to make treatment decisions on your behalf if you can no longer do so. The proxy should be someone you know

§Excerpted with permission. The Joint Centre for Bioethics Living Will was developed by Dr. Peter A. Singer. It is a guide to help you think about and express your wishes about future health and personal care decisions. The Living Will is not intended to be used in the absence of specific medical or legal advice. Neither the Joint Centre for Bioethics nor Peter Singer assumes liability for any loss or damage suffered by any person by reason of their reliance on the information contained herein. The University of Toronto and other institutions participating in the Joint Centre for Bioethics make no representations regarding the technical quality, accuracy or lawfulness of the material presented herein. You may download and print this Living Will, in its entirety (which includes legal information specific to each province, as well as further information on personal care decisions), free of charge, at <www.utoronto.ca/jcb/jcblw.htm>. If you have any suggestions for improving this Living Will, please send them to Peter Singer at the Joint Centre for Bioethics, University of Toronto, 88 College St., Toronto, Ontario M5G 1L4 (telephone 416-978-2709; fax 416-978-1911; e-mail peter.singer@utoronto.ca).

and trust, and who understands your way of thinking about your health care treatment and personal care. This could be your spouse, partner, family member, or close friend. This person should him/herself be capable of making health care decisions and be willing to act as your proxy. Because the proxy is responsible for carrying out your wishes, *it is important that you discuss your wishes with your proxy*. Otherwise, it may be difficult for your proxy to guess what your wishes might be. You may name more than one person to act as your proxy, but you should state whether they should make decisions together as a group, or whether they should be given authority individually. In addition, you may want to indicate how disagreements between your proxies should be resolved. You might also want to name different proxies to make different types of decisions. Taking these steps can help to avoid conflict in case your proxies disagree about your treatment. You may also wish, in your living will, to say whether you would want your doctors to follow the treatment decisions of your proxy, or your wishes as expressed in the instruction directive, if these two appear to be in conflict.

What Is an Instruction Directive?

An *instruction directive* specifies *what* health care or other personal care choices you would want your proxy to make in particular situations. This Living Will gives you information on which to base your health and personal care decisions. It also provides space for you to express, in your own words, the values and beliefs that should guide these decisions. Health care decisions are those made either by you, or by someone on your behalf, to consent or to refuse to consent to a treatment. Treatment refers to anything done for a diagnostic, therapeutic, preventive or palliative (comfort care) reason. Personal care decisions refer to decisions about those aspects of your daily life that are necessary for maintaining your health and well-being. These include shelter, nutrition, hygiene, clothing, and safety.

What Type of Living Will Should I Make?

Because instruction and proxy directives are complementary, your living will should, if possible, contain both of these directives. However, if you find that making decisions for a possible future illness is too difficult, then you may want to complete only the proxy directive. In this case, your proxy (or proxies) will make treatment and care decisions for you, based on their judgement as to what you would want, or would be best for you. Or, if you do not have someone you trust to make decisions on your behalf, then you may want to complete only the instruction directive. If you do that, persons making decisions for you will be guided by your instructions in making treatment and personal care decisions for you.

Do I Need to Complete the Living Will with My Doctor?

It is a good idea to review your living will with your doctor. The doctor can ensure that you have understood the choices in the living will and that the instruction directive is suitable for your own health situation.

Do I Need to Complete the Living Will with My Lawyer?

It is a good idea to consult a lawyer with experience in this area. A living will is a legal document with serious legal implications. A lawyer can ensure that your living will is legally valid in your province. A lawyer's assistance may be particularly helpful if your capacity to make a living will is likely to be challenged, or if there may be disagreement among your family or between your family and proxy. If you plan to consult a lawyer, use this information to help you discuss your wishes about health and personal care with your loved ones, but do not sign or witness the living will form on pages 342–343, because the lawyer may want to incorporate this into his or her own form.

What Should I Do with My Completed Living Will?

Since a living will speaks for you when you are no longer able to speak for yourself, other people must know that it exists. Give copies of your living will to your proxy, doctor, lawyer, and family members. If you review your wishes with these people and give them the opportunity to discuss your living will with you, they will be more likely to understand and follow your wishes. Do not put your living will in your safety deposit box, since it will not be easy to gain access to it when needed. You may photocopy the Living Will (pages 337–343) once you have completed it.

What If I Change My Mind About My Wishes or Proxy?

You can change your mind about your health care or other personal care decisions or your proxy at any time while you are still capable. If you change your mind, you should change your living will. Also, you should review your living will at regular intervals, such as once a year, and when there are important changes in your life, for example: if your medical condition changes, if you are admitted to hospital, if you marry or divorce, or if your proxy dies. If you change your living will, replace all copies of the old one with copies of the new one. You should destroy the old copies so they do not get mixed up with the new copies of your living will.

Will My Living Will Be Followed?

Yes, it should be followed. The Canadian Medical Association has endorsed a policy supporting living wills and most doctors favour them. In provinces with specific legislation, people may be legally required to follow your living will. However, there could be circumstances in which you would not want people to follow your living will, for example, if there is evidence that you have changed your mind but have not changed your living will, or there has been a medical advance that you did not know about when you completed the forms. In your living will, you can say how much leeway you want to give your proxy in following your wishes.

JOINT CENTRE FOR BIOETHICS
Living Will Form

Be sure to discuss your wishes with your proxy. You can use the descriptions of the health situations and treatments (pages 340–342), and the Living Will form, to help you with this discussion.

This living will is a legal document. Although you can complete this form without a lawyer, it is a good idea to consult a lawyer with experience in this area.

The living will contains medical information to help you make decisions. If you have questions about the descriptions of health situations or treatments, or about your own medical conditions and what might happen to you in the future, you should discuss these with your doctor.

Complete the living will using a black pen to make it easier to photocopy. When you have completed it, make copies to give to your proxy or proxies, doctor, and lawyer.

If you change your mind about who you want to be your proxy, or about your wishes regarding treatment, change your living will and give copies of the new one to anyone who has a copy of the old one. Then, destroy all copies of your old living will.

The Proxy Directive

The proxy must follow the wishes of the person making the living will. In situations for which the person has not specified a wish, the proxy would make the decision based on the person's best interests, taking into consideration the person's values and beliefs. If you name more than one person to act as your proxy, you should say how they will make decisions.

There are three options: First, you can have your proxies make decisions individually, in the order that you list them in your living will. If the first named proxy is unavailable, or has died, then the next proxy listed would make the necessary decisions on your behalf, and so on. Second, you can say that you want your proxies to make decisions as a group. If this case, you should indicate how you would like disagreements between your proxies to be resolved. This could be by majority vote or by giving your first named proxy the final say. Third, you can limit the authority of your proxies to make certain decisions. For example, you may have someone who you want to make decisions about your health care, and someone else to make other personal care decisions such as nutrition, clothing, hygiene, or shelter. The wishes contained in this Living Will are intended to help your proxy or proxies understand what you want. You can also say how much leeway your proxy should have in interpreting your wishes; i.e., do you want your instructions followed exactly or used only as a guideline?

Proxy Directive

I authorize the following person(s) to make health care and other personal care decisions on my behalf if I am no longer capable of making them for myself.

Proxy 1

Name: _____

Relationship: _____

Address: _____

Telephone: _____

If you want more than one person to be your proxy, add the additional name(s) below (or use further sheets of paper):

Proxy 2

Name: _____

Relationship: _____

Address: _____

Telephone: _____

Do you want your proxies to make decisions individually, or as a group?

☐ individually

☐ as a group

If you want your proxies to make decisions as a group, how do you want disagreements resolved?

☐ follow directions of proxy 1

☐ follow directions of the majority of my proxies

If you want particular proxies to make health care decisions, and others to make personal care decisions, specify here:

_____

_____

How much leeway do you want to give your proxies in interpreting your wishes? Specify here:

_____

_____

Instruction Directive

The first part of the instruction directive is the Treatment Table, below. Please refer to "Health Situations" and "Life-Sustaining Treatments" (pages 340–342) for the definitions of terms used in this directive. For each of the health situations (first column of table), imagine that you are in the situation described, and then you develop a further medical problem that requires some life-sustaining treatment (top row of table). If you do not receive this treatment, you would die. If you receive the treatment, the chance that you will live depends on the nature of the medical problem. Even if you recover fully from the medical problem, you would return to the health situation you were in before you developed the further medical problem.

As an example, imagine that, at some future time, you suffer from a severe stroke. Then, you develop pneumonia requiring life-saving antibiotics. Without the antibiotics, you would die. With them, your chance of surviving depends on the nature and severity of the pneumonia. Of course, even if the antibiotics were successful in treating your pneumonia, you would still have severe stroke. You should then decide whether you would want the particular treatment (antibiotics) if you were in this condition (severe stroke).

Write your treatment decision ("yes," "no," "undecided," or "trial") in the box for every combination of health situation and treatment.

	CPR	RESPIRATOR	DIALYSIS	LIFE-SAVING SURGERY	BLOOD TRANSFUSION	LIFE-SAVING ANTIBIOTICS	TUBE FEEDING
CURRENT HEALTH	yes	yes	yes	yes	yes	yes	yes
PERMANENT COMA	no	no	no	no	no	no	no
TERMINAL ILLNESS	no	no	no	undecided	yes	yes	undecided
MILD STROKE	undecided	trial	trial	yes	yes	yes	trial
MODERATE STROKE	no	no	no	no	no	no	no
SEVERE STROKE	no	no	no	no	no	no	no
MILD DEMENTIA	yes	yes	yes	yes	yes	yes	yes
MODERATE DEMENTIA	no	no	no	no	no	no	no
SEVERE DEMENTIA	no	no	no	no	no	no	no

Health Situations

Current health: This describes the way your health is now.

Permanent coma: You would be permanently unconscious. Permanent coma is usually caused by decreased blood flow to the brain, e.g., from the heart stopping. You would be unable to eat or drink and would need a feeding tube for nourishment. You would not have bowel or bladder control. You would need to be in bed and you would never regain consciousness. You could live at home with someone caring for you all day and night; otherwise you would probably need to be cared for in a chronic care hospital.

Terminal illness: You would have an illness for which there is no known cure, such as some types of cancer. It is likely that you would die within six months even if you received treatment.

Stroke: You would have damage to the brain causing permanent physical disability such as paralysis. You might also have trouble communicating because of impaired speech. These problems stay the same for the rest of your life. They do not get worse with time unless there is another injury to the brain, such as another stroke. Stroke can be described as:
- **Mild:** You would have mild paralysis on one side of the body. You could walk with a cane or walker. You would be able to have conversations, but might have trouble finding words. You could carry out most routine daily activities, such as work and household duties, dressing, eating, bathing, and using the toilet. You would have bowel and bladder control. You could live at home with someone caring for you for a few hours a day.
- **Moderate:** You would have moderate paralysis on one side of the body. You would be unable to walk and would need a wheelchair. You could carry out conversations, but might not always make sense. You would need help with routine daily activities. You may have bowel and bladder control. You could live at home with someone caring for you throughout the daytime; otherwise you would probably need to live in a nursing home.
- **Severe:** You would have severe paralysis on one side of the body. You would be unable to walk, and would need to be in a chair or bed. You would not have meaningful conversations. You would be unable to carry out routine daily activities. You would need a feeding tube for nourishment. You would not have bowel or bladder control. You could live at home with someone caring for you all day and night; otherwise you would probably need to be cared for in a chronic care hospital.

Dementia: You would have a progressive and irreversible deterioration in brain function. You would be awake and aware but you would have trouble thinking clearly, recognizing people, and communicating. The most common cause of dementia is Alzheimer's disease. Dementia gradually gets worse over months or years. Dementia can be described as:
- **Mild:** You could have conversations, but would be forgetful and have poor short term memory. You could carry out most routine daily activi-

ties, such as work and household duties, dressing, eating, bathing, and using the toilet. You would have bowel and bladder control. You could live at home with someone caring for you for a few hours each day.

- **Moderate:** You would not always recognize family and friends. You could carry out conversations but you might not always make sense. You would need help with routine daily activities. You may have bowel and bladder control. You could live at home with someone caring for you throughout the daytime; otherwise you would probably need to live in a nursing home.
- **Severe:** You would not recognize family and friends, and would be unable to have meaningful conversations. You would be unable to carry out routine daily activities. You would need a feeding tube for nourishment. You would not have bowel and bladder control. You could live at home with someone caring for you all day and night; otherwise you would probably need to be cared for in a chronic care hospital.

Life-Sustaining Treatments

In each of the health situations described above, you might need one or more of the following life-sustaining treatments:

- **Cardiopulmonary resuscitation** (CPR) is used to try to restart the heart if it has stopped beating. CPR involves applying pressure and electrical shocks to the chest, assisted breathing with a respirator (breathing machine) through a tube inserted down the throat and into the lungs, and giving drugs through a needle into a vein. It is usually followed by unconsciousness and several days in an intensive care unit. Without CPR, immediate death is certain. On average when hospitalized patients are given CPR, it is successful at restarting the heart in about 41% of patients (41 patients out of 100). However, about 14% (14 patients out of 100) will live to be discharged from hospital. Patients whose hearts are successfully restarted but who do not survive to hospital discharge spend several days in an intensive care unit before death. The chance that a person will live depends on the cause of the heart stopping and the seriousness of the person's other illnesses.
- **Respirator** (breathing machine) is used when a person cannot breathe; e.g., because of emphysema or a serious pneumonia. A tube is put down the person's throat into the lungs. The respirator is needed as long as the person's lungs are not working. Without the respirator, a person with respiratory failure will probably die within minutes to hours. With the respirator, the chance that a person will live depends on the cause of the respiratory failure, and the seriousness of the person's other illnesses.
- **Dialysis** (kidney machine) replaces the normal functions of the kidney. Dialysis removes excess potassium, water, and other waste products from the blood. Without dialysis, the potassium in the blood would build up and cause the heart to stop. Dialysis is needed as long as the person's kidneys are not working. Without dialysis, a person with kidney failure will die within 7 to 14 days. With dialysis, the chance that a person will live depends on the cause of the kidney failure and the person's other illnesses.

- **Life-saving surgery** may involve a wide range of procedures, e.g., removal of an inflamed gall bladder or appendix. Without surgery, a person with a serious illness may die within hours to days. With surgery, the chance that a person will live depends on why the person needed surgery and the seriousness of the person's other injuries or illnesses.
- **Blood transfusion** refers to blood given through a needle inserted in a person's vein. A person who is bleeding very heavily from a car accident, stomach ulcer, or during major surgery needs a blood transfusion. Without it, a person who is bleeding very heavily will probably die within hours. With a blood transfusion, the chance that a person will live depends on the seriousness of the person's other injuries or illnesses.
- **Life-saving antibiotics** refers to the drugs needed to treat life-threatening infections; e.g., pneumonia or meningitis. These drugs usually are given through a needle inserted in a person's vein. Without antibiotics, a person with a life-threatening infection will likely die in hours to days. With them, the chance that a person will live depends on the seriousness of the infection and of the person's other illnesses.
- **Tube feeding** involves putting a tube into a person's stomach (through the nose, or through a small hole in the abdomen). A person who cannot eat (e.g., someone in a coma) needs a feeding tube. Without tube feeding, a person who cannot eat or drink will die within days to weeks. With tube feeding, the chance that a person will live depends on the seriousness of the person's other injuries or illnesses.

Further Instructions

In the space below (or on a separate page), you may express in your own words the situations in which you would or would not want various life-sustaining treatments.

_____

_____

Statement by Person Completing This Living Will

I have read and understood all sections of this Living Will. All previous living wills made by me are revoked, and this directive is to be followed. The person(s) whom I have named as proxy (proxies) is/are authorized to give directions and make decisions on my behalf concerning my personal care and to give or refuse consent on my behalf to treatment, in accordance with the instructions found in this Living Will.

Name: _____

Address: _____

Signature: _____

Date: _____

Instructions for Witnesses

This document should be signed in the presence of two witnesses (although requirements in different provinces vary). The witnesses must be present together and sign immediately after the living will is signed by the person completing it. Neither witness should be the proxy or the proxy's spouse.

In Ontario, the following people may not be a witness: a child of the patient; anyone who him/herself has a legal guardian; and anyone who is less than 18 years old.

In Newfoundland, witnesses must be "independent."

Witness 1

Name: _____

Address: _____

Signature: _____

Date: _____

Witness 2

Name: _____

Address: _____

Signature: _____

Date: _____

Agreement to Act As Proxy

(Required in Newfoundland and Prince Edward Island)

I agree to act as proxy for _____ in the event that he/she becomes incapable.

Proxy 1

Name: _____

Signature: _____

Date: _____

Proxy 2

Name: _____

Signature: _____

Date: _____

Abortion. The interruption of a pregnancy either spontaneously or intentionally by means of medical intervention.

Action. A lawsuit or court proceeding in which an injured party asserts a claim for damages or some other remedial court order against a wrongdoer.

Actus Reus. The physical element of a criminal offence, i.e., the voluntary performance of a prohibited act that results in physical or other harm (e.g., assault causing bodily harm).

Adjudicate. In law, the functions of a court or administrative tribunal in hearing evidence in a legal controversy between two or more parties, assessing the evidence, making findings of fact and credibility, and rendering a decision (e.g., a verdict of guilty or not guilty in a criminal trial, or a finding of liability and assessment of damages against a defendant in a civil trial).

Administrative Tribunals. Government boards, agencies, councils, and commissions charged with administration of a particular area (e.g., property taxes, human rights complaints, energy rates, transport licences). These often operate like courts in that they decide claims before them, grant licences, etc.

Advance Directive. A document made and signed by a mentally competent adult detailing specific medical treatments that are to be administered or withheld in the event that the maker later becomes incapable of expressing such wishes owing to mental or physical illness (e.g., Alzheimer's disease, coma).

Affidavit. A written statement of facts made under oath or solemn affirmation.

Appeal. A legal proceeding in which a superior appellate court (cf.) is asked by one or more parties to the original proceedings to review those proceedings in order to determine whether the inferior court or administrative tribunal committed any errors of law, misconstrued the evidence before it, exceeded its powers, or otherwise acted contrary to law in adjudicating upon the matter. This is not a retrial, but a review of the proceedings at trial or at the hearing.

Appellant. The party to a court action (usually the party who loses at trial or against whom an unfavourable judgement is made) who brings an appeal of a trial decision in an appellate court.

Appellate Court. A court that hears appeals or reviews decisions of lower or inferior courts.

Applied Ethics. The application of particular ethical theories to actual problems or issues.

Assault. Conduct (such as a physical or verbal threat) that creates in another person an apprehension or fear of imminent harmful or offensive contact.

Assisted Insemination. A form of donor insemination (cf.), typically used when the male partner's sperm count is low, in which sperm are extracted and concentrated before being artificially introduced into the recipient's uterus.

Assisted Suicide. Any aid directed at terminating the life of persons who, due to severe physical limitations or illness, cannot act for themselves.

Autonomy. An ethical principle, founded on respect for persons, that assumes a capable and competent person is free to determine a self-chosen plan unless that plan interferes with the rights of others.

Bargaining Agent. In labour relations, a union certified by provincial statute and authorized to negotiate collectively on behalf of a group of employees.

Bargaining Unit. In labour relations, a group of employees who are members of a union and who are bound by the terms of a collective agreement (employment contract) negotiated by the union on their behalf with their employer.

Battery. Harmful or offensive and non-consensual contact with the person or clothing of another.

Beneficence. A principle that obliges us to act in such a way as to produce some good or benefit for another.

Bill. A draft or proposed law that is not yet passed and must be voted upon by Parliament or a legislature. Usually introduced by the government party, but any member of Parliament may introduce a bill.

Biomedical Ethics. A field of ethics that focusses on issues associated with science, medicine, and health care.

Burden of Proof. The obligation on a party to litigation (i.e., a criminal or civil lawsuit) to prove a certain fact or facts to a judge or jury.

Case Law. The law as set forth in decided cases. This is called jurisprudence in civil law systems. (See also "Precedent.")

Categorical Imperative. In Kantian ethics, a supreme principle that a law of morality must follow.

Certification. In labour relations law, the process whereby a given union is legally recognized as the official representative for collective bargaining and labour relations purposes of a certain group of employees in a given industry.

Chain of Causation. In negligence law, a series of related successive events, each of which is dependent upon the previous one, which ultimately result in damage or injury to persons or property. There must be links between all such events in that each must result from the preceding one.

Charter of Rights and Freedoms. A portion of Canada's written Constitution that sets out the fundamental rights and freedoms of all persons in Canada and limits the rights of the State to breach or infringe upon these rights. Laws or governmental action that violate these rights without proper justification are null and void.

Civil Code. A central written and formal source of civil law principles and rules.

Civil Law. A system of law based on Roman law, prevalent in most European countries and the Province of Quebec, in which legal principles and rules are codified or written in organized fashion into a central statute or code.

Closed Shop. In labour relations, a place of employment in which, as a condition of employment, a worker is required to belong to the union representing the employees.

Codification. The process of formally arranging legal rules and principles on any area into a central source of law known as a code.

Collective Agreement. A written contract of employment between an employer and a unionized group of non-managerial employees. It binds all employees, lasts for at least one year, and sets out conditions of employment (e.g., wages, hours of work, benefits, sick leave, pension, layoffs, termination, disciplinary action, arbitration of grievances).

Collective Bargaining. In labour relations, the process by which a union (the bargaining agent) negotiates the conditions of employment of a group of non-managerial employees (the bargaining unit) with an employer or group of employers.

Common Law. English system of law dating back to the 11th century, based on unwritten principles derived from judicial precedents.

Complainant. In professional disciplinary matters, a person who complains, through a formal disciplinary procedure, about the treatment accorded him or her by a member of a self-governing profession (e.g., a physician, nurse, dentist, lawyer).

Conciliator. In labour relations, a person usually appointed by the provincial minister of labour to intervene in a strike or other labour dispute in an attempt to work out a settlement agreeable to both sides, narrow the issues under dispute, and canvass possible solutions.

Consent. The permission given by a person to someone else to perform an act upon the person giving such permission. Consent can be explicit (expressed) or implied by the circumstances or the conduct of the person giving it.

Constitution. A written law that sets forth the fundamental rules and principles defining how a country is organized and its laws passed, and the extent of the government's powers and the powers of its courts.

Constitutional Convention. In British, Canadian, and Commonwealth constitutional law, a practice that is not a part of the legal written Constitution, yet is followed by tradition. For example, it is a convention that the Queen (or the Governor General, in Canada) always follows and accepts the advice of her ministers and will give Royal Assent to all legislation submitted to her (or her Governor General, in Canada). Although the Queen can legally decline to give such assent, to do so would create a constitutional crisis and political impasse.

Contempt of Court. The deliberate violation of a court order by a party who is subject to such order; or, conduct that is disrespectful or disruptive of court proceedings.

Contract. An oral or written agreement between two or more parties that creates legally binding, mutual obligations and rights.

Contributory Negligence. A situation in which a plaintiff, who has sued another for damages for negligence, is held partly responsible for the damage or injury sustained because the plaintiff is partly at fault.

Controlled Act. In Ontario (under the *Regulated Health Professions Act, 1991*, SO 1991, c. 18, section 27), a specific medical act or procedure that may be performed only by a person who is a member of a health profession (e.g., a nurse, doctor, dentist) and who is authorized by a health profession Act (e.g., the *Nursing Act, 1991*, SO 1991, c. 32) to perform such an act. (See Chapter Five for a list of controlled acts.)

Cooling-off Period. In labour relations, the period between the breakdown in negotiations and the time in which unionized employees may legally commence a strike against the employer or after which the employer may legally lock out the employees. Its purpose is to attempt to settle tensions between labour and management and assist in the resumption of negotiations.

Coroner's Inquest. An inquiry convened under the authority of a coroner to look into the circumstances of a death when that person has died in suspicious circumstances, as a result of wrongdoing, possible negligence, or accident (i.e., not through natural causes). The inquest is presided over by a deputy coroner, and determinations of fact and recommendations are made by a jury.

Costs. In legal proceedings, the lawyers' fees and other expenditures associated with the conduct of the proceeding from beginning to end.

Court of First Instance. (See "Original Jurisdiction.")

Criminal Code of Canada. An Act of Parliament that lists and defines all criminal offences, and sets out procedural rules for trying such offences and punishing convicted persons.

Criminal Law. The body of law that prohibits certain specified conduct or acts set out in a criminal code or other statute and includes sanctions (punishment), such as imprisonment or fines, for breach. It includes all rules of criminal procedure used in trying accused persons charged with offences; regulates relationships between the State (society) and the individual; and aims to keep and maintain order.

Criminal Negligence. Conduct in which the actor (the accused) has acted intentionally in a reckless or wanton manner, showing disregard for the rights or safety of others who might reasonably be expected to suffer harm or damage as a result of such conduct, and where damage or harm ensues.

Cryopreservation. The freezing of sperm or embryos for later use in assisted insemination.

Cultural Relativism. The view that individual and group responses to morality are relative to the norms and values of that particular culture or society, or to the specific situation. Also called normative relativism.

Custom. In law, practice or rules of a particular trade or industry given force of law by the courts in the absence of specific statute law, case law, or doctrine governing the particular area.

Damages. A sum of money awarded by a court at the end of a civil trial and claimed by the plaintiff against the defendant as compensation for an injury to person or property caused by the defendant.

Decertification. In labour law, the process whereby a union loses its right to represent a group of employees and to bargain collectively on their behalf, either through its failure to take steps to negotiate a collective agreement, or through a vote of the members themselves.

Defendant. A person or party against whom a lawsuit is brought; the party sought to be made responsible for the plaintiff's damages.

Delegation. The assignment to another person, by a health professional, of a certain act or procedure which that professional is authorized by law and by the professional regulatory body to perform. Delegation may be lawful if the person to whom the task is delegated is adequately trained to perform the act and properly supervised.

Democratic Rights. Rights enshrined in the *Charter of Rights and Freedoms,* which provide for democratic participation of citizens in government. These include: the right to vote, a maximum five-year term limit on the life of Parliament or a provincial legislature (i.e., an election at least every five years), and the requirement that Parliament or a legislative assembly sit at least once per year (i.e., no rule by decree or dispensing with legislative approval of laws).

Deposition. In Quebec, under the *Professional Code,* a written complaint of a complainant given under oath according to the procedures in such code.

Descriptive Ethics. A systematic explanation of moral behaviour or beliefs.

Detain. To hold in police custody or control without freedom to leave.

Directive. (See "Advance Directive.")

Disclosure. The obligation of each party to a lawsuit under the rules of civil procedure to reveal to the other party or parties all evidence, documents, reports, records, etc. that will be relied upon at trial.

Division of Powers. In Canadian Constitutional law, the allocation by the Constitution, as between the federal Parliament and the provincial legislatures, of the right to make laws in specific areas such as criminal law, civil law, defence, municipal law, etc.

Doctrine. Texts, journal articles, treatises, restatements of the law, and other learned writings of legal scholars on any legal subject; used by lawyers and judges as an aid in interpreting or developing the law.

Documentary Discovery. The right of each party in a lawsuit to obtain copies of all relevant documents possessed by or in the control of the opponent(s), and upon which the opponent(s) will rely at trial.

Donor Insemination. A therapeutic procedure in which sperm from a healthy donor (who may or may not be the woman's partner) are artificially introduced into a fertile woman's uterus.

Dual Procedure Offence. In criminal law, an offence that may be tried either as a summary conviction offence or an indictable offence at the option of the Crown attorney. The choice usually depends on the seriousness of the facts surrounding the laying of charges.

Due Process. The right of every citizen, regardless of race, sex, colour, creed, or religion, to receive fair treatment according to established procedures and rules of natural justice.

Duty. The legal obligation to perform some act or take a particular course of conduct that is owed towards an individual or individuals, or society as a whole. (See also "Obligation.")

Duty of Care. A legal obligation imposed on an individual to act or refrain from acting in a way such as to avoid causing harm to the person or property of another who might reasonably be affected and who ought to be in the actor's contemplation.

Ectogenesis. The maintenance of an embryo in an artificial womb.

Embryo Donation. The making available of surplus cryopreserved embryos that are no longer needed or wanted by the couple who originated them (i.e., by in vitro fertilization). The alternatives are to destroy the embryos or to use them for research purposes.

Equality Rights. The right to be treated equally by and before the law regardless of one's race, sex, religion, ethnic origin, physical or mental disability, age or skin colour. These rights are specifically enshrined in the Canadian *Charter of Rights and Freedoms.*

Ethical Dilemma. A situation in which the most ethical course of action is unclear, when there is a strong moral reason to support each of several positions, or when a decision must be made based on the most right or the least wrong choice of action.

Ethical Principles. A set of values based on ethical theory and intended to guide right action.

Ethical Theory. A framework of assumptions and principles intended to guide decisions about morality.

Ethics. The philosophical study of questions regarding what is morally right and wrong.

Examination for Discovery. A preliminary oral examination at which the lawyer for each party in a trial has the opportunity to ask relevant questions of the other party or parties, under oath, to obtain full disclosure of all evidence and facts that will be relied upon at trial.

Evidence. The material with which a party builds its case against another and proves a fact or set of facts. It may take the form of oral testimony from witnesses given under oath, documentary or real physical evidence such as DNA, blood samples, hair and clothing fibres, photographs, etc.

Fidelity. A principle that guides relationships and is based on loyalty, promise keeping, and truth telling.

Findings of Fact. In law, conclusions drawn by a trier of fact (i.e., a judge or jury) as to what actually occurred, and in what sequence, in a given case. These are based upon an examination and assessment of the evidence adduced at trial by the parties to the litigation (whether criminal or civil). For example, in a civil action in a motor vehicle accident case, one witness may testify that A. drove his vehicle through the intersection against a red light, while another witness may say that the light was green. The trier of fact will assess the evidence given by these two witness, determine which is more credible, and make a finding of fact as to which colour the light was when the accident occurred.

Fundamental Rights. Specific rights enshrined the Canadian *Charter of Rights and Freedoms* that are considered to be basic and necessary in every democratic society (e.g., the freedoms of religion, conscience, thought and expression, press, peaceful assembly, association).

Garnishment. A court-ordered procedure by which individuals or corporations owing money to a defendant debtor are required to pay a portion or all of it to the sheriff for distribution among the defendant's creditors, including the plaintiff.

Grantor. A person of sound mind and usually (in most provinces) over the age of majority who signs a document giving another power to make medical treatment decisions on that person's behalf or decisions respecting that person's property or finances. (See also "Power of Attorney for Personal Care.")

Health Disciplines Board. A provincial body that regulates a health profession with respect to licensing members and that ensures appropriate educational and professional qualifications, standards of practice, and ethical conduct by members. Such a body may have various names, depending on the province.

Hearsay Evidence. A statement given by a party under oath in court that another person, not present in court and not a party to the proceedings, made a statement as to a given state of affairs. This statement is then used by the party offering it in evidence to prove the truth of the facts asserted in such statement. Such evidence is generally inadmissible in court.

Hybrid Offence. In criminal law, an offence that can be tried either by indictment or summarily at the option of the Crown. (See also "Dual Procedure Offence.")

Indemnity Fund. A fund provided by a provincial nursing regulatory body to compensate clients or patients who have suffered injury or damage as a result of a member's professional or other misconduct or criminal or fraudulent acts. Such a fund has been established in Quebec, for example.

Indictable Offences. The most serious of criminal offences; usually triable by a jury, but only after a preliminary hearing at which the accused is ordered to stand trial. Punishment ranges from several years to life imprisonment and/or heavy fines.

Inferior Court. A lower level of court that is judicially subordinate to a superior one. Usually a trial court, which is bound by previous decisions of an appeal court.

Informed Consent. In health care, a legally capable patient's consent to a specific medical treatment, in which the patient is informed by the health practitioner of the nature and purpose of the treatment, all its material risks and benefits, and the material risks of not proceeding with treatment. A material risk is one that a patient would reasonably wish to know prior to making the decision of whether to undergo or forgo the proposed treatment.

Injunction. A court order obtained by one party against one or more other parties that directs those others to refrain from a specific conduct or to perform a specified act.

In Vitro Fertilization. A process whereby fertilization occurs outside the body and without intimate human contact.

Judgement Debtor. A person who has been sued and against whom a court has issued a judgement finding him or her liable to pay a sum of money to the plaintiff.

Judgement Debtor Examination. An oral examination at which the defendant gives answers under oath to questions by the plaintiff's lawyer concerning his or her finances, sources of income, and ability to pay the judgement against him or her.

Jurisdiction. The authority of a court to hear and decide a legal dispute (e.g., civil or criminal) in a particular territory, as well as the types of orders and judgements it may make.

Jurisprudence. Judges' written decisions in past court cases, which serve as precedents for future decisions in civil law systems; not binding, but seen as evidence of how past courts have interpreted a civil code provision or legal principle. (See also "Case Law.")

Jurors. Members of a jury.

Jury. A group of 12 (in criminal juries) or six (in civil juries) citizens over the age of majority who are convened to hear evidence, make findings of fact, and ultimately deliver a verdict in a criminal or civil trial.

Justice. A principle that focusses on the fair treatment of individuals and groups within society.

Lawsuit. (See "Action.")

Legal Rights. Rights of all persons resident in Canada, which are invoked upon arrest or detention and when such persons are charged with a criminal offence. These are enshrined in the *Charter of Rights and Freedoms* and include: the right to life, liberty and security of the person (i.e., the right not to be compelled to give evidence against oneself in a police investigation, or the right to remain silent); the right to be secure against unreasonable search and seizure (e.g., having one's home searched without permission by the police without good reason and without a warrant issued by a justice of the peace); the right not to be arbitrarily detained or imprisoned; the right to be informed of the reason for one's arrest and to be informed of the charge; the right to speak to a lawyer in private and to be informed of this right; and the right to have the legality of one's detention determined by an impartial court and to be immediately released if that detention is judged to be unlawful. These rights also include the right to be tried within a reasonable time by an impartial court, to be presumed innocent until proven guilty, to reasonable bail, and to a jury trial if the punishment for the offence with which one is charged is five or more years' imprisonment. If acquitted or convicted of a criminal offence, a resident of Canada has the right not to be tried again for the same offence (the "double jeopardy" rule). Residents have the right, when punished for an offence of which they have been convicted, not to be subjected to cruel or unusual punishment (i.e., torture or degrading punishment and treatment, inhumane treatment or living conditions while in prison, and arguably, capital punishment).

Legislative Assembly. A provincial parliament consisting of only one house. Also called "the legislature."

Liability. The legal responsibility owed by a party at fault to another for damages incurred or injury suffered by that other.

Licensing. The granting by a nursing regulatory body, such as a College of nurses or provincial nursing association, to an otherwise qualified nurse, of the right to practise within the province in accordance with recognized standards of care and ethics and subject to any restrictions specified in the licence.

Litigant. A person or corporation who is a party to a lawsuit.

Living Will. A written document signed by a mentally competent person setting forth specific instructions regarding medical treatments to be applied or withheld in the event that the maker later becomes incapable of expressing those wishes. For example, the document might indicate whether resuscitation should be attempted in the event of a cardiac arrest.

Lockout. In labour relations, the employer's equivalent of the strike, in which the employer locks out its unionized employees from the workplace, or refuses to continue to employ them, in an effort to pressure them to concede during contract negotiations or in labour disputes. In most provinces, a lockout, like a strike, may occur only after the expiry of a collective agreement and only after a cooling-off period has elapsed under the applicable provincial labour statute.

Malfeasance. In law, doing an act that is one's duty to perform, but doing it poorly, incorrectly, or negligently.

Malpractice. The failure of a health professional or other specialist to observe and adhere to the appropriate standards of care for a given act or procedure; the negligent performance of a procedure or act requiring a reasonable degree of professional skill and ability. (See also "Negligence.")

Mens Rea. The mental element of a criminal offence, that is, the accused's state of mind when he or she is alleged to have committed a crime; the requirement that he or she was aware and intended wilfully to commit it, knew that the action was wrong, or was reckless as to the consequences of the action.

Metaethics. A philosophical focus on the meaning and nature of morality and ethics.

Misconduct. (See "Professional Misconduct.")

Mobility Rights. The rights of all persons legally resident in Canada to move in and out of Canada and between various provinces and cities; to take up residence anywhere in the country in order to pursue employment or educational and other opportunities. These rights are enshrined in the *Charter of Rights and Freedoms*.

Moral Distress. Stress that results when moral conflict is not addressed or satisfactorily resolved.

Negligence. The non-intentional category of tort law wherein one person has, through carelessness, failed in a duty of care towards another such that that other has sustained injury to person or property.

New Reproductive Technologies. Techniques to promote pregnancy by overcoming or bypassing infertility, including donor insemination, assisted insemination, in vitro fertilization, cryopreservation, ovum and embryo donation, and surrogacy. Advanced genetic technologies have also been developed that include sex selection, embryo research, prenatal diagnosis, and human embryo cloning.

Non-feasance. Failing to do that which is one's legal duty or obligation to do.

Non-maleficence. A principle that obliges us to act in such as way as to prevent causing harm to others.

Notwithstanding Clause. A provision in the Canadian Constitution that permits Parliament or a legislature to exempt a given law from being subject to certain rights enshrined in the *Charter of Rights and Freedoms*. This clause provides that a law may continue to apply for up to five years, even if it contravenes a provision of the Charter. The five-year limit is designed to ensure that rights are not permanently infringed (violated) by a law. After five years, the notwithstanding clause expires insofar as it applies to that particular law, unless it is invoked again.

Nursing Ethics. The study of moral questions that fall within the sphere of nursing practice and nursing science.

Objective Standard. The standard of the reasonable or "average" person against which someone's particular conduct in a given situation is judged. For example, a nurses performing a given task in a particular manner will have their methods of doing such task measured against the manner in which one would expect a reasonably competent and skilled nurse to perform it.

Obligation. In law, some act or course of conduct that the law requires an individual or individuals to perform, either for the benefit of another party or parties or that of society in general. (See also "Duty.")

Open Shop. A place of employment in which union membership is not mandatory (cf. "Closed Shop").

Order-in-Council. Subordinate legislation passed by the Cabinet, usually in the form of regulations made to supplement and provide further detail to a particular statute. Such orders are usually passed pursuant to authority contained in the statute. In the event that the regulation or order goes farther than the statute authorizes, the order may be declared *ultra vires*, or beyond the power of the Cabinet to enact.

Original Jurisdiction. The first court to hear a criminal or civil case, i.e., the court in which the litigation process begins.

Originating Process. A document issued out of a court that begins a legal proceeding and must be formally served upon (delivered to) a defendant or responding party or parties. (See also "Statement of Claim" and "Writ of Summons.")

Parliament. A body of elected lawmakers (Members of Parliament or MPs) entrusted with the power to make laws for the country or a province. The federal Parliament consists of two houses (the Senate and the House of Commons) and the Queen (the Head of State).

Plaintiff. The party who brings a lawsuit and seeks damages against another for breach of contract or other wrong done to that party.

Pleadings. The court documents filed by each party to the lawsuit outlining the nature of the claim, the defence to the claim, and the issues to be tried in the action.

Power of Attorney. Generally in Canada, a document in which a legally capable person appoints another to manage the maker's financial affairs and make decisions on the maker's behalf in the maker's absence or unavailability. In Ontario, under the *Substitute Decisions Act, 1992,* SO 1992, c. 30, two types of powers of attorney are recognized in law: a power of attorney for property (as above), and a power of attorney for personal care (see below).

Power of Attorney for Personal Care. In Ontario, a legal document in which the maker appoints someone to make decisions on his or her behalf regarding medical treatment, care, feeding, clothing, shelter, hygiene, etc., in the event that he or she becomes incapable owing to physical or mental illness. This document takes legal effect only on the maker's becoming incapable of making treatment decisions and giving consent for himself or herself. (See also "Grantor.")

Precedent. A previous judge's decision that serves as a guide or basis for deciding future cases having similar facts or legal issues. A higher-court precedent is usually binding on an inferior court. (See also "Case Law.")

Preliminary Inquiry. In criminal law, a hearing held before a provincial court judge at which the Crown prosecutor is required to show that the evidence presented is such that a reasonable jury properly instructed could convict the accused. If the evidence is found insufficient in this regard, the accused must be discharged.

Presumption of Innocence. The principal of law that holds that a person charged with a criminal offence is not guilty until and unless proven guilty of the offence at trial. The Crown (i.e., the prosecution) is obliged to prove that the accused committed the offence beyond a reasonable doubt; the accused need not prove that he or she did not commit the offence.

Pre-trial Conference. A conference of all parties and their lawyers held a few weeks before trial in the presence of a judge other than the one who will hear the trial. The judge reviews the facts of the case and the positions of each party, as well as the strengths and weaknesses of each party's case. Then the judge advises the litigants how the case might be decided. This is a last attempt to reach a settlement without a lengthy and expensive trial.

Prima Facie Duties. Those duties that one must always act upon unless they conflict with those of equal or stronger obligation.

Principles. (See "Ethical Principles.")

Procedural Law. Law that regulates how individual rights are asserted and enforced in the judicial system, such as which court hears the matter, what documents must be filed and when, etc.

Professional Code. In Quebec, a code of conduct that regulates the behaviour and practice of various professions in that province, including nursing.

Professional Liability Coverage. Insurance coverage provided to licensed members of a provincial nursing College or association to insure such members against possible professional negligence claims brought against them by patients arising out of any acts or omissions in the course of providing treatment.

Professional Misconduct. In the regulation of the nursing profession, any conduct by a licensed or certified nurse that specifically contravenes the ethical and professional standards or rules of conduct set out by the provincial regulatory body.

Professions Tribunal. In Quebec, an administrative tribunal that hears appeals (with leave) from disciplinary decisions involving members of the Ordre des infirmières et infirmiers du Québec, and other professional regulatory bodies in the province.

Program Management. A style of health care governance in which individual programs or health care units collaborate to fulfil the agency's mission, vision, and goals. Decision making is decentralized, consumer focussed, and information based.

Proximate Cause. A concept of causation wherein damage, injury, or other resulting event must not be too remote or unforeseeable a consequence of a particular act or omission.

Proxy. In health care, a person appointed or otherwise authorized by law to give consent to a specified medical treatment or procedure on behalf of another where the patient is unable to give such consent owing to physical or mental incapacity.

Proxy Consent. In health care, the person legally authorized or appointed to give consent to medical treatment on behalf of an incapable patient.

Reasonable Doubt. The standard of proof in a criminal case. This means that the Crown (the prosecution) must satisfy the trier of fact (either a judge or a jury) that the accused committed the offence with which he or she is charged, giving sufficient evidence such that no real or logically compelling reason exists in the trier's mind that the accused did not commit such act.

Recertification. The process wherein a health professional may be required to take further training and undergo further examination to demonstrate proficiency in certain professional skills or to maintain such proficiency as a condition of being licensed or certified to practise.

Registration. In the regulation of nursing practice, the recording of a nurse's name and other particulars and enrolment of that person as a member of a provincial nursing regulatory body.

Regulations. Detailed secondary laws passed by a federal or provincial Cabinet pursuant to a specific statute. The statute usually gives the Cabinet the power to make detailed rules to carry out the intent and purpose of the Act but which are too detailed and time-consuming for Parliament to enact.

Remedies. The judgements and orders that a court may grant under the law in favour of a plaintiff to correct a wrong done to his or her person or property by a liable defendant. These include damages, an order that the defendant do or refrain from doing a particular action, an order reversing a transaction or contract, etc.

Reprimand. In nursing disciplinary matters, a penalty awarded against a member of the profession by the provincial nursing regulatory body for contravention of the body's regulations or professional misconduct, in which the member is admonished before the body orally or in writing (in public or private) not to engage in such conduct or to refrain from breaching professional or ethical standards.

Respondent. The party to a court action (usually the successful party) against whom an appeal of a trial decision is brought in an appellate court.

Responsible Government. A form of government in which ministers of the Crown (the Cabinet and Prime Minister) are elected members of Parliament and are accountable to it for the exercise of governmental power. This is unlike a presidential system (as in the United States), in which the executive branch of government (the President and Cabinet) is completely separate from and form no part of the legislative branch.

Revocation. In nursing disciplinary matters, the cancellation of a nurse's licence or certificate to practise nursing in the province. This is usually a penalty awarded against the nurse for violation of the regulatory body's professional or ethical standards and rules of conduct.

Right. A claim or privilege to which one is justly entitled, or what one can do, either legally or morally.

Rules of Civil Procedure. Detailed rules and regulations that govern procedure in the commencement and conduct of court actions, trials, the gathering of evidence, documentation, and the enforcement of court orders and judgements.

Sanctity of Life. A principle that emphasizes the continuation of life at all cost.

Sexual Harassment. Any unwanted conduct, language, or behaviour of a sexist or sexual nature directed by one person against another.

Sheriff. An officer of the court in a particular county or judicial district who is responsible for enforcing court orders, carrying out judicial sales of real estate or other property, and serving court documents on witnesses.

Standard of Care. Legal yardstick against which a person's conduct is measured to determine whether that person has been negligent.

Stare Decisis. Rule of English common law whereby courts are legally bound to follow previous court decisions, which have the force of law. Usually, courts will follow precedents whose facts and legal issues are similar or identical to the case they are deciding. (See also "Precedent" and "Case Law.")

Statement of Claim. A document prepared and filed by a plaintiff in a lawsuit that initiates the court action. It sets out the damages and other relief sought from the court and the bare facts (but not the evidence) upon which the plaintiff relies to support a claim against a defendant.

Statement of Defence. A document prepared and filed by the defendant in a lawsuit. It sets forth the defendant's version of the facts (but not the evidence) giving rise to the action and the legal grounds or reasons why the defendant is not liable for the plaintiff's damages.

Statute Law. A formal written law passed by Parliament or a provincial legislature, which takes precedence over and supersedes common law case law. Also found in civil law systems.

Substantive Law. Law that sets out detailed rights and obligations of citizens in private dealings with one another and with society in general.

Summary Conviction Offences. In criminal law, offences of a less serious nature that are tried without a jury in a fairly rapid, straightforward way and for which the maximum punishment is six months' imprisonment or a fine of up to $2000, or both.

Surrogacy. An arrangement whereby a woman bears a child for another couple or individual. The gestational mother may be the biological mother (through sperm donation of either the male partner or a donor), or may carry the embryo of the couple, an embryo donated by another couple, or one created from a donor egg and donor sperm.

Tort. An intentional or non-intentional (i.e., negligent) wrongful act that causes damage or injury to another's person, reputation, or property.

Trial Court. (See "Original Jurisdiction.")

Union. In labour law, a group of non-managerial employees in a common trade or industry organized in association with a constitution and membership for the purpose of advancing the common interests of its members respecting employment relations with a common employer or group of employers.

Utilitarian Theory. An ethical theory that considers an action to be right when it leads to the greatest possible balance of good consequences or to the least possible balance of bad consequences.

Utilization Management. In health care, a system of reviewing the efficiency with which scarce resources are used, and instituting and maintaining strategies to improve their day-to-day management.

Value. An ideal that has significant meaning or importance to an individual, a group, or a society.

Veracity. A moral principle that emphasizes truth telling.

Vicarious Liability. In negligence law, the liability of a principal (an employer) for the negligent or tortious acts of the principal's agent (an employee) done within the scope of the agent's authority or employment.

Victim Impact Statement. A statement given by a person against whom criminal or unprofessional behaviour (in the case of nurses) has been directed (e.g., sexual or physical abuse by a nurse against a patient), in which the person describes the emotional and physical effects that the conduct has had upon him or her. This is usually used in criminal trials as part of the determination of an appropriate sentence, and in professional disciplinary matters, in determining the appropriate sanction or penalty to be assessed against an offending member.

Vitiate. In law, to cancel a given legal act or render it null and void.

Volenti Non Fit Injuria. Latin phrase meaning, "He who consents cannot receive an injury." (See also "Voluntary Assumption of Risk.")

Voluntary Assumption of Risk. In negligence law, a situation in which an injured plaintiff is in possession of sufficient information or has knowledge of dangerous conditions or a state of affairs, but assumes the risk that he or she may be injured as a result of such conditions, despite this knowledge. For example, a participant at a hockey game assumes the risk that he or she may be injured during the game. This may reduce the liability of a defendant in a subsequent negligence suit.

Writ of Summons. (See "Statement of Claim.")